PHONOLOGY
Assessment and Intervention
Applications in Speech Pathology

PHONOLOGY
Assessment and Intervention Applications in Speech Pathology

Robert J. Lowe, Ph.D.
Associate Professor
Bloomsburg University
Bloomsburg, Pennsylvania

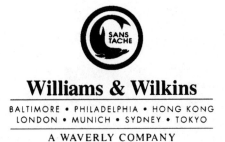

Williams & Wilkins

BALTIMORE • PHILADELPHIA • HONG KONG
LONDON • MUNICH • SYDNEY • TOKYO

A WAVERLY COMPANY

Editor: John P. Butler
Managing Editor: Linda S. Napora
Copy Editor: Richard H. Adin
Designer: Ann Feild
Illustration Planner: Ray Lowman
Cover Designer: Dan Pfisterer

Accurate indications, adverse reactions, and dosage schedules for drugs are provided in this book, but it is possible that they may change. The reader is urged to review the package information data of the manufacturers of the medications mentioned.

Printed in the United States of America

Library of Congress Cataloging in Publication Data

Lowe, Robert J.
    Phonology : assessment and intervention applications in speech pathology / Robert J. Lowe.
      p.   cm.
    Includes index.
    ISBN 0-683-05205-5
    1. Speech therapy.   2. Phonetics.   I. Title.
RC423.L69   1994
616.8'55—dc20
                           94-6201
                           CIP

94 95 96 97 98
1 2 3 4 5 6 7 8 9 10

*To Bonnie S. Lowe, my wife of seventeen years
and main supporter in all that I do and try to do. All my love, always.*

Preface

WHEN I WAS FIRST APPROACHED about writing a textbook on the topic of phonology, my initial thought was, why? How could I improve upon the fine texts that are already available? The books that I have used have worked well for my undergraduate classes, but what about a graduate-level text? A graduate-level text could focus on current approaches to assessment and intervention, provide a much needed foundation in phonological theory, and discuss the implications of cultural diversity that have not even been considered until recently. At the graduate level there would be no need to cover the various traditional approaches used in assessment and intervention. Instead, the book could concentrate on presenting techniques in linguistic analysis and language-based intervention. Writing such a text made sense.

Phonology: Assessment and Intervention Applications in Speech Pathology was developed with an orientation to graduate students and professionals who already have a background in the more traditional aspects of articulation. Its purpose is to upgrade the information and skills of the professional and to provide the graduate student with a solid base in the practical application of phonology to the assessment and intervention of speech disorders.

The field of speech-language pathology has seen a revolution in how articulation/phonology is viewed. Since the late 1960s we have continually moved from viewing speech errors as a separate entity treated at the surface level through ear training, drill, and phonetic placement to phonology, where speech errors are assessed and treated as part of the language system. For some of us, the change has been difficult because it has meant learning new terminology, mastering the application of new assessment instruments, and incorporating treatment approaches that require time and thought in development and implementation. For others, the change has been a natural occurrence that follows similar changes in philosophy that have influenced the area of language in general. As such, it has been a welcome change. Besides, it has made the treatment of speech errors a lot more interesting than drill work!

In the development of this book I tried to keep two main objectives in mind. First, I strongly believe that the purpose of education is to prepare the student for future education. Learning is a life-long process and formal learning (school) only provides a foundation that will allow the acquisition of new information. As such, I wanted to present the student with the nuts and bolts of phonology that would enable the future professional to understand and assimilate new information encountered in this rapidly growing field. As a result, the book includes chapters on basic phonological principles, phonological theory, normal phonological development, the basics of distinctive features and phonological rules, and phonological processes. The book also includes information on current practices in assessment and intervention and on implications of cultural diversity. This information provides the student with a strong foundation for future learning.

My second objective was to be practical. The vast majority of professionals in speech-language pathology are actively employed as clinicians, and clinicians want practical information. Chapters 4 and 5, Distinctive Features and Phonological Processes, include exercises to promote learning of the basic definitions. Chapter 6 includes forms and a speech sample for practice analysis. Chapter 7, Intervention, provides guidelines for selection of intervention targets and specific guidelines for development of language-based activities. Chapter 8, Phonology and Cultural Diversity, acquaints the clinician with practical considerations for assessing and working with clients of a cultural heritage that is not your own.

At the completion of this text I believed that my objectives had, for the most part, been accomplished. The book provides the foundation information needed for future learning and the practical aspects needed to apply the information today. Certainly, more could have been written. Already, I have considered additions to cover assessment and intervention of special populations (e.g., infants, mentally disabled, hearing impaired) and, possibly, a chapter on empowering parents as clinicians. I'm sure other areas will surface with time and the further development of this fascinating field of phonology.

Robert J. Lowe

Acknowledgments

THE DEVELOPMENT OF THIS text was a major undertaking and could not have been accomplished without the help and support of many individuals. They all have my heartfelt gratitude. To my children, Ryan, Garrett, Shawn, and Rachel, who have had a part-time father this past year, thank you for putting up with a busy schedule and for the understanding you have shown. A special thanks to my past teaching assistants, Heather Daubert, Felicia Gurzynski, Tiffiany Jancuska, and Dina Pachence, who were tremendously helpful in collecting research, editing, and tracking down references. Thank you to Frank Parker, Adele Proctor, Jackie Bauman-Waengler, and Julia Mount Weitz, whose chapter contributions made this text far better than what I could have done on my own. Working a full-time job while writing a text makes life very tense; thanks to Ron Champoux and Dianne Angelo for the comic relief and their much appreciated friendship. Thank you to John Butler, Linda Napora, and Crystal Taylor of Williams & Wilkins. Your continuing encouragement and support along the way made a big difference. And finally, a special thank you to Jean Blosser who suggested my name for this project. Thanks Jean, I hope we get to meet someday!

Robert J. Lowe

Contributors

Jacqueline Bauman-Waengler, Ph.D., CCC-SP
Associate Professor
Department of Speech Pathology and Audiology
Clarion University
Clarion, Pennsylvania

Frank Parker, Ph.D.
Professor
Department of English
Louisiana State University
Baton Rouge, Louisiana

Adele Proctor, Sc.D
Associate Professor
Department of Speech and Hearing Science
University of Illinois at Urbana-Champaign
Champaign, Illinois

Julia Mount Weitz, Ph.D.
Assistant Professor
Bloomsburg University
Bloomsburg, Pennsylvania

Contents

Phonology: An Overview

Chapter 1

Robert J. Lowe

THE HUMAN VOCAL TRACT is capable of a wide variety of sounds from grunts and squeals to pops and hisses. Among those sounds is a relatively small group that appear uniquely qualified to be used in the production of speech. The study of these speech sounds is called phonology.

Phonology is the subdiscipline of linguistics that focuses on speech sounds and sound patterns. It is the study of spoken language. Speech sounds refer to linguistically relevant sounds used in the formation of syllables, words, and sentences. Sound patterns refer to the sets of sounds that occur in a given language, permissible arrangements of these sounds, and the processes for adding, deleting, or changing the sounds (Sloat, Taylor, and Hoard, 1978).

Each language has its own unique system of sound patterns. The goal of phonology is "to study the properties of the sound systems which speakers must learn or internalize in order to use their language for communication" (Hyman, 1975, p. 1). This goal includes (*a*) describing the sound patterns of languages, (*b*) describing the organization of speech sounds in the mind, (*c*) describing how languages differ from one another in this organization, and (*d*) discovering phonological universals—common properties shared by the various sound systems of the world's languages.

This book, however, is not about phonology for linguistics majors. The focus of this book is on the clinical application of phonology in the field of speech-language pathology. The speech-language pathologist (SLP) is not a phonologist, although the two professionals do share a common interest in the sound systems of languages. The phonologist is interested in all languages and usually focuses on the study of intact language systems and the development of theories to explain the acquisition of language. The SLP, although grounded in normal language development, is most concerned with the analysis and remediation of impaired language systems and devotes little time to theories explaining how language systems are acquired.

Despite the differences in focus, the field of speech-language pathology has gained much from the field of linguistics and in particular phonology. Many of the concepts used by SLPs

1

have their origins in the field of linguistics. Examples include concepts of the phoneme, distinctive features, phonological processes, deep and surface structures, and phonological rules.

Procedures and concepts borrowed from linguistic analysis of phonology are being used with increasing frequency in the field of speech-language pathology as evidenced by such texts as Ingram's (1976) *Phonological Disability in Children*, Grunwell's (1982) *Clinical Phonology*, and Stoel-Gammon and Dunn's (1985) *Normal and Disordered Phonology in Children*. The influence also can be seen in the growth of assessment instruments making use of phonological analysis. Examples here include the *Compton-Hutton Phonological Assessment* (Compton and Hutton, 1978), *The Assessment of Phonological Processes-Revised* (Hodson, 1986), the *Khan-Lewis Phonological Analysis* (Khan and Lewis, 1986), the *Assessment Link between Phonology and Articulation (ALPHA)* (Lowe, 1986), and the *Bankson-Bernthal Test of Phonology* (Bankson and Bernthal, 1990).

This textbook will cover the basic principles of phonology as applied to the clinical analysis and remediation of speech disorders. Chapter 1 focuses on concepts of phonology that underlie phonological assessment. These concepts are important to an understanding of phonological analysis. Chapter 2 provides a study of phonological theory, reviewing major theories and their impact on the profession of speech-language pathology. Chapter 3 reviews the literature on normal phonological development. Distinctive features and phonological rule writing are covered in Chapter 4. Chapter 5 presents an in-depth review of processes including hands-on exercises to sharpen this important tool of assessment. Chapter 6 is a step-by-step guide to analysis and assessment of phonological disorders. Language-based intervention is covered in Chapter 7. Chapter 8 looks at the growing area of cultural diversity and the need for culturally sensitive phonological assessment.

PRINCIPLES OF PHONOLOGY

PHONOLOGY AND PHONETICS

Students in speech-language pathology are well acquainted with phonetics. Most have had at least one course in transcription and hands-on experience in transcribing speech samples. Exposure to phonology is typically in a developmental language acquisition course where students are exposed to the phonological component of language. Traditionally the two disciplines have been considered separate, autonomous areas of study with some overlap. Phonetics is seen as focusing on the physiological and physical nature of sounds without regard to how those sounds function in a language. As expressed by Ohala (1990, p. 154), "As a part of the speech universe, phonetics is thought to be the 'hardware' that implements the control signals from the phonological component." On the other hand, phonology is viewed as the study of how sounds are organized and function in communication. Phonology is much more concerned with the system of contrastive speech sounds and how they are used in conveying meaning.

The difference between phonetics and phonology hinges on their relationship to the other language components. The phonetics of a language can be studied without regard to the language's syntax and semantics. The phonology of a language, however, must take into consideration these other language components in order to describe how speech sounds are organized and function for communication.

Despite the differences in emphasis, the two fields have much overlap, particularly in areas where phonology tries to explain regularities seen in speech patterns. Ohala (1990) notes the growing body of literature showing that phonological units and processes (phonological domain) occur because of the physical nature and structure of the speech mechanism (phonetic domain). An example of this is the cross-language tendency for fricatives, affricates, and stops to lose voicing in word-final position. This "natural pattern" is likely due to the aerodynamic conditions of the phonetic environment, thus we have a phonetic "cause" for a phonological rule. As presented by Ohala (1990) there is much to be gained from an integrated view of phonetics and phonology.

Levels of Representation

Generative phonology and other theories of phonology suggest that there are levels of representation in the organization of language. The concept of levels of representation is necessary as there does not appear to be agreement between labels attached to sounds and their actual production. For example, we can agree that the vowels in the words "pat" and "pad" are the same, but at the same time we also note that the vowel in "pat" has a shorter duration than the vowel in "pad." So how do we explain this situation where the vowels are the same but also different? By considering levels of representation we can show that at one level the vowels are the same but when realized (spoken) they are different.

The level where they are the same is the phonological or underlying level of representation. At this level the segments are stored as phonemes. Phonemes are realized as allophones at the surface or phonetic level of representation. But we still have not answered our question of how the two productions of the vowel can be different. The difference is due to phonological rules that connect the two levels of representation. The rules function to translate segments on one level into segments on the other level. One of those rules states that vowels preceding a voiced consonant will be lengthened. Thus we find that the vowel in "pad" has a longer duration than the vowel in "pat" but they are still the same vowel.

In summary, a simple description of the levels of representation in phonology includes an underlying level where segments are stored as phonemes, a phonetic level where the phonemes are produced as allophones, and phonological rules that join the two levels. Chapter 2 reviews the major phonology theories and presents some alternative views on representation.

Underlying Representation and Speech Errors

There are two main positions concerning the relationship between the underlying level of representation and speech production. The first position is that the child's underlying representation is identical to the adult surface form whether or not the child produces that form correctly. The second position is that the underlying representation may be identical to the adult surface form in some cases of speech errors, but might differ from the adult surface form in others. Most approaches employing phonological process descriptions assume the first view. Approaches making use of generative phonology tend to assume the second position.

The importance of these two positions to the clinician is in determination of rules connecting the two levels. The rules would be different depending upon the assumed nature of the underlying representation. If in two children the underlying representations that result in the same surface form are different, then the phonological rules required to derive the surface form would have to be different as well. As these rules may be used to determine treatment goals, assumptions made about underlying representation are important. For a more detailed discussion of these two positions see Maxwell (1984).

PHONOLOGY AND LANGUAGE

Language has traditionally been studied as consisting of three interacting systems: semantics, syntax, and phonology. The phonological component, as described by Edwards and Shriberg (1983) has two levels: covert and overt. The covert level contains the language user's knowledge of phonology including phonetic and phonemic inventories, phonotactic rules, morphophonemic rules, and allophonic rules. The overt level is the level of articulation and involves the planning and execution of motor movements of the articulators during speech production.

As noted the systems are viewed as interacting. Edwards and Shriberg (1983, pp. 36–37) describe the interaction between phonology and the other language components:

> The phonological component of a language is that portion concerned with sounds. It interacts with the other components of language—the semantic and the syntactic, and also with pragmatic functions. These other components and functions are concerned with choice and ordering of words in accordance with appropriate social contexts and individual histories, needs, and intentions. These inputs to the phonological component provide the message. The task of the phonological component is to translate this message into manifest speech.

This model of phonology provides a general guideline for how phonology will be viewed in this text. Speech output is considered the result of a complex series of interactions that includes not only language inputs but also inputs from domains that influence language (i.e., cognitive and environmental). These inputs have an influence on the speaker's phonological knowledge that in turn will influence speech output. Speech output is also influenced by motor and physiological factors that control the physical articulation of speech sounds.

PHONEME

One of the key concepts to the study of phonology is the phoneme. The introduction to this chapter indicated that phonology was interested in the study of linguistically relevant speech sounds. Linguistically relevant speech sounds are those that contrast and are called phonemes. Let us clarify this with an example. We could agree that the words pat, bat, mat, and cat all have different meanings. We also could agree that the words differ from each other by only the first sound or segment. The other segments "a" and "t" are the same. At the phonetic level then, we find that the sounds representing p, b, m, and k affect meaning. In other words we could not take any of these sounds and use them in place of one of the others without also changing the meaning of the word it began. The sounds contrast word meaning which gives them phonemic status.

Phonemes are contrastive—the exchange of phonemes will change word meaning. In fact, the phoneme system is a system of contrasts but, as noted, phonemes can have more than one representation at the surface level. In fact, every production of a phoneme will be unique in some way from every other production of that phoneme. So how is it that some sounds at the phonetic level contrast and others at this level do not? The answer leads us into a discussion of what constitutes an allophone.

Allophones are variations of a phoneme as produced at the phonetic level. To qualify as allophones of a phoneme, sounds must meet certain characteristics. First, allophones must be phonetically similar, meaning that the sounds are generally produced with the same place, manner, and voicing features. Second, allophones do not contrast with one another. This lack of contrastiveness is due to either free variation or complementary distribution.

Allophones of a phoneme are in free variation if they can be exchanged in a word without changing word meaning. An example would be [t] versus [tʰ]. Aspirated [t] usually occurs in word-initial position in English. The unaspirated version occurs in /s/ clusters. However, the two versions could be exchanged without any effect on word meaning. In other words, we could use the unaspirated version in word-initial position one time and the aspirated version the next time without any effect on the meaning conveyed by the word.

Not all allophones of a phoneme are in free variation. Some occur in complementary distribution. Complementary distribution means that two allophones do not occur in the same phonetic environment—they complement each other. MacKay (1987, p. 182) explains:

> Things that are complementary go together to make a coherent whole, and indeed the environments of each of the allophones go together to make up the environment for the entire phoneme. As an example, we could say dark and light /l/ are in complementary distribution in English. That is, all of the environments of [l] plus all of the environments of [ɫ] are mutually exclusive; they, along with the environments of syllabic [l̩], make up the environment of all English /l/s.

Free variation and complementary distribution are language dependent. In English, aspirated and unaspirated stops are not contrastive, but this is not true of Hindi where aspiration signals a meaning difference. In Hindi, [t] and [tʰ] are allophones of two different phonemes and they cannot be exchanged without changing word meaning.

Just as the allophones of a phoneme can differ with the language so can the phonemes. Languages may not even share the same phonemes. German for example has no /θ/ sound, Berber has no /p/ or /v/ and Finnish has a /t/ but no /d/. Languages also may vary in the distribution of phonemes. In English, the [ʒ] occurs in word-medial and final position. This sound in French occurs in all three word positions.

In summary, we find that a phoneme is represented by a family of sounds called allophones. These allophones are phonetically similar and will not contrast word meaning with one another but will be contrastive with allophones of other phonemes. Phonemes and their allophones are language specific with each language having a unique set of phonemes and patterns of distribution. (For a description of the English consonants and vowels refer to the Appendix.)

In working with child language systems the clinician will find that children do not necessarily use speech sounds as required by the adult standards. The child's system is still developing and as such, sounds may occur in free variation or complementary distribution (being used as allophones) that would normally contrast in the adult language. For example, a child might freely interchange [t] and [d] in word-initial position (free variation) until he/she realizes the contrastive value of the voicing feature. At that point the two sounds take on phonemic status and function to contrast words in the child's system.

NATURALNESS

Naturalness of phonological phenomena refers to what is simple or plausible in a phonetic sense. Certain regularities occur often in languages due to the influence of context on sound production. For example, a natural syllable shape is the CV. This shape is found in every known language and thus it is considered more natural than the CVC shape that is found in a limited number of languages.

Edwards and Shriberg (1983, pp. 87–88) describe natural speech phenomena as ones that occur more often than others—they are more widespread in the languages of the world, are less likely to be lost historically, and are acquired earlier by children. These speech phenomena could refer to segments, sound classes, syllable shape, phonological rules, or processes.

Naturalness leads us into a discussion of markedness. In describing related speech phenomena such as voicing cognates (e.g., [t] and [d]), the sound that is more natural is referred to as the unmarked member (Sloat, Taylor, and Hoard, 1978). The other member is marked. Toombs, Singh, and Hayden (1981) present the markedness values for common substitutions in child speech (Table 1.1).

They describe the unmarked member of a sound pair as the one that

1. requires less articulatory effort,
2. is less acoustically complex,
3. is less perceptually ambiguous,
4. is acquired developmentally earlier,
5. occurs more often in the languages of the world.

Another means of determining naturalness is to look at implicational laws. Sloat, Taylor, and Hoard (1978, p. 101) note "Where the presence of a given sound in a sound system nearly always implies the presence of another sound, we say an implicational law holds between the sounds." In comparing [t] and [d] they observe that there are languages that have [t] without the occurrence of the [d], but there are no languages that have [d] without also having the [t]. In other words, presence of [d] implies [t] but [t] does not imply the presence of [d]. Here the [t] would be more natural—unmarked.

The following observations from Sloat, Taylor, and Hoard can be made about naturalness:

1. Voiced obstruents are more marked than voiceless.
2. Obstruents are less marked than sonorants.
3. Stops are more natural than fricatives.
4. Fricatives are more natural than affricates.
5. [n] is the most natural nasal.
6. [s] and [h] are the most natural fricatives.
7. Low front vowels appear to be the most natural vowels.
8. CV syllable is the least marked followed by CVC.

Elbert and Gierut (1986) discuss implicational relationships and their impact on generalization in the treatment of phonological disorders in children. This will be discussed further in Chapter 7.

TABLE 1.1. Markedness Values for Specific English Phonemes

	Nasal	Labial	Voice	Sonorancy	Sibilancy	Continuancy	Front/Back
p	U	U	U	U	U	U	U
b	U	U	M	U	U	U	U
t	U	M	U	U	U	U	U
d	U	M	M	U	U	U	U
k	U	M	U	U	U	U	M
g	U	M	M	U	U	U	M
f	U	U	U	U	U	M	U
g	U	U	M	U	U	M	U
θ	U	M	U	U	U	M	U
ð	U	M	M	U	U	M	U
s	U	M	U	U	M	M	U
z	U	M	M	U	M	M	U
ʃ	U	M	U	U	M	M	M
ʧ	U	M	U	U	M	U	M
ʤ	U	M	M	U	M	U	M
w	U	U	(U)	M	U	(U)	U (flexible)
r	U	U	(U)	M	U	(U)	U
l	U	M	(U)	M	U	(U)	U
j	U	M	(U)	M	U	(U)	M
m	M	U	(U)	(U)	U	(U)	U
n	M	M	(U)	(U)	U	(U)	U
ŋ	M	M	(U)	(U)	U	(U)	M

LANGUAGE UNIVERSALS

A concept related to naturalness is that of universals. Language universals are linguistic features that are shared by all languages. For example, all languages have the vowel [a] in their phonetic inventories (Hyman, 1975). The vowel [a] is a true universal. Linguists study universals in an attempt to learn what general properties of language would account for the similarities (Parker, 1986).

Some features are common to most languages, but not all, and these are called near universals as opposed to true linguistic universals (Sloat, Taylor, and Hoard, 1978). For example, most languages have the sound [n] in their inventories, but not all languages. The [n] sound is a near universal.

DISTINCTIVE FEATURES

A feature is a subphonemic characteristic that can be used to describe phonemes. The characteristic is usually an acoustic or articulatory property associated with a sound. For example, a place of articulation like the front of the mouth, or a manner characteristic like nasality. These features are thought to occur together during sound production much like the notes of a musical chord. A feature is distinctive if it can be used to distinguish between speech sounds. As defined by Grundy (1989, p. 37), a distinctive feature "refers to any phonetic characteristic of a group of sounds which serves to distinguish that group from another group of sounds."

Phonemes can be described by collections of features. Each phoneme is evaluated on a two-value (binary) system with respect to various features. If the feature is present a "+" or a "1" is assigned to the feature. If the feature is absent a "−" or "0" is scored. The collection of features that describes a phoneme is called a feature bundle.

There are many systems of distinctive features and not all systems use binary scoring. Some assign graduated values to the features. The Irwin-Wong (1983) system, for example, uses a four point scaling for the feature of oral-nasality, ranging from complete orality, where the velopharyngeal valve is completely closed, to complete nasality, where it is open and the oral passageway is closed.

The first complete distinctive feature system was developed by Jakobson, Fant, and Halle (1952). It was their intent to develop a set of subphonemic features that could be used to describe the phonological components of all languages. Their system contained 12 features described in terms of acoustic and articulatory characteristics and given binary values.

Many feature systems have been developed since Jakobson, Fant, and Halle's. The system developed by Chomsky and Halle (1968) has seen the most application in speech-language research. This system is based on 13 binary features that can be used to describe the phonemes of any language. Other systems used by SLPs include Singh and Polen (1972), Ladefoged (1975), and Blache (1989).

One of the values of distinctive features is that they can be used to describe groups of sounds based on common characteristics. This provides a convenient means for investigating speech behaviors as most sound changes (processes) do not involve random sets of sounds but are based on sounds that are linked in terms of phonetic classes (Sloat, Taylor, and Hoard, 1978). Both features and phonological processes allow the analysis of this type of sound change.

In the early 1970's distinctive features saw considerable application in the analysis of speech disorders. Early advocates of distinctive features, like McReynolds and Bennett (1972), McReynolds and Huston (1971), Pollack and Rees (1972), and Singh and Singh (1972), viewed distinctive features as a practical means for analyzing articulation disorders. In particular, distinctive feature analysis was seen as a means to describe multiple misarticulations in an economical manner. With respect to remediation, feature approaches appear to capitalize on generalization so that training of one feature may positively affect production of other sounds containing that feature (McReynolds and Bennett, 1972).

Walsh (1974) has pointed out several inadequacies of feature analysis and the trend in the field has been toward use of phonological process descriptions. However, recent work with autosegmental phonology and consonant inventories has shown promise for a resurgence in the use of distinctive feature analysis (Chin and Dinnsen 1990; Chin and Dinnsen, 1991; Dinnsen, Chin, Elbert, and Powell, 1990) and distinctive features continue to have utility in the writing of phonological rule descriptions of sound changes.

PHONOLOGICAL PROCESSES

David Stampe (1979) developed the concept of processes in his theory of Natural Phonology. As conceptualized by Stampe, phonological processes are mental operations present at birth that act to restrict a child's speech productions. All children are born with these processes and must learn to eliminate or suppress those processes that are inappropriate to his/her native language. Natural Phonology assumes that the child's underlying representation closely resembles that of the adults and the processes act upon the underlying representation to derive the surface form. Initially, the surface forms are very simple, but as the child matures inappropriate processes are suppressed or in some way eliminated so that more complex productions can be made.

Stampe considers "natural" processes as those that are innate and phonetically motivated so that their occurrence is common across languages and seen as a part of the normal acquisition of the sound system. He makes a distinction between processes and rules. Whereas processes are innate, the rules are "imposed by the language" meaning they have to be learned. Learning to aspirate voiceless stops word-initially and not to aspirate in /s/ clusters would be a rule specific to English. Devoicing in word-final position, on the other hand, would be a natural phonological process as it is phonetically motivated and commonly seen across languages and in language acquisition.

Edwards and Shriberg (1983, pp. 33–34) make a different distinction between processes and rules. They define a phonological process as referring "to any systematic sound change that affects a class of sounds (e.g., velars, fricatives) or a sound sequence, such as /s/ plus sonorant clusters (/sw, sl/, etc.)." A rule is defined as a more or less formal statement of the phonological process. In these two definitions processes and rules refer to the same speech phenomena but differ in the degree of specificity in which they are described with the phonological rule providing a more detailed description of the sound changes.

Application of processes to the field of speech-language pathology is due largely to Ingram's (1976) book, *Phonological Disability in Children*. Ingram first applied the use of processes to the analysis of children's speech errors. In examining child phonology it can be observed that errors are typically not random but are systematic variations of the adult models. These regularities often involve whole classes of sounds and phonological processes can be used as descriptors of these sound change patterns.

It should be noted that this use of processes differs from Stampe's original definition. Stampe viewed the processes as psychologically real and thus actively applied to the underlying representation. The field of speech-language pathology typically employs processes as descriptors of regularities seen in child phonology and makes no claims about the role that processes play in deriving the surface form.

Phonological processes are categorized into two or three types. Bernthal and Bankson (1988) suggested two categories: (*a*) whole word processes, which operate to simplify word or syllable structure, and (*b*) segment processes, which involve some form of substitution for specific segments or types of segments. Ingram (1976) categorized phonological processes into three main types: (*a*) syllable-structure processes, in which the syllabic shape of the target word is changed;

(*b*) substitution processes, in which one class of sounds substitutes for another class; and (*c*) assimilation processes, in which one sound assimilates to another sound in the same word.

PHONOLOGICAL RULES

The concept of phonological rules was introduced with Generative Phonology in *The Sound Pattern of English* (Chomsky and Halle, 1968). Generative phonology posited an underlying (phonological) level of representation and a phonetic representation that were connected by phonological rules. Phonological rules described the derivations that occurred to the underlying representation for the surface form to be realized.

Sloat, Taylor, and Hoard (1978, p. 159) note that there is some controversy about whether phonological rules reflect rules actually used by speakers in producing utterances. They suggest, however, that what is most important is that it is possible to find regularities in data from real language and to represent these regularities by means of phonological rules. As such, typical use of rules in speech-language pathology parallels that of phonological processes—as descriptors of patterns observed in the speech behaviors of children. This view is reflected by Bernthal and Bankson (1988, p. 48) who define a phonological rule as "a formal expression of some regularity that occurs in the phonology of a language or in the phonology of an individual speaker."

Although in recent years the use of phonological processes in assessment has increased, there has been little use of phonological rules by speech-language pathologists. The few exceptions (e.g., Dinnsen, 1984; Elbert and Gierut, 1986; Powell, 1991) come from researchers/clinicians taking a generative approach to describing sound systems. Results from these studies are opening doors to some interesting possibilities in both assessment and intervention (see Chapters 6 and 7). As such, clinicians would be well advised to be familiar with the basic concepts of phonological rules and rule writing as these may become the future tools of the profession.

The use of rules has another advantage that can be used by those who prefer phonological process descriptions. Processes are appropriate to capturing general sound changes affecting classes of sounds and sound sequences, but sound changes can be influenced by phonetic context. For example, stopping may only occur in word-initial position or only with lingual fricatives. These specifics can be described using phonological rules. They provide a much more accurate description of what occurs in a speaker's phonology and may point out some regularities that would be missed by process descriptions. In the author's view, the use of phonological processes is very useful for analyzing sound changes that affect classes of sounds or sound sequences, but phonological rule descriptions are needed to specify how the processes are applied.

REFERENCES

Bankson N, Bernthal J. Bankson-Bernthal Test of Phonology. San Antonio: Special Press, Inc., 1990.
Bernthal J, Bankson N. Articulation and phonological disorders. Englewood Cliffs: Prentice-Hall, 1988.
Blache S. A distinctive feature approach. In Creaghead N, Newman P, Secord W, eds. Assessment and remediation of articulatory and phonological disorders. 2nd ed. Columbus: Merrill Publishing Company, 1989:361–382.
Chin S, Dinnsen D. Consonant clusters in disordered speech: correspondence strategies and constraints. Paper presented at the Fifteenth Annual Boston University Conference on Language Development, Boston, MA, 1990.
Chin S, Dinnsen D. Feature geometry in disordered phonology. Clinical Linguistics and Phonetics 1991;5(4):329–337.
Chomsky N, Halle M. The sound pattern of English. New York: Harper and Row, 1968.
Compton A, Hutton S. Compton-Hutton phonological assessment. San Francisco: Carousel House, 1978.

Dinnsen D. Methods and empirical issues in analyzing functional misarticulation. In Elbert M, Dinnsen D, Weismer G, eds. Phonological theory and the misarticulating child (ASHA Monograph No. 22). Rockville, MD: ASHA, 1984: 5–17.

Dinnsen D, Chin S, Elbert M, Powell T. Some constraints on functionally disordered phonologies: phonetic inventories and phonotactics. Journal of Speech and Hearing Research 1990;33:28–37.

Edwards M. Phonological assessment and treatment in support of phonological processes. Language, Speech, and Hearing Services in Schools 1992;23:233–240.

Edwards ML, Shriberg LD. Phonology: applications in communicative disorders. San Diego: College-Hill Press, 1983.

Elbert M, Gierut J. Handbook of clinical phonology: approaches to assessment and treatment. Boston: College-Hill Press, 1986.

Grundy K. Linguistics in clinical practice. London: Taylor and Francis, 1989.

Grunwell P. Clinical phonology. 2nd ed. Baltimore: Williams and Wilkins, 1987.

Hodson B. The assessment of phonological processes-revised. Danville, IL: Interstate Press, 1986.

Hyman L. Phonology: theory and analysis. New York: Holt, Rinehart and Winston, 1975.

Ingram D. Phonological disability in children. New York: American Elsevier Publishing Co., Inc., 1976.

Irwin J, Wong S. Phonological development in children: 18 to 72 months. Carbondale: Southern Illinois University Press, 1983.

Jakobson R, Fant G, Halle M. Preliminaries to speech analysis. Cambridge, MA: MIT Press, 1952.

Khan L, Lewis N. Khan-Lewis phonological analysis. Circle Pines, MN: American Guidance Service, 1986.

Ladefoged P. A course in phonetics. New York: Harcourt Brace Jovanovich, 1975.

Lowe R. Assessment link between phonology and articulation (ALPHA). Moline, IL: LinguiSystems, Inc., 1986.

Lowe R. Workbook for the identification of phonological processes. Austin: Pro Ed, 1989.

MacKay I. Phonetics: the science of speech production. Boston: College-Hill Publication, 1987.

Maxwell E. On determining underlying phonological representations of children: a critique of the current theories. In Elbert M, Dinnsen D, Weismer G, eds. Phonological theory and the misarticulating child (ASHA Monograph No. 22). Rockville, MD: ASHA, 1984:18–29.

McReynolds L, Bennett S. Distinctive feature generalization in articulation training. Journal of Speech and Hearing Disorders 1972;37:462–471.

McReynolds L, Huston K. A distinctive feature analysis of children's misarticulations. Journal of Speech and Hearing Disorders 1971;36:155–156.

Ohala J. There is no interface between phonology and phonetics: a personal view. Journal of Phonetics 1990;18:153–171.

Parker F. Linguistics for non-linguists. Boston: College-Hill Publication, 1986.

Pollack E, Rees N. Disorders of articulation: Some clinical applications of distinctive feature theory. Journal of Speech and Hearing Disorders 1972;37:451–461.

Powell T. Planning for phonological generalization: an approach to treatment target selection. American Journal of Speech-Language Pathology 1991;1(1):21–27.

Singh S, Polen S. Use of a distinctive feature model in speech pathology. Acta Symbolica 1972;3:17–25.

Singh S, Singh K. A self-generating distinctive feature model for diagnosis, prognosis, and therapy. Acta Symbolica 1972;3(2):89–99.

Sloat C, Taylor S, Hoard J. Introduction to phonology. Englewood Cliffs: Prentice-Hall, Inc., 1978.

Stampe D. A dissertation on natural phonology. New York: Garland, 1979.

Stoel-Gammon C, Dunn C. Normal and disordered phonology in children. Baltimore: University Park Press, 1985.

Toombs M, Singh S, Hayden M. Markedness of features in the articulatory substitutions of children. Journal of Speech and Hearing Disorders 1981;46:184–191.

Walsh H. On certain practical inadequacies of distinctive feature systems. Journal of Speech and Hearing Disorders 1974;39:32–43.

Appendix 1.1 | English Consonants and Vowels

ONE OF THE EARLIEST systems for the description of consonants in disordered speech involves the use of place, manner, and voicing characteristics. These descriptors still provide a useful analysis system for speech disorders. In addition, many of the phonological processes described in Chapter 5 are based on changes in place, manner, and voicing, so a review at this time will have benefits later when defining processes.

Any English consonant can be identified by its place, manner, and voicing characteristics. Place refers to where in the vocal tract the sound is produced. Manner refers to modifications of the airstream during sound production and voicing refers to the presence or absence of vocal fold vibration. Figure 1.1 shows a breakdown of English consonants based on their place, manner and voicing features.

PLACE OF ARTICULATION

Place is determined by where in the vocal tract the point of most closure or constriction occurs in production of the speech sound (Lowe, 1989). Places of articulation occur at various points along the vocal tract from the lips to the glottis.

Bilabial. The term "bilabial" means two lips. Bilabial is the most anterior of the places of articulation and includes the consonants /b/, /p/, /m/, and /w/.

Labio-dental. This place of articulation refers to sounds made with the lips and teeth. Labio-dental productions involve the upper incisors contacting the lower lip during sound production. The labio-dental consonants are /f/, and /v/.

Lingua-dental. The lingua-dentals are also referred to as interdentals and are made with the tongue tip touching the inside margin of the upper central incisors. The lingua-dental consonants are /θ/ and /ð/.

Lingua-alveolar. The alveolar ridge lies immediately behind the upper central incisors. Sounds made with the tongue contacting or almost contacting the alveolar ridge include /t/, /d/, /s/, /z/, /n/, and /l/.

Palatal. The palatal area lies directly behind the alveolar ridge near where the vault of the mouth roof angles upward. The palatal consonants are: /j/, /r/, /ʃ/, /ʒ/, /tʃ/, and /dʒ/. The anterior portion of the palatal area and the posterior of the alveolar ridge are sometimes referred to as the palato-alveolar area.

Velar. The velum or soft palate lies immediately anterior to the uvula and is the place of articulation for the following sounds: /k/, /g/, and /ŋ/.

Glottal. The most posterior place of articulation is the glottis. The /h/ is the only English

Manner

	Stop-Plosives		Nasals	Fricatives		Affricates		Liquids	Glides
	VL	V		VL	V	VL	V		
Bilabial	p	b	m						w
Labio-Dental				f	v				
Lingua-Dental				θ	ð				
Lingua-Alveolar	t	d	n	s	z			l	
Palatal						tʃ	dʒ	r	j
Velar	k	g	ŋ						
Glottal	ʔ			h					

(Place is labeled vertically on the left.)

FIGURE 1.1. Place, manner, and voicing characteristics of English consonants.

consonant made at the glottis, but the glottal stop [ʔ] also is made at this location and is used in many word productions often substituting for the /k/.

MANNER OF ARTICUATION

As noted, manner refers to how the speech sounds are produced, or more exactly, how the airstream is modified as it travels through the vocal tract. The divisions of manner vary in the degree of constriction required during sound production and range from complete closure to a very open vocal tract.

Stop-Plosives. During production of a stop-plosive the vocal tract is completely blocked either by the tongue or the lips. The velopharyngeal port is closed at this time which allows the build-up of air pressure behind the point of closure. In plosive production the airstream is released abruptly causing a pop (explosion). The stop-plosive consonants include /p/, /b/, /t/, /d/, /k/, and /g/.

Fricatives. Fricatives are produced by directing the airstream through a narrow constriction in the vocal tract. Again the velopharyngeal port is closed during production. The forcing of the air through the constriction results in a turbulence or friction. The nine fricative consonants are /f/, /v/, /θ/, /ð/, /s/, /z/, /ʃ/, /ʒ/, /h/.

Affricates. These sounds are considered a combination of a stop and a fricative. Their production involves a closure (stop) followed by a homorganic (same place) fricative. The two English fricatives are: /tʃ/ and /dʒ/. These sounds are also symbolized as /č/ and /ǰ/ respectively.

Nasals. These sounds are produced with closure of the vocal tract while the velopharyngeal port remains open. Airflow is through the nasal cavity giving the sounds their nasal quality. The three nasals are /m/, /n/ and /ŋ/.

Liquids. These sounds are vowel-like consonants that have a very open vocal tract during their production. The liquids include /l/ and /r/.

Glides. The glides are made with a very open vocal tract much like the liquids. The production of a glide includes a rapid movement or shift of articulation as it is made. The two glides are /w/ and /j/.

Obstruents. At times subgroups of sound classes function together in sound changes. The class known as obstruents is one such group. It is made up of stops, continuants, and affricates. Obstruents are generally defined as sounds that are articulated with a greater degree of obstruction in the vocal tract than would be associated with vowels or semivowels.

VOICING

Voicing refers to the action of the vocal folds during production of speech sounds. If the folds are vibrating during production, the sound is voiced. If the folds are not vibrating during production then the sound is voiceless. The plosives, fricatives, and affricates all have both voiced and voiceless members. Pairs of sounds that agree in place and manner but differ in voicing are called voicing cognates. The nasals, liquids, and glides are all voiced.

ENGLISH VOWEL SYSTEM

The English vowel system consists of about 15 monophthong vowels. MacKay (1987) notes that these vowels are typically classified using three dimensions:

Height: The vertical dimension is height and refers to how high the tongue is placed during production of the vowel. Height categories include high, upper-mid, mid, lower-mid, and low.

Frontness: The horizontal dimension of frontness refers to how far forward or back the tongue is in the oral cavity during vowel production. Frontness is described by the categories of front, central and back.

Roundness: This dimension refers to lip-rounding. If lip-rounding occurs during production of the vowel it is called a rounded vowel. Only the back vowels in English are rounded. Other categories of rounding include unrounded and spread.

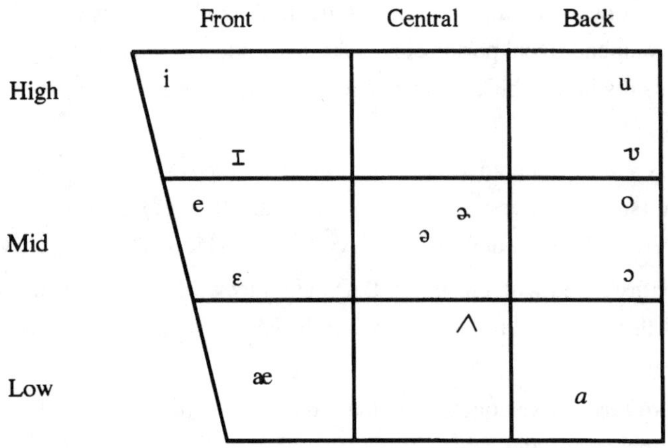

FIGURE 1.2.   Vowel quadrangle.

Tongue position during production of vowels is illustrated using a vowel quadrangle (see Figure 1.2). The quadrangle positions the vowels with respect to tongue height and frontness. The display mirrors tongue position in the vocal tract during vowel production.

MacKay (1987, p. 69) includes the dimension of tense-lax in his description of vowels. "The terms tense and lax refer to a number of phonetic features that appear together, including tongue root position, tongue body position and lip position." Tense vowels tend to have the tongue root and body advanced and the lips either more rounded or more spread in comparison to lax vowels.

MacKay (1987, p. 72) provides the following vowel descriptions for monophthongs. The word examples were added:

Vowels	Descriptions	Examples
[i]	high, front, tense (spread)	bee
[ɪ]	high, front, lax (unrounded)	bit
[e]	(upper-)mid, front, tense (unrounded)	bait
[ɛ]	(lower-)mid, front, lax (unrounded)	bet
[æ]	low, front (unrounded)	bat
[u]	high, back, tense (rounded)	boot
[ʊ]	high, back, lax (unrounded or slightly rounded)	book
[o]	upper-mid, back (rounded)	boat
[ʌ]	lower-mid, back (or central) (unrounded)	but
[ɔ]	lower-mid, back (rounded)	caught
[ɑ]	low, back (unrounded)	*fa*ther
[ə]	mid-central	*a*bove
[ɚ]	central, rhotic {unstressed}	moth*er*
[ɝ]	central, rhotic {stressed}	bird

DIPHTHONGS

In addition to the pure vowels, the English system also has a number of diphthongs. "A diphthong is a vowel whose quality or timbre changes considerably during its articulation" (MacKay, 1987, p. 73). Diphthongs are produced with the vocal tract shaped for one vowel and then shifting into production of a second vowel. The following are the English diphthongs:

Diphthong	Examples
[aɪ]	buy, my, sigh
[aʊ]	now, how, cow
[ɔɪ]	boy, toy, joy

Another term used in describing vowels is *rhotic*. Rhotic vowels are those that sound like an "r." The major rhotic vowel in English is the *schwar* as heard in the final syllable of the word "beaver." There are also rhotic diphthongs which are formed with a monophthong paired with the schwar. Some of the common rhotic diphthongs are

Vowel	Examples
[ɪɚ]	deer, steer, fear
[ɔɚ]	door, more, store
[ɑɚ]	car, star, bar
[ɛɚ]	care, stair, dare
[ʊɚ]	poor, jury

Chapter 2 | Phonological Theory

Frank Parker

PHONOLOGY AS PSYCHOLOGY

As IT IS PRESENTLY CONCEIVED, phonology is the study of the *unconscious knowledge* that underlies a human being's ability to pronounce his or her language. It is not the study of speech itself (articulatory phonetics), nor the speech signal (acoustic phonetics), nor hearing (auditory phonetics). Instead, it is the study of mind; in particular, the part of the mind that accounts for a person's ability to judge a particular pronunciation as acceptable or unacceptable in his or her native language. Consider, for example, the phrases in (1).

(1a) a history book
(1b) *an history book
(1c) a historical novel
(1d) an historical novel

First, note that all of the phrases in (1) are perfectly acceptable except for (1b) *an history book*. (The unacceptability of (1b) is indicated by the asterisk in front of it.) That is, all of the phrases in (1) would go completely unnoticed in normal conversation or reading, except for (1b).

Second, note that you do not have to be a linguist to judge (1b) *an history book* as unacceptable. Virtually *any* native speaker is able to judge instantaneously that all of the phrases in (1) are perfectly normal English except for (1b). The fact that these judgments are discrete ((1b) is bad; the others are good) and can be made by any native speaker suggests that human beings possess knowledge that allows them to make such judgments. Quite simply, it is the job of the phonologist to make this knowledge explicit.

Let's now try to articulate the knowledge that would account for the acceptability judgments

Note: Since phonology is a branch of linguistics (as opposed to speech-language pathology), a linguist has written this chapter on phonological theory. Consequently, the notation and terminology of this chapter may vary slightly from that used in the rest of this book.

in (1). One thing English speakers know is that *a* appears only before a word beginning with a consonant (C) and *an* appears only before a word beginning with a vowel (V). This distribution of *a* and *an* has a clear phonological basis: languages tend to prefer CVCV syllable structure, where C's and V's alternate, and to avoid a series of C's or V's (e.g., CCV or CVV). Thus, the use of *an* before a word beginning with a V amounts to inserting a C (*n*) between the two V's, as in *a eye* (VV) → *an eye* (VCV). We can state this generalization in the form of a rule, which we'll call *n*-Insertion. Specifically, we will stipulate that *n*-Insertion adds an *n* to the singular indefinite article (*a*) if that article precedes a word beginning with a vowel.

This rule correctly predicts that (1a) *a history book* and (1c) *a historical novel* are acceptable, since a V (*a*) appears before a word beginning with a C. It also correctly predicts that (1b) **an* *history book* is unacceptable, since *an* appears before a word beginning with a C. What this rule does not predict, however, is the acceptability of (1d) *an historical novel*. Instead, the *n*-Insertion rule predicts that (1d) should be unacceptable, since *an* appears before a word beginning with a C. Thus, the phonologist's task is now not to explain why (1b) is bad (the *n*-Insertion rule takes care of that) but rather to explain why (1d) *an historical novel* is good.

Another thing speakers know is that *h* can be deleted under certain circumstances in English. Note, for example, that the *h* in *her* can be optionally deleted, as in *Give 'er the book*. Let's call this rule *h*-Deletion. Note, too, that this rule is sensitive to stress. That is, an *h* beginning a stressed syllable cannot be deleted (e.g., *hóspital*), but an *h* beginning an unstressed syllable can be (e.g., *hospítable*). (Try this yourself. Saying *hóspital* without the *h* is much odder than saying *hospítable* without the *h*.) It's worth mentioning that we could have inferred the *h*-Deletion rule directly from form (1d) *an historical novel*. That is, the fact that *an* appears before *historical* is evidence in itself that the *h* has been deleted.

Now that we have the two rules of *n*-Insertion and *h*-Deletion, we are in a position to explain the acceptability of form (1d) *an historical novel*. In the word *histórical*, *h* begins an unstressed syllable and thus can be optionally deleted via *h*-Deletion. Once it is deleted, *histórical* now begins with a V (*i*). The *n*-Insertion rule now inserts an *n* to preserve the alternation of C's and V's. The derivation of *an historical novel* is given below. (A derivation is essentially a record of the rules that transform one linguistic form into another.)

	a histórical novel
h-Deletion:	*a istórical novel*
n-Insertion:	*an istórical novel*

Note, too, that these rules must apply in the order given above (*h*-Deletion first and then *n*-Insertion). If they apply in the opposite order, they yield an unacceptable form (**a istórical novel*), as follows.

	a histórical novel
n-Insertion:	cannot apply
h-Deletion:	*a istórical novel*

Note, too, that the two rules we have postulated, and their relative ordering, account for *all* of the judgments in (1), not just for the seemingly anomalous form (1d). The derivations of all four forms are given below.

	(1a) *a history book*	(1b) **an history book*	(1c) *a historical novel*	(1d) *an historical novel*
	a hístory book	a hístory book	a histórical novel	a histórical novel
h-Deletion:	cannot apply	cannot apply	does not apply	a istórical novel
n-Insertion:	cannot apply	cannot apply	cannot apply	an istórical novel

Note that (1b) **an history book* cannot be derived: *h*-Deletion cannot apply; therefore, *n*-Insertion cannot apply. Note, also, that both (1c) *a historical novel* and (1d) *an historical novel* can be derived because *h*-Deletion is an optional rule: it optionally does not apply in (1c), thereby blocking the application of *n*-Insertion, and it optionally does apply in (1d), thereby creating the environment for *n*-Insertion.

Let's stand back from this example for a minute and consider what we have done. We started off with the pronunciation of four phrases and noted that three were acceptable and one was unacceptable. We then speculated on what a speaker would have to know (unconsciously) to make these judgments. We hypothesized that a speaker would have to know, first, that an *h* in an unstressed syllable could be optionally deleted; second, that the singular indefinite article *a* has an *n* attached to it when it appears before a word beginning with a V; and, third, that if both processes apply to the same form, *h*-Deletion must apply before *n*-Insertion. We then showed that anyone possessing these three pieces of knowledge would make exactly those judgments in (1) above; namely (1a) *a history book*, (1b) **an history book*, (1c) *a historical novel*, and (1d) *an historical novel*. In short, we have constructed a **theory**: "a cohesive explanation of a set of phenomena, which has the capacity to predict events" (Schwartz, 1992, p. 269).

The most important thing to understand from this example is that the phonologist's primary goal is to discover the unconscious knowledge that speakers have about the pronunciation of their language. Facts about the physiology and acoustics of speech and hearing are of importance to the phonologist only insofar as they further provide insight concerning this unconscious knowledge.

COMMON PROPERTIES OF PHONOLOGICAL THEORIES

All phonological theories rely on four fundamental theoretical constructs: segments, features, levels of representation, and rules.

SEGMENTS

Consider the following explanation of segments.

When we listen to someone talk, we *hear* speech but we *perceive* segments, psychological units which correspond more or less to "speech sounds." It is necessary to make this distinction because the sound waves produced by the vocal tract are *continuous* (not divided neatly into individual sounds); however, our interpretation of these sound waves is *discrete* (we perceive distinct sounds, one following the other). For example, if someone utters the word *war* within our hearing, what we actually hear is a sound that gradually changes shape through time. What we perceive, however, is a series of three discrete segments *w-a-r*. This distinction between hearing and perceiving is fundamental to an appreciation of phonology, although it is not an easy concept to grasp. In particular, it is not immediately evident that speech is a gradually changing sound. In order to grasp this concept, you might try a simple experiment: Take some recorded speech (e.g., an audio tape) and play it at half speed. You'll notice that the "speech sounds" blur one into the other. An experiment such as this illustrates quite dramatically that what we perceive as discrete segments is actually a continuous, gradually changing, physical signal. (Adapted from Parker, 1986, p. 86)

The point to keep in mind is that *all* theories of phonology make the fundamental assumption that the continuum of speech is interpreted and organized in terms of phonological segments.

FEATURES

Segments are not thought to be the minimum units of phonology. Rather, segments are assumed to be made up of independent properties called *features*. For example, the feature [±labial] can be used to divide English consonants into two groups, as follows.

[+labial]:   *p, b, f, v, m, w*
[−labial]:   all others

Defining segments according to their feature content allows the phonologist to capture the fact that *groups* of segments behave similarly in a given language. For example, English does not allow two labial consonants to begin a syllable. We have words like *quick*, which begins with *kw*; *Gwen*, which begins with *gw*; and *twin*, which begins with *tw*. But we don't have words like *pwin* or *bwik*, both of which begin with two labial consonants.[1] This generalization would be impossible to capture without features. Instead, we would have to say that *w* can appear after *k*, *g*, and *t* but not *p* or *b*. Likewise, features allow us to make other generalizations, such as saying that vowels are lengthened before voiced consonants. In this case, we cannot identify "vowels" and "voiced consonants" without the features [±vocalic], [±consonantal], and [±voice]. Similarly, without the feature [±nasal], we cannot capture the generalization that vowels become nasalized before nasal consonants; and so on. The point to keep in mind is that *all* theories of phonology make the fundamental assumption that segments are composed of features.

LEVELS OF REPRESENTATION

All forms of rational inquiry require the analyst to be able to describe two entities as both the "same" and "different" at the same time. This may sound like a paradox, but consider the following letters of the alphabet: A, a, *a*. On the one hand, they are all the "same" in that they are all instances of the first letter of the alphabet (in contrast, say, to b, the second letter of the alphabet). On the other hand, they are all "different" in that A is a capital letter, but a and *a* are lower case. Likewise, A and a are block letters, whereas *a* is cursive. In other words, from one point of view all three letters are the same; from another point of view they are different.

Linguists call these different "points of view" *levels of representation*. Consider, for example, the words *cap* and *cab*. Any native speaker of English can tell you that they have the same

---

[1]Apparent exceptions are words such as *pueblo* and *bwana*, which begin with labial clusters. Note, however, that both words are borrowed from other languages (*pueblo* from Spanish and *bwana* from Swahili) and English speakers tend to pronounce them with a schwa between the labials. The effect of the schwa is to break up the cluster and avoid the violation.

vowel. This is uncontroversial. It is equally uncontroversial, however, that the vowel in *cab* is longer than the vowel in *cap*. That is, within the speech of any native speaker of English, the vowel in *cab* will be systematically longer than the vowel in *cap*. Phonologists resolve this apparent paradox, where two entities are both the same and different at the same time, by claiming that the vowels in *cap* and *cab* are identical on one level of representation (i.e., the underlying level), but that the vowel in *cab* is longer than that in *cap* on another level of representation (i.e., the surface level). The point to keep in mind is that *all* theories of phonology make the fundamental assumption that segments will have to be described on different levels of representation.

PHONOLOGICAL RULES

Segments on different levels of representation are related to each other by way of phonological rules. Such rules are simply generalizations about phonological processes that apply within a given language. Consider once again our *cap/cab* example discussed above. On the underlying level of representation the vowels in these words are identical; on the surface level the vowel in *cab* is longer. These two descriptions can be related by way of the following generalization about English: vowels are lengthened before voiced consonants. Thus, vowels on the underlying level of representation are related to vowels on the surface level by means of this phonological rule. Other familiar phonological rules of English are such generalizations as "Voiceless stops are aspirated in syllable-initial position," "Vowels are nasalized before a nasal consonant," and so on. The point to keep in mind is that *all* theories of phonology make the fundamental assumption that segments on different levels of representation are related systematically by way of phonological rules.

In this section, I have tried to clarify the four fundamental concepts that all theories of phonology rely upon: segments, features, levels of representation, and phonological rules. You will also notice that I have avoided using such terms as *phonemic* as well as any sort of phonemic transcription. This is because such concepts are not common to all theories of phonology, but instead enter into particular theories. The following sections address specific theories of phonology, including phonemic theory, linear phonology, autosegmental phonology, and metrical phonology.

PHONEMIC THEORY

The essence of phonemic theory is the recognition that the speech sounds in a particular language can be grouped into classes called *phonemes*. Phonemes, in turn, are defined in terms of contrast.

Phonemic theory grew out of the need to organize large numbers of sounds in a language into a smaller number of more manageable groups. Linguists in the early twentieth century began investigating the phonologies of a variety of exotic and unfamiliar languages. Among these were American Indian languages, which (like all languages) contained hundreds of different sounds. In order to make the analysis of these sounds more manageable, the phonologists tried to organize these sounds into groups. This in essence was the driving force behind phonemic theory.

To get some sense of their task, consider the problem faced by someone trying to investigate English for the first time, but who, at the same time, cannot speak English. After hundreds of hours of work, this investigator might record numerous tokens of the following words: *pin*, *spit*, and *pig*. The investigator might then make the following observations: the *p*'s in *pin* and *pig* are aspirated; the *p* in *spit* is not aspirated; the vowels in *pin* and *pig* are long; the vowel in *spit* is not long; the vowel in *pin* is nasalized; the vowels in *spit* and *pig* are not nasalized. This would give the analyst the following inventory of speech sounds.

aspirated *p*	long *i*
unaspirated *p*	short *i*
	long, nasalized *i*

Now, if you imagine this type of analysis carried throughout the entirety of English, the analyst would end up with a huge inventory of sounds. In order to impose some sort of order on this situation, phonemic theorists categorized these speech sounds, which they called *phones*, into contrasting groups which they called *phonemes*. Phonemicists developed the convention of using slashes (//) for phonemes and brackets ([ ]) for phones. The phones associated with a particular phoneme were called *allophones* of that phoneme. Thus, using this notation, they were able to say that English, for example, has one phoneme /p/ which has two allophones [p] and [pʰ]. Likewise, English has one vowel /ɪ/ which has three allophones [ɪ], [ɪ:], and [ĩ:].

Theorists defined phonemes in terms of **contrast**. Phones are said to contrast, or belong to different phonemes, if the substitution of one for another causes a change in meaning. For example, [n] and [ŋ] contrast in English because when [ŋ] in *sing* is replaced with [n] a change in meaning occurs; that is, *sing* becomes *sin*. Thus [n] and [ŋ] are allophones of different phonemes in English, namely /n/ and /ŋ/, respectively. On the other hand, [m] and [ɱ] do not contrast in English because when [m] in *comfort* is replaced by [ɱ] (a labio-dental nasal), no change of meaning occurs; that is, *comfort* remains *comfort*. Thus, [m] and [ɱ] are allophones of the same phoneme in this case, namely /m/.

Accordingly, phonemic theory admits of two levels of representation: the **phonemic level**, which embodies all of the phonological properties of a language that are capable of contrast, and the **phonetic level**, which embodies all phonological properties of that language, whether contrastive or not. For example, in English the phoneme /ɪ/ and its three allophones [ɪ], [ɪ:], and [ĩ:] would be represented on the phonemic and phonetic levels as follows.

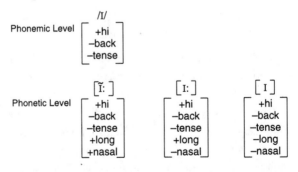

These two levels of representation are related by phonological rules (which phonemic theorists called **distribution statements**), as in the following example.

/ɪ/ :   [ĩ:]   before nasal consonants
        [ɪ:]   before voiced consonants
        [ɪ]   elsewhere

Phonemicists, however, divided sharply over the nature of phonemes. The empiricists conceived of phonemes as physical entities, directly discoverable in the speech signal. Leonard Bloomfield, who was representative of this viewpoint, states,

> Only two kinds of linguistic records are scientifically relevant. One is a mechanical record of the gross acoustic features, such as is produced in the phonetics laboratory. The other is a record in terms of *phonemes, ignoring all features that are not distinctive in the language.* (1933, p. 85; emphasis added)[2]

Bloomfield implies that phonemes are essentially a physical record of speech sounds *minus* the non-distinctive elements. Non-distinctive elements would include predictable or redundant properties of this physical record. For example, the aspiration of voiceless stops is predictable from the fact that they are in syllable-initial position before a stressed vowel; thus, aspiration is non-distinctive.

In contrast to empiricists like Bloomfield were the mentalists. They conceived of phonemes as psychological entities, which were inferable from the speech signal but not directly observable in it. Edward Sapir, who was representative of this viewpoint, states,

> In the physical world the naive speaker and hearer actualize and are sensitive to sounds, but what they feel themselves to be pronouncing and hearing are 'phonemes.' . . . *what the naive speaker hears is not phonetic elements but phonemes.* (1933/1972, p. 23; emphasis added)

Sapir illustrates his conception of the phoneme as a psychological entity with the following anecdote. Sapir was doing field work on Southern Paiute, an American Indian language spoken in western Utah and Arizona. As a pastime, he tried to teach his interpreter, an Indian named Tony, how to write Paiute phonetically. On one occasion he wanted Tony to write the word [paβa] 'at the water.' ([β] is a voiced bilabial fricative.) He told Tony to break the word into syllables and write down what he heard. Sapir was amazed when Tony syllabified the word as [pa]-pause-[pa]. In other words, the consonant Tony perceived in the second syllable was not [β] but rather [p]. Thus, Sapir realized the distinction between phones (e.g., [β]) and phonemes (e.g., /p/). Phonemes are psychological entities that exist independently of the physical speech signal. They are not simply the aggregate of the physical features of speech minus the predictable or redundant properties, as materialists like Bloomfield believed.

This debate over the nature of the phoneme lasted into the 1960's, but the psychological interpretation eventually won out and became a basic building block of linear phonology. The behaviorist bias, however, still manifests itself occasionally in applied fields, where it is not uncommon to encounter phrases such as "the phoneme /p/ is *articulated* with the lips."

Phonemic theory is still useful today for representing segments that contrast within a given speaker's repertoire. For example, consider the following exchange between a father and his 3-year-old daughter about nursery school.

FATHER: What is the name of the dog at your school?
CHILD: Way.

---

[2]One of Bloomfield's colleagues, W. Freeman Twaddell, is typical in his rejection of any sort of psychological interpretation of the phoneme. He states, ". . . In so far as he occupies himself with psychical, non-material forces, the scientist is not a scientist" (1935, p. 57).

FATHER: Way?
CHILD: No, Way.
FATHER: Did you say Way?
CHILD: No. (Angrily) I said WAY!
FATHER: (Suddenly catching on) Oh, you mean Ray?
CHILD: Yes, that's what I said—Way!

In this example, the child is not able to produce the relevant distinction between [r] in *Ray* and [w] in *Way*. However, she is able to perceive the distinction in her father's output. In other words, [r] and [w] contrast for this child and thus represent two separate phonemes in her inventory, even though she may produce them identically.

LINEAR PHONOLOGY

Linear phonology, perhaps better known as **generative phonology**, has two essential characteristics. First, it developed as a reaction to phonemic theory; in particular, it rejected the phonemic level of representation. Consequently, linear phonology admits of two levels of representation: morphophonemic and phonetic. Second, it allows more than one phonological rule to apply to a form between the underlying level of representation and the surface level.

Linear phonology was first laid out by Morris Halle in *The Sound Pattern of Russian* (1959). Chomsky and Halle further developed the theory in *The Sound Pattern of English* (1968). These revolutionary treatments essentially argued that the phonemic level of representation, which was crucial to phonemic theory, was not abstract enough to capture all phonological generalizations. Instead, linear phonologists argued that the relevant phonological levels of representation were the morphophonemic and the phonetic.

In order to understand this argument, we need to define some terms. A **morpheme** is the minimal unit of phonological form associated with a constant meaning. The word *wives*, for example, is made up of two morphemes *wife* 'female spouse' + *−s* 'more than one.' The **morphophonemic** level gives each morpheme a unique phonological representation. Thus, the root form of *wife/wives* would have to be represented either as //waɪf// or //waɪv//, since they both represent the same morpheme. (Morphophonemes are indicated by double slashes.) The **phonemic** level, however, gives each contrasting segment (or phoneme) a unique representation. Thus, the final segment in *wife* would have to be represented as /f/, but the corresponding segment in *wives* would be represented as /v/, since /f/ and /v/ contrast. The **phonetic** level, as in virtually all phonological theories, gives the predictable detail associated with each segment. Thus, the vowel in *wife* would be represented as [aɪ], but the vowel in *wives* would be represented as [aɪ:], since vowels in English are systematically longer before voiced consonants. In other words, the morphophonemic level preserves the identity of morphemes; the phonemic level preserves the identity of phonemes; and the phonetic level provides predictable detail. These generalizations are illustrated in the following chart. (+ = morpheme boundary.)

	wife	*wives*
Morphophonemic Level	//waɪf//	//waɪf+z//
Phonemic Level	/waɪf/	/waɪvz/
Phonetic Level	[waɪf]	[waɪ:vz]

Linear phonologists, however, argued that the only relevant levels of phonological representation are morphophonemic and phonetic. Although Halle's original argument against a phonemic level used Russian examples, for simplicity's sake I will discuss an analogous example from English. The words *impossible* and *intolerable* contain the same negative prefix, represented morphophonemically as //ɪn//. The nasal segment undergoes the phonological rule of Nasal Assimilation, which changes the place of articulation of the nasal to that of the following consonant. Thus, the //ɪn// prefix in *impossible* becomes labial (i.e., /m/) because it precedes a labial consonant (i.e., //p//). Likewise, the //ɪn// prefix in *intolerable* remains dental (i.e., /n/) because it precedes a dental consonant (i.e., //t//); and so on. This is illustrated in the following chart.

	impossible	*intolerable*
Morphophonemic Level	//ɪn + p. . .//	//ɪn + t. . .//
Nasal Assimilation	↓	
Phonemic Level	/ɪmp. . ./	/ɪnt. . ./

Now consider the word *invaluable*, which may also undergo Nasal Assimilation whereby the //ɪn// prefix becomes labio-dental (i.e., [ɱ]) because it precedes a labio-dental consonant (i.e., //v//). Note, however, that [ɱ] is not a separate phoneme in English; in this case it is simply an allophone of /n/. Thus, in order to preserve the phonemic level of representation (i.e., a level on which there are only phonemes), we would have to allow the rule of Nasal Assimilation to apply *twice*: once *above* the phonemic level, turning //ɪn// into /ɪm/ in *impossible*, and once *below* the phonemic level, turning /ɪn/ into [ɪɱ] in *invaluable*. This is illustrated in the following chart.

	impossible	*intolerable*	*invaluable*
Morphophonemic Level	//ɪn + p. . .//	//ɪn + t. . .//	//ɪn + v. . .//
Nasal Assimilation	↓		
Phonemic Level	/ɪmp. . ./	/ɪnt. . ./	/ɪnv. . ./
Nasal Assimilation			↓
Phonetic Level	[ɪmp. . .]	[ɪnt. . .]	[ɪɱv. . .]

Linear phonologists claimed that this kind of analysis missed a significant generalization solely to preserve a phonemic level of representation. They argued that to preserve the generalization that there was a single rule of Nasal Assimilation in English, the theory would have to dispense with the phonemic level. A linear analysis of the same data is given in the following chart.

	impossible	*intolerable*	*invaluable*
Morphophonemic Level	//ɪn + p. . .//	//ɪn + t. . .//	//ɪn + v. . .//
Nasal Assimilation	↓		↓
Phonetic Level	[ɪmp. . .]	[ɪnt. . .]	[ɪɱv. . .]

The linear analysis is much simpler, but it requires the rejection of the phonemic level.

Another innovation of linear phonology was to allow more than one phonological rule to apply in the derivation of a particular form. You will recall that phonemic theorists handled phonological rules by way of distribution statements. As we discussed earlier, the words *pin*, *pig*, and *spit* have three different vowels: [ɪ̃ː], [ɪː], and [ɪ], respectively. Accordingly, phonemicists would represent these facts in terms of the following distribution statements.

/ɪ/   :[ĩ:] before nasal consonants
      [ɪ:] before voiced consonants
      [ɪ]   elsewhere

These types of statements can be interpreted as allowing only one rule to apply between the underlying phonemic form and the surface phonetic form. Consider, for example, the first distribution statement above, which can be interpreted as something like /ɪ/ becomes long and nasalized before a nasal consonant. This distribution statement is formalized below as a phonological rule.

	pin
Phonemic Level	/pɪn/
Vowel Lengthening and Nasalization	pĩ:n
Phonetic Level	[pĩ:n]

The linear phonologists thought that such an analysis conflated two generalizations: (*a*) that the vowel is long because the following consonant (/n/) is voiced and (*b*) that the vowel is nasalized because the following consonant (/n/) is a nasal. Thus, they factored out the contribution of each property and put them into separate rules, as follows.

	pin
Morphophonemic Level	//pɪn//
Vowel Lengthening	pɪ:n
Vowel Nasalization	pĩ:n
Phonetic Level	[pĩ:n]

The establishment of the morphophonemic level as the most abstract level of phonological representation and the concomitant rejection of the phonemic level has become a mainstay of phonological theory to this day. Likewise, the concept of multistep analysis, where more than one rule applies in the derivation of a single form, is fundamental to current phonological theory.

Linear phonology is most useful for illustrating surface variation in a single morpheme. Consider, for example, a child who says [dɔ:] for *dog* and [dɔ:gi] for *doggie*. The fact that the [g] appears in at least one of the two related words is evidence for representing the morpheme *dog* in this child's lexicon as //dɔg//. The surface forms would be derived from this form by way of two phonological rules: (a) Vowel Lengthening—a vowel is lengthened before a voiced consonant, and (b) Final Consonant Reduction—a consonant is deleted at the end of a word. The derivation of each word is illustrated below.

Morphophonemic Level	//dɔg//	//dɔg+i//
Vowel Lengthening	dɔ:g	dɔ:gi
Final Consonant Reduction	dɔ:	cannot apply
Phonetic Level	[dɔ:]	[dɔ:gi]

Linear phonology is still capable of handling the vast majority of phonological phenomena that practitioners in applied fields deal with today.

Before leaving the subject of linear phonology, let's consider two theories that fall within its domain: David Stampe's Natural Phonology, first published in ''The Acquisition of Phonetic Representations'' (1969), and Joan Hooper's Natural Generative Phonology, comprehensively treated in *An Introduction to Natural Generative Phonology* (1976). It is worth emphasizing that there are more theories of *phonological acquisition* than theories of *phonology*.

Stampe's **natural phonology** essentially claims that children do not acquire the phonological rules of the language to which they are exposed, but rather are born with an innate, universal set of rules (Stampe calls them *processes*) and learn to suppress those that do not apply in their own language. Consider, for example, German and English. German has a rule of Final Devoicing whereby an obstruent (i.e., stop, fricative, or affricate) is devoiced in word-final position. English does not have such a rule. The conventional position would be that neither German nor English speakers are born with this rule, but that German speakers learn it because they are exposed to examples that support it. In contrast, natural phonology assumes that both German and English speakers are born with the rule, but that English speakers learn to suppress it because they are not exposed to examples that support it. This situation is illustrated in the diagram below.

	Conventional Position	*Natural Phonology*
Germans	learn Final Devoicing	do not suppress Final Devoicing
English	do not learn Final Devoicing	suppress Final Devoicing

Hooper's **natural generative phonology** essentially claims that the only phonological rules that a child can learn are those that express exceptionless surface generalizations. Consider, for example, the words *writer* [ráɪɾər] and *rider* [ráɪːɾər]. The [ɾ] in *writer* is a manifestation of /t/ and that in *rider* is a manifestation of /d/. The conventional explanation of the length contrast is as follows: The vowel in *writer* is short because it preceded voiceless /t/ and the vowel in *rider* is long because it preceded voiced /d/, at an earlier stage in the derivation. The conventional treatment would be to posit the underlying representation //raɪt+ər// for *writer* and //raɪd+ər// for *rider*, then derive the surface forms via the rules of Vowel Lengthening and Flapping. This solution, however, would not be allowed in natural generative phonology, because the Vowel Lengthening rule does not express an exceptionless surface generalization. This is because the same voiced consonant ([ɾ]) is preceded by both a short vowel in *writer* [ráɪɾər] and a long vowel in *rider* [ráɪːɾər]. Thus, because of this one single exception to the generalization that all vowels are long before voiced consonants, natural generative phonology would be forced to reject this generalization and posit the underlying representation //raɪt+ər// for *writer* (with a short vowel) and //raɪːd+ər// for *rider* (with a long vowel).

Natural phonology and natural generative phonology have had an impact on the development of phonological theory during the past 20 years, especially in terms of "learnability theory" (i.e., what is a human being capable of learning about a language based on samples of that language?). Both of these theories, however, have always been firmly grounded in the linear framework.

AUTOSEGMENTAL PHONOLOGY

Linear phonology derives its name from the fact that a phonological representation is conceived of as a single, linear string of segments, each composed of a number of feature specifications. Autosegmental phonology essentially claims that some features can be factored out of this linear arrangement of segments and represented independently.

This extension of linear phonology was first proposed by John Goldsmith in his MIT dissertation, *Autosegmental Phonology* (1976). Goldsmith proposed this theory to account for tonal phenomena; but before getting into tone, let me try to illustrate the essential problem he was working on with an English example. Linear phonology does not allow *sequences* of features within one segment. In other words, the phonological properties represented by feature specifications are defined as extending *throughout* each segment. For example, consider the representation of the feature [±voice] in the word *pea:*

/p/   /i/[3]
[−vce]   [+vce]

In this linear representation, the *entire* segment corresponding to /p/ is [−vce] and the *entire* segment corresponding to /i/ is [+vce].

Now consider an affricate such as /č/, the initial consonant in *chip*. Affricates, by definition, begin like a stop and end like a fricative. The feature that differentiates stops and fricatives is [±continuant]. (Stops are [−continuant] and fricatives are [+continuant].) However, since a single segment cannot be designated both [+continuant] and [−continuant] at the same time, linear phonologists constructed the feature [±delayed release] solely to designate affricates. That is, an affricate is [+delayed release] to indicate two states of the vocal tract: the pre-release state (i.e., a stop) and the release state (i.e., a fricative). As shown in the diagram below, linear phonology would represent /č/ as on the left, where the feature [+delayed release] is used solely to avoid the contradictory feature specification on the right.

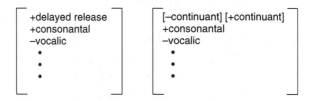

A feature such as [±delayed release], however, violates feature theory in that we now have a property (i.e., complete closure of the vocal tract) that does not extend throughout an entire segment.

The solution proposed by Goldsmith was essentially to factor out the property that changes within the boundaries of one segment (in this case [±continuant]) and put it on another "tier." Consider how /č/ would be represented in autosegmental phonology.

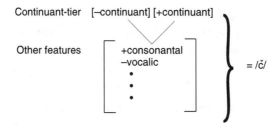

Note how the autosegmental treatment gets around the problem of having a property change within the boundaries of a segment. According to Goldsmith, the one-tiered representation of

---

[3]Do not be confused by the use of single and double slashes. Most phonologists, regardless of the theory they subscribe to, use single slashes to designate underlying forms, whether phonemic or morphophonemic. The one notable exception, of course, is when the point of the discussion is to *distinguish* between phonemic and morphophonemic levels of representation.

linear phonology should be split into several tiers. Each tier can then have a different number of segments. Thus, a single segment on one tier (e.g., [+consonantal, −vocalic] . . .) can be associated with more than one segment on another tier (e.g., [+continuant] and [−continuant]). In fact, the term *autosegmental* derives from the phrase *autonomous segments*. According to Goldsmith, autonomous segments are segments on one level that do not match one-for-one those on another level. (Actually, since many autosegments contain a single feature, it might have been less confusing if Goldsmith had called his theory *autofeatural phonology*, indicating that individual features are what can be factored out of a linear representation and put on a different tier.)

Now let's consider how autosegmental phonology can be extended to tone, since tone is what originally motivated the theory.[4] English has three tones: High, Mid, and Low. They are assigned to words (in isolation) according to the following rules.

(a) High tone is assigned to the vowel with primary stress.
(b) Low tone is assigned to the final vowel and to any vowels preceding it, back to the stressed vowel.
(c) Mid tone is assigned to any vowels preceding the stressed vowel.

According to these rules, all words in isolation will have one High tone and one or more Low tones, but some words will not have a Mid tone (i.e., words having primary stress on the first syllable).

Let's now consider two problems that argue for an autosegmental treatment of tone. The first is the case where two tones must be associated with a single vowel. Consider the names *Patricia*, *Trisha*, and *Trish*. In *Patricia* the second syllable has primary stress so it is assigned High tone; the final vowel is assigned Low tone; and the vowel preceding stress is assigned Mid tone, as follows.

This example does not present a problem for linear phonology since there is a one-to-one correspondence between vowels and tones.

In *Trisha* the first syllable has primary stress so it is assigned High tone; the final vowel is assigned Low tone; but since there are no vowels preceding stress, no Mid tone is assigned. This is illustrated in the following diagram.

Again, this example does not present a problem for linear phonology since there is a one-to-one correspondence between vowels and tones.

Now consider the name *Trish*. There is only one syllable so it has primary stress and is

---

[4]Systematic tonal phenomena do occur in English, even though most people outside of phonology do not realize it. Schwartz, for example, writing in a speech pathology journal, stated that "this particular feature [i.e., tone] is not relevant for English" (1992, p. 272).

assigned High tone. But what about Low tone? According to our rules, Low tone is obligatory and is assigned to the final vowel, as follows.

/tríš/

H L

There are two things to note about this example. First, this representation accounts for the fact that when this name is spoken it has a High tone followed by a Low tone. (It is particularly noticeable when it's sung: Imagine a father going out in the yard and calling his daughter by this name; it would come out something like *Tri-ish.*) Second, this example, where two tones are associated with one vowel, *requires* an autosegmental treatment. That is, tone has to be removed from the segmental representation of the vowel and placed on a separate tier; otherwise the only vowel in the word would have to be specified as [+high] and [+low] at the same time—a specification that is essentially uninterpretable.

The second problem that argues for an autosegmental treatment of tone is a case where two or more vowels must be associated with a single tone. Consider, for example, the word *Indianapolis.* The *nap* syllable has primary stress so it is assigned High tone; the following vowels are assigned Low tone; and the preceding vowels are assigned Mid tone, as follows.

/Indiə nǽpəlɪs

M   H   L

This example, where two or more vowels are associated with a single tone, does not *require* an autosegmental treatment. Each vowel could in fact be assigned a Mid, High, or Low tone depending on its relation to primary stress, as follows.

/ɪ n d i ə n ǽ p ə l ɪ s/
[+M]   [+M] [+M]   [+H] [+L] [+L]

This linear solution, however, clearly fails to capture the generalization that Mid tone is assigned to *all* vowels preceding the stressed vowel and that Low tone is assigned to *all* vowels from the final vowel to the stressed vowel, *regardless of their number.*

In short, autosegmental phonology was originally conceived to account for cases where a single segment is associated with two mutually exclusive properties. Examples are affricates, which are necessarily associated with both [+continuant] and [−continuant], and stressed monosyllables, which are necessarily associated with a High tone and a Low tone. It is also useful in cases where a single property is associated with a number of segments.

One practical application of autosegmental theory is to feature spreading. Consider, for example, the feature [±round]: the vowels /u, ʊ, o, ɔ/ and (in most dialects) the consonants /r, w, š, ž/ are all [+round]; all other segments in English are [−round]. There are two rules for "spreading" the feature [±round]. First, [±round] spreads from a vowel to adjacent consonants. Thus, we have the following feature spreading in *stout.* (A solid line = an inherent feature specification; a dotted line = a spread feature specification.)

stout

[s t a ʊ t]

[−rnd][+rnd]

Second, [±round] spreads from a consonant to an adjacent consonant up to a vowel. Thus, we have the following spreading in *quaint.*

$$[kwent]$$

[+rnd][−rnd]

Feature spreading in English also occurs with such features as [±voice] and [±nasal], which makes them amenable to an autosegmental treatment.

METRICAL PHONOLOGY

The primary innovation of metrical phonology has been to extend the hierarchical conception of linguistic structure from syntax to phonology, as follows.

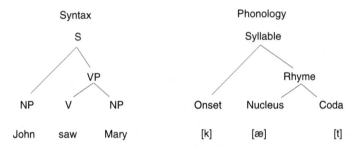

This innovation essentially allows phonologists to deal with two problems that had resisted solution in linear phonology: (*a*) the analysis of stress and (*b*) a representation of syllables.

Metrical phonology was first conceived by Mark Liberman in his MIT dissertation, *The Intonational System of English* (1975), to account for stress. The theory was refined and expanded in Liberman and Prince, "On Stress and Linguistic Rhythm" (1977). Liberman and Prince objected to the treatment of stress in linear phonology on two grounds. First, stress was one of the few non-binary features. That is, most other features were two-valued (e.g., [±voice], [±nasal]), but there are an infinite number of values for stress in linear phonology. Consider the following phrases and the stress values assigned in linear phonology. (1 = heaviest stress.)

(2a) *French Lit* 'French literature'
　　　　2　1
(2b) *French Lit teacher* 'teacher of French literature'
　　　　3　1　2
(2c) *old French Lit teacher* 'teacher of French literature who is old'
　　　　2　4　1　3

In (2a) *French* is assigned a stress value of 2; in (2b) it is assigned a value of 3; and in (2c) it is assigned a value of 4. This analysis is paradoxical given the fact that the word *French* is used in exactly the same sense in each one of these phrases. The point is that there are a potentially infinite number of stress values in linear phonology and that they change depending upon how many other words are in the phrase.

In contrast, a basic tenet of metrical phonology is that stress should be seen as a relation between two units instead of a feature assigned to a segment. As such, stress patterns are represented in terms of a binary branching tree where one branch is labelled *S* (for "stronger") and the other is labelled *W* (for "weaker"). Thus, every tree in metrical phonology must be of one of the following two basic types.

For example, *French Lit, French Lit teacher,* and *old French Lit teacher* would have the following structures in metrical phonology.

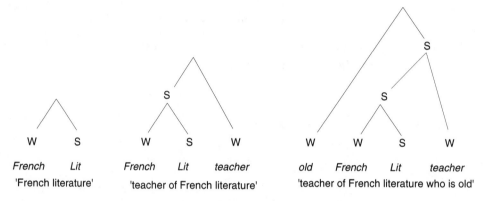

| French | Lit | | French | Lit | teacher | | old | French | Lit | teacher |

'French literature'   'teacher of French literature'   'teacher of French literature who is old'

Note that in these representations stress is binary in that there are only two values for stress (S and W) and the stress assignment for *French* does not change with the addition of words to the phrase. In all three phrases it is W.

The second objection Liberman and Prince had to the treatment of stress in linear phonology was that the patterns assigned by the rules implied a relationship between words that in fact were unrelated in terms of stress. Consider again the phrase *French Lit teacher.*

   French Lit teacher 'teacher of French literature'
      3   1   2

This representation implies that *French* and *teacher* have a stress relation in that *French* (3) has weaker stress than *teacher* (2). Likewise, it implies that *Lit* and *teacher* have a stress relation in that *Lit* (1) has heavier stress than *teacher* (2). Liberman and Prince, however, argue that there are only two relevant stress relations: *Lit* has stronger stress than *French,* and *French Lit* has stronger stress than *teacher.* The following hierarchical structure captures exactly these generalizations.

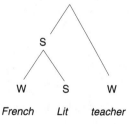

   French   Lit   teacher

That is, *Lit* is stronger than *French,* and *French Lit* is stronger than *teacher.* Unlike linear phonology, this metrical representation implies absolutely no stress relation between *French* or *Lit* and *teacher.*

A second innovation of metrical phonology was to introduce the concept of syllable to phonology for the first time. As Clements and Keyser state,

> Until very recently, generative [i.e., linear] phonology was premised on the notion that phonological representation consists of linear strings of segments with no hierarchical organization other than that provided by syntactic phrase structure. In particular, the notion syllable was thought to play no role in phonological organization. (1983, p. 1)

Consider, for example, the representation of the word *extended* in linear phonology: //ɛkstɛndəd//. Note that there is no indication of syllable boundaries.

Contrast this linear representation with that in metrical phonology, as illustrated below. (The Greek letter *sigma* (σ) = syllable.)

Note that this metrical representation not only indicates syllables, but also which consonants are associated with which syllable. The general rule for syllabification in English is to associate consonants with the *following* vowel, unless it violates a **phonotactic** constraint (i.e., a restriction on the number and kinds of segments that can occur in sequence). Take, for example, the second vowel /ɛ/ above. We begin by trying to associate each of the preceding consonants with it. Thus, /tɛ/ is a possible syllable in English, and so is /stɛ/; however, /kstɛ/ is not, since /kst/ is not a possible cluster. Therefore, we associate /st/ with the following vowel and /k/ with the preceding vowel.

In short, metrical phonology has extended hierarchical structure to phonology. From this, phonologists have been able to construct a very simple theory of stress: every binary branching tree has a weaker branch and a stronger branch. Likewise, hierarchical structure has allowed for linguists to incorporate the concept of syllable into phonology.

For practical purposes, this metrical representation can be extended to include a morphological representation of a word as well as its syllabic representation, as illustrated below with *extended*. (The Greek letter *mu* (μ) = morpheme.)

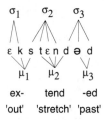

This type of metrical representation captures quite nicely the fact that syllable boundaries do not always coincide with morphological boundaries.

SUMMARY

Let me try to summarize the main points of this chapter. First, phonology is primarily the study of mind (i.e., psychology) rather than speech (i.e., physiology). Second, all theories of phonology incorporate four fundamental concepts: segments, features, levels, and rules. Third, we have looked at four basic theories of phonology: phonemic theory, linear phonology, autosegmental phonology, and metrical phonology. These four theories, however, should not be seen as mutually exclusive. Rather, they should be viewed as evolutionary steps in phonological thought. Phonemic theory is responsible for the insight that speech sounds have to be described on at least two different levels of representation—phonemic and phonetic. Phonemes, in fact, are the best theoretical construct available for representing segments that *contrast* in a speaker's inventory. Linear phonology is responsible for the insight that the function of phonology is not to relate phonemes to phones, via distribution statements, but rather to relate morphemes to phones via phonological rules. Linear phonology, in fact, is the best theoretical construct available for handling the vast majority of phonological phenomena. Autosegmental phonology is responsible for the insight that one or more features can be factored out of a linear representation and put on separate tiers. An autosegmental treatment is required when a single segment is associated with two mutually exclusive properties (e.g., affricates). An autosegmental treatment is desirable when more than one segment is associated with a single property (e.g., rounding). Metrical phonology is responsible for the insight that phonological representations have hierarchical structure much as do syntactic representations. This insight has led to theories of stress and the syllable.

ACKNOWLEDGMENTS

I want to thank Tom Walsh and Kathryn Riley for their invaluable help with this chapter.

REFERENCES

Bloomfield L. *Language.* New York: Holt, Rinehart and Winston, 1933.
Chomsky N, Halle M. *The sound pattern of English.* New York: Harper and Row, 1968.
Clements GN, Keyser SJ. *CV phonology.* Cambridge, MA: MIT Press, 1983.
Goldsmith J. *Autosegmental phonology.* MIT Doctoral Dissertation (1976). New York: Garland Press, 1979.
Halle M. *The sound pattern of Russian.* The Hague: Mouton, 1959.
Hooper JB. *An introduction to natural generative phonology.* New York: Academic Press, 1976.
Liberman M. *The intonational system of English.* MIT Doctoral Dissertation, 1975.
Liberman M, Prince A. On stress and linguistic rhythm. *Linguistic Inquiry* 1977;8:249–336.
Parker F. *Linguistics for non-linguists.* Boston: Little, Brown, 1986.
Sapir E. The psychological reality of phonemes. *Journal de Psychologie Normale et Pathologique* 1933;30:247–265 (in French). Reprinted in Makkai B, ed. *Phonological theory.* New York: Holt, Rinehart and Winston, 1972:22–31.
Schwartz RG. Clinical applications of recent advances in phonological theory, *Language, Speech, and Hearing Sciences in Schools* 1992;23:269–276.
Stampe D. The acquisition of phonetic representation. *Papers from the 5th Annual Meeting of the Chicago Linguistic Society,* 1969:443–454.
Twaddell WF. *On defining the phoneme* (Language Monograph, 16). Baltimore: Linguistic Society of America, 1935.

Normal Phonological Development

Chapter 3

Jacqueline Bauman-Waengler

THE LAST DECADE has witnessed considerable changes in terminology within the field of speech pathology. The much needed influence of linguistics, for example, replaced several familiar terms. We now read about phonological disorders, phonological processes, and clinical phonology. Within this context we also experienced a shift from sound or speech sound development to phonological development. To some this signaled only a difference in wording. Actually, though, the basic concept had undergone a fundamental transformation. Speech sound development refers primarily to the gradual articulatory mastery of sound productions within a given language. Thus, the proficiency of a child to produce adult-like speech sounds is measured. Phonological development, on the other hand, implies the acquisition of a sound system intricately connected to the child's overall growth in language. Phonology refers to the language-specific function of speech sounds, to their ability to establish, when arranged in certain ways, meaningful units of the language in question, namely "words." Speech sound production is certainly one portion of phonological development, however, it is not its entirety.

The purpose of this chapter is first to examine some of the available information in articulatory and phonological development. This examination will range from the babbling stages of a child's so-called prelinguistic development to the near completion of the child's phonological system during the early school years. In reviewing the literature an attempt will be made to discuss the various studies so that the student and practitioner will become aware of the differences in design and purpose which have often resulted in rather contrasting outcomes.

Another goal of this chapter is to show interdependencies between language and phonological development. Developing phonology cannot be meaningfully separated from other aspects of emerging language. It is an integral part of the child's total language acquisition process. Hence, while cognitive and motor abilities play important roles in the unfolding of phonology, the child's acquisition of semantic, morphosyntactic, and pragmatic skills influence it as well.

Language development is a truly amazing process, the phonological portion is one of its most important aspects.

Finally, this chapter will provide the reader with approximate ages for the various stages of phonological development. These guidelines will become important when we try to separate normal from abnormal development.

Over the years many investigators have tried to determine when individual sounds were "mastered" in specific groups of children. Such group findings will be discussed, however, the large role of individual variation and its impact on the child's phonological development will be emphasized. Each child develops her or his language in a particular manner. Recent findings (Stoel-Gammon and Cooper, 1984; Vihman, 1992) underline that although general trends across children can certainly be identified, individual variation is more the rule than the exception.

BABBLING

The beginning of phonological development is often associated with the child's first meaningful words. Therefore, specific sounds and sound combinations have been verified that occur more or less frequently in these initial words. Is this, however, actually the beginning of an emerging phonological system? Do not these words actually prove that the productional and perceptual development of the phonological system is well on its way?

Within the area of child language a division is made between linguistic development, or the appearance of the first real words, and prelinguistic behavior, including vocalizations prior to this one-word stage. This division could be substantiated by the use of meaningful versus non-meaningful productions. However, in effect, one major cause for this separation was the so-called discontinuity hypothesis formulated by Roman Jakobson (1941/1968). According to this viewpoint, babbling was a random series of vocalizations during which a multitude of sounds were produced with no apparent order or consistency. Such behavior was to be clearly separated from the following systematic sound productions evidenced in the first words. The division between prelinguistic and linguistic phases of sound production was, according to Jakobson, often so complete that the child might actually undergo a period of silence between the end of the babbling period and the first real words.

Research since that time (e.g., Oller, Weiman, Doyle and Ross, 1976; Stark, 1979) has repeatedly documented that (a) babbling behavior is not random; rather, the child's productions develop in a systematic manner, (b) not all sounds are randomly produced during this babbling stage but a subset of phones occur more often, and (c) the transition between babbling and first words is not abrupt but continuous; late babbling behavior and the first words are very similar in respect to the sounds used and the way they are combined. It also appears that the child's perceptual abilities are rather developed before the first meaningful utterances. For example, some word comprehension is evident at approximately 9 months of age. In respect to phonology, the discrimination between phonetic speech sound categories has often been shown in infants within the first few months of life (see Jusczyk, 1992, for a review of these studies). The presence of phonemic contrasts in very young children has also been documented (Shvachkin, 1973). Although this acquisition is gradual, more general contrasts begin at approximately 1 year of age. Findings like these suggest that the child's language system starts to develop prior to the first spoken meaningful words.

The beginning of a child's phonological system seems often to hinge on the observations by adults that the child demonstrates phonemic distinctions such as those seen in the words [noʊ] versus [goʊ]. However, this observation may only reflect our understanding of and preoccupation with the phoneme rather than the actual beginning of a phonological system. Traditionally, the phoneme is defined as the smallest unit that distinguishes meaning. Therefore, we know that /h/ and /s/ are American-English phonemes as they distinguish meaning in such words as "hat" versus "sat." However, this phoneme concept represents only the end product of an analysis, a minimal unit that still can signal a difference in meaning. Yet larger units can function contrastively as well. Within the context of language development these larger constructs may play an important role. For example, two words can be dissimilar in the totality of their sound constituents: "foot" versus "car." Due to this difference, they are appropriate signs to signal differences in meaning linguistically. Early European structuralists of the Prague School of linguistics have called such signs phonological units (Trubetzkoy, 1939, 1969).

According to the structuralists, phonological units can be quite variable in size, ranging in length from multisyllabic words to phonemes, their minimal form. For example, phonological units could be multisyllabic, such as in "elephant" versus "calendar." They can also be reduced to a single syllable, as in "mo-ther" versus "fa-ther." The actual sound distinction here occurring between the first word syllables /mʌ/ versus /fɑ/. Phonological units can even be smaller than that; they can go down to the single sound level. Although such single sounds are not meaningful in themselves, they can nevertheless establish differences in word meaning such as in [tɑp] versus [pɑp]. If sounds serve this function in a given language, they are said to be **phonemes** of that language. Phonemes, then, are the smallest of all phonological units.

Applying this concept to the beginning stages of phonological development in children, we could propose that the child first perceives, distinguishes, and produces larger phonological units, perhaps at the word or syllable level. Only later might the child learn to differentiate between the smallest phonological units at the phoneme level. Similar ideas have been generated by Ferguson (1978), Kiparsky and Menn (1977), Menn (1975, 1980), and Waterson (1971). This is also a viable thought within the attunement-refinement theory outlined by Ingram (1989). Originally proposed by Oller (1980), this theory sees the child as an active participant in his/her development. Although all children have certain basic abilities, they build on them through interaction with the environment. Categorical skills acquired through this interaction at one stage will lead to greater differentiations at a later stage. Thus, the child could well begin with distinguishing relatively large phonological units, then progress to the differentiation of smaller and smaller ones. The phoneme distinction could be the end product of this distinction, occurring sometime during the stage of the first 50 words (Ingram, 1989).

With this in mind, one could argue that phonological development begins before its manifestation in the use of the first words. How much before? Only at approximately 6–8 months of age does the child's vocal tract approximate its later adult shape, a prerequisite for sound production as we know it. These physiological changes coincide with the beginning of the babbling period. Most authors agree that the babbling at this stage is already closely related to the first words. It shows refined perception and productions which are similar to those later used in the first 50 words. Following this reasoning, the discussion of phonological development will commence at the beginning of the babbling stage.

Forms of Babbling

Babbling usually begins abruptly around 6 months of age and extends until the child's first words appear at age 10–13 months. Most children continue to babble into the time when they say their first words. The initial portion of babbling is known as **reduplicated babbling**. At this stage basically similar strings of consonant-vowel productions occur. There might be slight quality variations in the vowel sounds of these strings of babbles, however, the consonants will stay the same from syllable to syllable. An example of this might be [mamə]. During the second portion of the babbling era, at approximately 9 months of age, **nonreduplicated** or **variegated babbling** begins. Now, as the child babbles, consonants and vowels may vary from syllable to syllable. An example of this might be [mabə]. These two types of babbling have often been collapsed into one single stage called **canonical babbling**.

From the previous description one has the impression that they are sequential in nature, a child first going through reduplicated babbling and then later nonreduplicated babbling. This has been documented by Elbers (1982), Oller (1980), and Stark (1979), to mention a few. However, more recent investigators have questioned this pattern. For example, Mitchell and Kent (1990) assessed the phonetic variation of multisyllabic babbling in eight infants at 7, 9, and 11 months of age. Their findings showed that (*a*) nonreduplicated babbling was present from the point in time the infant began to produce multisyllabic babbling, not evolving out of an earlier period of reduplicated babbling, and (*b*) no significant difference was found between the amount of phonetic variation for the vocalizations when the infants were 7, 9, and 11 months old. These and other findings (Holmgren, Lindblom, Aurelius, Jalling, and Zetterstrom, 1986; Smith, Brown-Sweeney, and Stoel-Gammon, 1989) call into question widely accepted models of clearly defined stages in infants' prelinguistic behavior. It could also be that the children in this and other studies demonstrated examples of individual variation. One child in the Mitchell and Kent study, for example, increased phonetic variation across the age range in question while another subject showed the exact opposite tendency, i.e., a decrease in phonetic variation from 7–11 months.

One factor which may account for the seemingly oppositional findings is the method of data collection/analysis. The phonetic transcription of infants' babbling behavior is not an easy task. Without phonemic boundaries to aid in establishing perceptual categories, the transcriber is forced to rely on phonetic variation between utterances. Phonetically no two natural productions can ever be exactly the same. Therefore, how much phonetic variation was accepted as being the "same" babble and when were two babbles considered to be "different"? In addition, the investigators' criteria for data analysis always varied somewhat.

With these methodological difficulties in mind, let's try to examine the child's segmental productions towards the end of the canonical babbling stage. Since the productions cannot yet be said to be true vowels and consonants of a particular language system, they will be referred to as **vocoids** and **contoids.** These are terms which were used by Pike (1941) to indicate non-phonemic function of speech sounds within a language system.

Vocoids

One of the earliest series of investigations with a large number of children were those carried out by Irwin and colleagues in the 1940s and 50s. According to these data on 57 children from

13–14 months of age, there was still a continued predominance of the [ɛ], [ɪ] and [ʌ] vocoids. Thus, front and central vocoids were found to be favored over back vocoids.

If we compare Irwin's data to Kent and Bauer's (1985), similarities as well as differences arise. While Kent and Bauer also report high percentages of [ʌ] and [ɛ] vocoids, other vocoids such as [ɪ] and [u] were utilized far less often by the infants in the Kent and Bauer study. The rank order of the six most prevalent vowels from the two investigations are

Irwin (1948) ɛ ɪ ʌ ʊ ɑ u
Kent and Bauer (1985) ʌ ɛ æ ɑ ʊ

Although some differences can be observed, one could generalize from these findings that central and front vocoids do seem to show a higher frequency in the later babbling of infants.

Contoids

Several authors have investigated the contoids which predominate in the late babbling stage. Locke (1983) provides an excellent overview of the results for three major investigations (Table 3.1).

As can be seen, the most frequent contoids were [h] [d], [b], [m], [t], [g], and [w]. Although some differences again exist between the findings, the amazing agreement is that the 12 most frequent contoids produced represent about 95% of all the contoids transcribed in the three

TABLE 3.1. Relative Frequency of English Consonant-like Sounds in the Babbling of 11–12-Month-Old American Infants[a]

More Frequent Consonants				Less Frequent Consonants			
Sound	A[b]	B	C	Sound	A[b]	B	C
h	31.77	21.0	18.3	v	1.03	1.0	0
d	20.58	30.0	13.5	l	.96	1.0	1.6
b	9.79	5.0	10.0	θ	.85	0	.4
m	6.69	1.0	7.2	z	.56	0	0
t	4.34	0	3.6	f	.37	0	0.4
g	4.15	12.0	8.4	ʃ	.37	0	0
s	3.45	0	.4	ð	.34	0	0.8
w	3.39	17.0	8.4	ŋ	.33	1.0	3.2
n	2.65	1.0	4.4	ʒ	.10	0	0
k	2.12	1.0	6.3	r	.10	0	0
j	1.77	9.0	11.6	tʃ	0	0	0
p	1.63	0	1.6	ʤ	0	0	0
Totals	92.33	97.0	93.7		5.01	3.0	6.4

[a]The three investigations represented are: A: Irwin (1947); B: Fisichelli (1950); C: Pierce and Hanna (1974).
[b]The A columns total less than 100% because the difference (2.66%) represents several sounds in Irwin's original tabulations that have no phonemic equivalent in American English phonology (e.g., [ʔ ç χ]).

studies. These findings stand in contrast to earlier statements that babbling consisted of a great multitude of sounds, with sounds from languages all over the world being represented. On the contrary, these and other investigations suggest that only a rather limited set of phones are babbled.

Looking at Table 3.1 it appears that there were no non-English sounds utilized by the infants studied. This is partially conditioned by the investigative methods employed and by the perceptual limitations inherent in phonetic transcription. As to the methodology, in the Irwin studies only three non-English sounds were transcribed, the rest were ignored. The Fisichelli study considered exclusively English sounds. The Pierce and Hanna investigation, on the other hand, did document that the infants produced several non-English sounds with some frequency. Other investigations (e.g., Stockman, Woods, and Tishman, 1981) have confirmed the occurrence of non-English sounds in this late babbling period, although not to any high degree.

The second difficulty encountered with non-English sounds pertains to the perceptual basis of phonetic transcription. Someone not trained in listening for and transcribing non-English sounds certainly will encounter grave problems recognizing and categorizing them. Locke (1983, p. 5) summarizes this difficulty appropriately by stating "there might have been more (non-English sounds) if the listeners were themselves non-English, or more effectively oriented to non-English sounds and modes of symbolization."

During the later babbling periods open syllables are still the most frequent type of syllables. In Kent and Bauer (1985), for example, V, CV, VCV, and CVCV structures accounted for approximately 94% of all syllables produced. While closed syllables were present, they were found to be very limited in the repertoire of the infant at this age.

We have discussed some aspects of babbling in children. However, one important question should still be addressed. Does babbling have anything to do with later language development? If so, we might be able to predict the linguistic development of children based on their prelinguistic productions. Several researchers have suggested that both the (a) quantity and (b) diversity of vocalizations do indeed play a role in later language development.

As to their quantity, attempts have been made (e.g., Camp, Burgess, Morgan, and Zerbe, 1987; Kagan 1971; Roe 1975, 1977) to correlate the quantity of vocalizations at a certain babbling age to later language performance. Here quantity was defined as the number of vocalizations during a specific time period. Although somewhat different criteria were used in the various studies, the results showed that the amount of prelinguistic vocalizations was positively related to later language measures. For example, a positive correlation was found for the verbalization scores on the Bayley Scales of Infant Development at 1 year of age (Camp, et al., 1987), vocabulary size at 3 years, and reading performance measures at 5 years of age (Roe, 1977).

Diversity of vocalizations was measured by the number of different consonant-like sounds heard in the babbling of infants (Stoel-Gammon and Otomo, 1986), the number of structured CV syllables (Menyuk, Liebergott, and Schultz, 1986), the proportion of vocalizations containing a true consonant (Vihman and Greenlee, 1987), and the ratio of consonant-like sounds to vowel-like sounds (Bauer, 1988; Bauer and Robb, 1989). A Danish investigation (Jensen, Boggild-Andersen, Schmidt, Ankerkus, and Hansen, 1988) utilized both quantity and diversity of vocalizations to predict later language skills. Summarizing the results of these methodologically varying studies, it appears that the diversity of contoid productions can be taken as an indicator of when speech begins. They also seem to predict the phonological as well as the degree of later language proficiency. While certain questions remain to be answered, a possibility to relate prelinguistic performance to later language skills would have exciting implications for the diagnosis and treatment of speech/language impaired children.

SUPRASEGMENTAL FEATURES

One way to look at spoken language is to refer to segmental versus suprasegmental elements. Segmentals pertain to the vowels and consonants which combine to produce syllables, words, and sentences. However, during their articulation our pronunciation varies in several different ways. We make use, for example, of a wide range of pitch and loudness variables. **Suprasegmentals** or **prosodic features** consist of those elements of speech which do not belong to the distinct vowels and consonants per se but accompany them. While segmentals relate to what we say, suprasegmentals refer to how we say it.

The linguistically most relevant suprasegmentals are the pitch, loudness, and tempo variations we use in speech. They have specific functions and may be analyzed separately. If combined they constitute the rhythm of a particular language or utterance.

The development of suprasegmentals or prosodic features in infants has gained considerable importance in the last years. Recent literature (Bonvillian, Raeburn, and Horan, 1979; Fernald, Taeschner, Dunn, Papousek, Boysson-Bardies, and Fukui, 1989; Jacobson, Boersma, Fields, and Olson, 1983; Stern and Wasserman 1979; Whalen, Levitt, and Wang, 1991) supports the viewpoint of close interaction between prosodic features, early child-directed speech (motherese), and early language development. Clearly, far more information is available in the area of segmental development. However, a better understanding of suprasegmental features and their development may offer us valuable insights into the transition from babbling to the first words and the close interconnection of segmental and suprasegmental acquisition.

Coinciding with the canonical babbling stage, or starting at approximately 6 months of age, the infant utilizes apparent patterns of prosodic behavior. Certain features are now employed consistently, primarily intonation, rhythm, and pausing (Crystal, 1986). Although these babbled utterances do not convey any meaning, the intonation patterns seem to the listener to be those of questions, statements, or exclamations. These prosodic patterns continue to diversify toward the end of the babbling period to such a degree that names such as "**expressive jargon**" (Gesell and Thompson, 1934) or "**prelinguistic jargon**" (Dore, Franklin, Miller, and Ramer, 1976) have been applied to them.

ACROSS LINGUISTIC BOUNDARIES/UNIVERSALS

So far we have examined the babbling behavior of children raised in English speaking environments. One question that has intrigued researchers for years is whether children of different language environments babble in a similar manner. If verified, this would point to prelinguistic universals of language acquisition. Such a position has been called the **independence hypothesis**. It states that prelinguistic vocalizations are limited by physiological maturational processes and are, thus, universal in nature. Therefore, the child's babbling does not depend on the linguistic environment. The opposing position, the **interactional hypothesis**, sees the babbling stage as the time span when a perceptual motor mechanism begins to operate. Thus, during this time the articulatory development is influenced by the auditory input signal: the child begins to produce language-oriented sounds. The interactional hypothesis reflects the ''babbling drift'' which had already been mentioned by Roger Brown in 1958. He thought that babbling drifted more and more in the direction of the speech which was heard by the infant. Thus, the language environment would definitely play a role in the babbling of the child. Children of varying language backgrounds would, therefore, also show differences in their later babbling productions.

Research findings have supported both viewpoints. Several investigators (e.g., Mehler, 1971; Weir, 1966) have reported discernible differences in babbling when children of various language backgrounds were analyzed. However, these differences were often just based on a listener's perception of the babbling in question. For example, one of the earlier studies by Weir (1966) concludes that differences could be noted between the babbling of Chinese, Russian, and American infants. These tentative results (the investigation was never concluded due to Weir's untimely death) were supported by other findings. However, as Locke (1983, p. 14) counters, ''if there were reliable differences among infants, they might represent dissimilarities in babbling stage rather than language environment.''

Other investigators found different results (e.g., Oller and Eilers, 1982; Olney and Scholnick, 1976). When Weir's original data were reanalyzed (Atkinson, MacWhinney, and Stoel, 1968) and again subjected to listener's judgments, the results were not significant. The percentage of listener's perceiving language differences in babbling was no greater than chance would predict. Similar investigations followed with slightly altered methodologies. The babbling of children from Thai, Spanish, Japanese, Mayan, and Dutch language environments, to mention a few, were recorded and judgments made as to whether differences could be established. In most cases the answer was no, listeners did not hear characteristic babbling for a Dutch child, for example, versus a non-Dutch child. To further emphasize this point, a summary of investigations from Locke (1983) is provided in Table 3.2. When contrasting consonantal productions, more similarities than differences can be noted between the babbling of children from various language environments.

More recently other researchers have argued that contoid descriptions and counts are not a valid basis for cross-linguistic comparisons. Actually, babbling is noted for the appearance of syllable productions with varied vocoids and contoids. Phonotactic patterns or suprasegmental variables such as intonation or rhythmic units might be far more representative than sound productions per se. Also, acoustic analyses might provide valuable information for cross-linguistic comparisons. To this end, several investigations have ascertained differences in the occurrence of vowels in Spanish and English infants (Oller and Eilers, 1982), significantly different vowel formant frequencies in infants of four different language backgrounds (de Boysson-Bardies, Halle, Sagart, and Durand, 1989), and intonational differences between the babbling of French and English infants (Whalen, Levitt, and Wang, 1991).

The verdict is simply not in yet. Even more importantly, an answer to this question—language drift or not in babbling—may not be possible at all. Although children of similar ages are, of course, compared, does this necessitate the conclusion that these children are all at similar stages of canonical babbling? Until now, at least, the children have been selected according to age; little control has been used to assure similarities in their prelinguistic development. Also, how much are the individual differences between children—which might play an extremely important role in answering this question—actually eliminated by the statistical procedure used? These and other problems are left to further research.

CONCLUSIONS

In this section the canonical babbling of infants has been discussed. This babbling stage can be understood as a portion of the phonological development due to (*a*) the presence of adult-like syllable structures and (*b*) suprasegmental patterns which seem to approximate those seen in the native language. Both contoid and vocoid productions seem to show definite patterns for all children. Although similarities, thus universals, have been noted across linguistic boundaries, newer investigations point more to specific differences based on the language environments of the infants. Certain measurements of babbling, especially quantity and diversity of sound production, have been correlated to later linguistic development.

TRANSITION TO FIRST WORDS

In this section the transition from variegated babbling to the first meaningful words will be treated. This transition is especially important as this is the time when the child moves from the prelinguistic to the linguistic phases of phonological development. Precursors of this transition which draw from previous developmental stages include, first, the formation of adult-like syllables with regular consonant- and vowel-like segments. These adult-like syllables have been accounted for since the onset of canonical babbling (Vihman, 1988a). A second element pertains to the incorporation of several different vocoids and contoids into the same production unit. This is a mark of variegated babbling, the last babbling stage. Both phenomena prepare the child for the production of first words.

In opposition to what has been proposed by the discontinuity model, it has been observed that children use the same sounds and syllable structures at the end of babbling and at the beginning of the first-words period (Ferguson, 1978; Ingram, 1974; Vihman, Macken, Miller, Simmons, and Miller, 1985). Structurally, therefore, the first words and late babbles are very similar. The decisive difference is that some of them now become meaningful.

If we were to isolate the period from babbling to the first words, i.e., from the end of variegated babbling to the first 10–20 words, would specific patterns emerge that might separate the two productionally? To substantiate such a claim longitudinal information would be needed tracing infants during this transitional period. This section will discuss selected longitudinal research endeavors which deal with this relatively short time span between the end of variegated babbling to the acquisition of the very first words.

SEGMENTAL DEVELOPMENT

Several investigators (e.g., Ferguson and Farwell, 1975; Oller, Weiman, Doyle, and Ross, 1976; Stark, 1980; Vihman, Ferguson, and Elbert, 1986) examined the phonetic characteristics of late babbling and early words. These studies suggest that babbling and early words have much in common. In fact, they were often so similar that difficulties arose differentiating the two.

In spite of these similarities, certain dissimilarities have been observed. If the longitudinal

TABLE 3.2. Consonantal Babbling Repertoire in 15 Language Environments

Environment	Afrikaans	Mayan	Luo	Thai	Japanese	Hindi	Chinese	Slovenian	Dutch	Spanish	German	Arabic	Norwegian	Latvian	English
Infant N	1	2	2	1	6	1	1	2	1	2	4	3	1	—	2
Age in Months	11–12	9	12	10–11	9–12	9–10	8–11	11	11	9	10–12	6–10	0–12	6–12	1–15
English repertoire															
h	*	*	*			*	*		*	*		*		*	*
d	*	*	*	*	*					*	*	*	*	*	*
b	*	*	*	*	*	*	*	*	*	*	*	*	*	*	*
m	*	*	*	*	*	*	*	*	*	*	*	*	*	*	*
t	*	*		*	*	*	*	*		*	*		*	*	
g			*		*	*	*	*	*				*	*	*
s	*												*		
w					*		*	*	*	*		*	*	*	
n	*	*	*	*	*		*	*		*	*		*	*	*
k	*					*	*		*		*	*	*	*	*
j			*	*				*		*	*	*	*	*	
p	*	*		*	*	*	*	*	*	*	*	*	*	*	*
Total	9	7	7	7	8	7	9	8	7	8	8	7	11	11	8

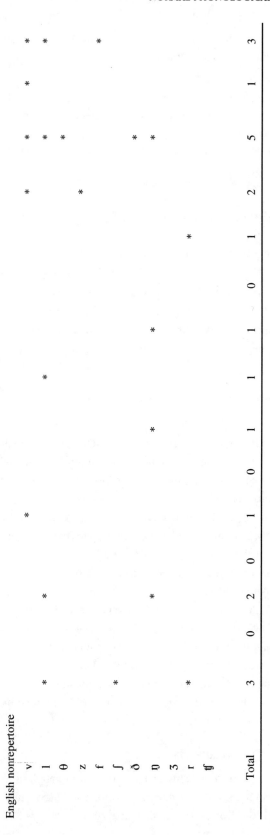

data from Vihman, et al. (1986), are analyzed at the first three levels of comparison, namely when the children had 0 words, 4 words, and 15 words, certain distinctions could be pointed out:

1. A large diversity existed between the children's productions in each of the three areas investigated (phonetic tendencies, consonant inventory, and word selection). So much so that the authors stated "the prevalence of individual variation was the strongest lesson to be learned" (p. 29). The more words the children acquired the more this diversity seemed to diminish.
2. Neither liquids nor consonant clusters appeared to any significant degree in the transition from late babbling to first words.
3. Eight of the 10 children utilized voiced stops in babbling but not in words; [g] was the most prominent example of this.
4. Labial sounds were the most frequent consonants of early words.
5. All children showed a preference for short vocalizations, especially monosyllables.

Again, this transitional period seems to be characterized by a great deal of individual variation. Also, there appears to be a significant use of specific sounds by particular children. It is important to recognize, however, that this time span may not be as continuous with late babbling as we have often felt. Certain contoids may belong more to the babbling era than to the subsequent phase of meaningful communication through words.

SUPRASEGMENTAL DEVELOPMENT

As the child moves from the end of the babbling period to first words, we do see, however, a continuation of previously noted intonational contours. These suprasegmental features, which at first occur only briefly, become more frequent and can be maintained over a longer period of time. The segmental productions at this time are shorter, more one-word like, and more phonetically stable (Crystal, 1986). Thus, when a babbled utterance of one or two syllables is produced with a specific prosodic pattern, the result is going to sound very much like an attempt at a meaningful utterance. Understandably, then, at this stage parents often try to interpret what the infant is actually "saying" on the basis of the prosodic-production unit heard.

There is not a lot of information on this short time interval between the end of babbling and the first few words. It does seem clear that by the end of variegated babbling the child produces specific prosodically oriented units or what has been called a **prosodic envelope**, **matrix** (Bruner, 1975), or **frame** (Dore, 1975). These units have both a segmental and a suprasegmental dimension. It appears from several observations that the prosodic features are the more stable of the two (Crystal, 1986; Menn, 1975). Therefore, while segmental variations can often be noted from production to production, the intonational pattern for the unit remains perceptually the same. From the information presently available to us, the period from late babbling to the first words is not signaled by suprasegmental changes.

ACROSS LINGUISTIC BOUNDARIES/UNIVERSALS

Several different hypotheses have been proposed concerning the period from babbling to early words. First, it was suggested that babbling has its foundation in a biological base which is common to all children (Jakobson, 1941/1968; Kent, 1984; Lenneberg, 1967; Locke, 1983).

Under this supposition we should see similarities between infants from different language backgrounds during the interval from late babbling to the first few words. A second hypothesis postulates that the infants' productions have already begun to be shaped by their native language prior to the first words (de Boysson-Bardies, et al., 1989). If that is the case we would see production differences between infants coming from differing language backgrounds. A third line of thought is that the children follow their own individual developmental paths. According to this hypothesis each child moves from babbling to first words in a characteristic manner (Stoel-Gammon and Cooper, 1984; Vihman, et al., 1986). If this is so, then children no matter what language environment they grow up in, would show idiosyncratic production patterns from babbling to their first words.

To examine these hypotheses Vihman (1992) reported the findings of a longitudinal cross-linguistic study. The data analyzed came from three separate studies which provided information on two groups of children from English speaking backgrounds, one group of children learning Swedish, one group of children learning French, and one group learning Japanese. Similar investigative methods and principles of data collection were employed for all of the studies.

First, the composition of "practiced" syllables was established for all groups of children. These practiced syllables were actually babbled baseline measures at the ages of 9-, 10- and 11-months. (It has to be pointed out that the range actually extended from 9–14 months of age, the Japanese children being clearly older at the time of the data collection.) These so-called practiced syllables were then compared to recordings made when the same children spontaneously produced 4, 15, and 25 words.

The analysis of the prelinguistic utterances demonstrated certain cross-linguistic similarities. The six top-ranked syllables were [da], [ba], [wa], [də], [ha], and [hə]. These data correspond to those summarized by Locke (1983) showing a high prevalence of [h] and [d] contoids in babbling.

French, of course, does not have an [h] sound in its phonological inventory. While h-type CV syllables were present in the babbling of French infants, they dropped considerably in frequency of usage at the 4- and 15-word levels. This apparent influence of the linguistic environment, however, does not account for a similar drop in [h] productions by the Swedish children in which [h] is a part of their consonant inventory. Syllables produced more frequently by children of different language environments included the use of [ko/go] by Japanese and [ti/di] by Swedish infants.

When prelinguistic utterances were compared to later word productions, the syllables used in early words were found to be primarily drawn from the practiced syllables of the prelinguistic sessions. However, eight of the 23 subjects failed to show this correspondence. Although a plausible explanation is tentatively applied to this inconsistency, the fact remains that over one-third of the subjects did not show a continuity between the practiced syllables of babbling and their use in first words. This lack of continuity did not apply to any one language based group but was evidenced by at least one child in each of the groups mentioned.

Clearly more information is needed before definite conclusions can be drawn. There does seem to be evidence that certain babbled sounds and syllables are common cross-linguistically. However, overwhelming support of one of the previously stated models is still outstanding at the present time.

CONCLUSIONS

It seems that for some children the first words are composed of syllable structures and speech sounds already present during the last babbling stages. While this might describe the transitional period for a number of children, it does not really explain them. Similar materials are apparently used at the end of babbling and at the beginning of the first words. That seems only natural, especially in light of the fact that babbling events regularly continue into the new period of first word productions, but why the sudden change from meaningless to meaningful phonological productions? That is, after all, the point. A great deal still needs to be explained about the transition of productional units and the child's cognitive understanding before the discontinuity hypothesis of old can be fully and safely discarded.

FIRST FIFTY WORDS

Around a child's first birthday a new developmental era begins—the linguistic phase. It starts with the moment when the first meaningful word is produced. That sounds plain enough, but there are some problems which exist in defining the first meaningful word. Must it be understood and produced by the child in all applicable situations and contexts? Must it have an adult-like meaning to the child? Must it be pronounced correctly or nearly so to be considered an actual word? What about those utterances which do not resemble our adult representation but are, nevertheless, used as words by the child in a consistent manner?

Most authors define the first word as an entity of relatively stable phonetic form which is produced consistently by the child in a particular context. This form must be recognizably related to the adult-like word form of that particular language. Thus, if the child says [ba] consistently in the context of being shown a ball then this form would qualify as a "word." If, however, the child says [dodo] when being shown the ball then this would not be accepted as a "word" because it does not approximate the adult form.

Children often invent words. They also use these "invented words" (Locke, 1983) in a consistent manner, thereby demonstrating that they seem to have meaning for the child. These vocalizations, used consistently but without a recognizable adult model, have been called **proto-words** (Menn, 1978), **phonetically consistent forms** (Dore, et al., 1976), **vocables** (Ferguson, 1978), and **quasi-words** (Stoel-Gammon and Cooper, 1984).

The time of the initial productions of words is typically called the **first 50 word stage**. This stage encompasses the time from the first meaningful utterance at approximately 1 year of age to the time when the child begins to put two "words" together at approximately 18 months. Whether this stage is actually a separate developmental entity might be questioned. Also, the strict 50 word cut-off point is, according to several studies, purely arbitrary (Ferguson and Farwell, 1975; Nelson, 1973). Nevertheless, it appears that the child produces approximately 50 meaningful words before the next generally recognized stage of development begins, the **two-word stage**.

During this "first 50 word stage" there seems to be a large difference between the productional and the perceptual capabilities of the child. For example, at the end of this stage, when the child can produce approximately 50 words, he/she is typically capable of understanding around 200 words (Ingram, 1989). This fact must have an effect upon the development of semantic meaning as well as on the phonological system. It must be clearly understood that by primarily analyzing productions of this stage we are only looking at one aspect of language development. The child's perceptual, motor, and cognitive growth, as well as the influence of the environment, all play indispensable roles especially in this stage of language acquisition.

In examining the course of phonological development during this period we see that it is heavily influenced by the individual words the child is acquiring. Children are not just learning sounds which are then used to make-up words but, rather, they seem to learn word units that happen to contain particular sets of sounds. Ingram (1976a) calls this a **presystematic stage** in which contrastive words rather than contrastive phones (i.e., phonemes) are acquired. The presystematic stage can be related to Cruttenden's (1981) **item learning** and **system learning** stages of early phonological development. In item learning the child first acquires word forms as unanalyzed units, as a productional whole. Only later, characteristically after the first 50 word stage, system learning occurs during which the child acquires the phonemic principles which apply to the phonological system in question.

The early portion of this stage is known as the **holophrastic period**. Holophrastic refers to the concept that the child uses one word to indicate a complete idea. During this phase the child does not have linguistic signs as we know them. Rather, the link between the object and its sign—both on the production as well as the conception levels—is not yet firmly established. A child might produce [da] to indicate a dog. The next day we could see that the production has changed somewhat to, perhaps, [do]. But this time the production may not refer to a dog alone but also to a cow or horse. According to Piaget, the child is still within the sensorimotor period of development. At this point the child has not yet achieved full imitative ability or object permanence. Thus, sounds and meanings drift and change. It is not until the end of the sensorimotor period, at approximately age 1;6 , that the child enters the true language period or the ability for representational thought.

SEGMENTAL DEVELOPMENT

Several authors (e.g., Ferguson and Farwell, 1975; Ingram, 1989) have pointed out factors which predominate productionally during the first word stage. These include: (*a*) phonetic variability and (*b*) a limitation of occurring syllable structures and sound segments.

The phonetic variability refers to the rather unstable pronunciations of the child's first 50 words. While this has been well documented (e.g., Farwell, 1976; Kiparsky and Menn, 1977; Menyuk and Menn, 1979; Stoel-Gammon and Cooper, 1984) it appears that some productions are more stable than others. Ferguson and Farwell (1975) refer to this category of words as **stable forms**. However, the authors do not provide a measure for this stability, and from their examples it is often not clear why certain words are considered more stable than others. To complicate matters, it seems that some children have a tendency to produce more stable articulations than others from the beginning of this stage. Stoel-Gammon and Cooper (1984) and French (1989) provide data on children whose phonetic realizations were stable from the first real word on.

Although phonetic variability has often been demonstrated in children during the first 50 word stage, it does not follow that all children will show comparable degrees of variability. For a particular child certain word forms may be more variable than others. Also, between children more or less variability in word pronunciation can be observed.

The second characteristic of this stage is the limitation of syllable structures and segmental productions utilized. From their relatively small repertoire of words it would seem logical to conclude that children do not produce a large array of syllable structures and sound segments. However, what are the actual limitations that we are seeing in the first 50 words?

First, certain syllable types clearly predominate. These are CV, VC, and CVC syllables. When CVCV syllables are present, they are full or partial syllable reduplications. This, of course, does not mean that other syllable types do not occur. Looking, for example, at the data from Ferguson and Farwell (1973), French (1989), Ingram (1974), Leopold (1947), Menn (1971), Stoel-Gammon and Cooper (1984), and Velten (1943), we see that these syllables are, indeed, the most frequently occurring. However, the children produced other syllables as well. Menn's Daniel, for instance, produced CCVC [njaj], Leopold's Hildegard a CCVCV [priti], and Ferguson and Farwell's T a CVCVVC [wakuak]. Also, if the individual children are examined to see if patterns emerge, we find differences. Certain children seem to favor specific types of syllables. For example, some children have the CVC structure present to a moderate degree from the very beginning of this stage. With others this syllable structure appears only later and does not constitute any major part of the child's phonology until after the 50 word stage (Ingram, 1976).

Second, what are the speech sound limitations which can be observed during the first 50 word stage? More specifically, what vowels and consonants are present, and which ones are not? Two publications which have had a large impact on this question are those presented by Jakobson (1941/1968) and Jakobson and Halle (1956). After studying several diary reports of children from varying linguistic backgrounds it was concluded that the first consonants are labials, most commonly [p] or [m]; these initial consonants are followed by [t] and later [k]; fricatives are present only after the respective homorganic stops have been acquired; the first vowel is [a], followed by [u] and/or [i].

Over the years these postulated universals have undergone a good deal of scrutiny. Although most of the investigators (e.g., Oller, et al., 1976; Stoel-Gammon and Cooper, 1984; Vihman, et al., 1986) have concentrated on consonant inventories, Ingram (1976) has attempted to grapple with the acquisition of vowels. He cited four case studies (Ingram, 1974; Leopold, 1947; Menn, 1971; Velten, 1943) and compared the vowels utilized in the first 50 words. All four of the children had an [a] vowel in their first words. Also, all four of the children had [u] and/or [i] within their inventories. This trend can be noted in Ferguson and Farwell's (1975) case study of T as well. However, analyzing the first 50 utterances presented by French (1989), an [a] vowel is frequently present but both [i] and [u] are absent from the child's inventory. A valid answer to the question of which vowels are really utilized and in which order is probably not as forthright as we would wish. Taking all variables into account, this is hardly surprising. General trends can certainly be noted, but the attempt to establish rules at this time is probably unrealistic.

Consonant inventories follow the same pattern. Although certain similarities have been verified, several investigations (e.g., Ferguson and Farwell, 1975; Stoel-Gammon and Cooper, 1984; Vihman, 1992; Vihman, et al., 1986) have pointed out the wide range of variability between individual subjects. If one wants to generalize, then the marked use of voiced labial and dental stops and nasals has to be underlined. Ferguson and Garnica (1975) make the point that [h] and [w] are also among the first consonants acquired. Findings substantiating these generalizations from five different investigations are summarized in Table 3.3.

TABLE 3.3. Comparison of Word Selection at 15-word-point (7 Stanford Subjects) and Initial Consonant Production by 19 Other English-speaking Children with 50-word Vocabularies[a]

	Stanford	Others		Stanford	Others[a]
p	×	+	ʃ	+	+
b	×	×	ʒ	0	0
t	×	+	ʧ	−	−
d	×	+	ʤ	−	−
k	×	+	m	×	×
g	+	+	n	×	+
f	+	−	ŋ	−	−
v	−	0	l	−	−
θ	+	−	r	+	−
ð	+	−	w	+	+
s	−	−	j	+	−
z	−	−	h	+	+

[a]Data derived from Ferguson & Farwell (1975), Shibamoto & Olmsted (1978), Leonard, et al. (1980), and Stoel-Gammon & Cooper (1984).

Note: × = all children in study; + = over half but not all children in study; − = more than one but less than half children in study; 0 = none of the children.

This table compares the consonant inventory of seven children labeled "Stanford" (Vihman, et al., 1986) to 19 other children which are from research studies noted in the table. As can be seen, all children have words containing [b] and [m]. There is a large percentage of children with [p], [t], [d], [k], [g], [ʃ], [n], [w], and [h] consonants.

These data reduce the individual variation among children considerably. For example, if child A produces two words with [n] versus child B producing 43 words with [n] initially, then both of those children will be counted for [n] use in this table even though the use of this particular sound in the two children's inventories is hardly comparable.

The next phase of this discussion follows almost automatically: Does the child show individual acquisition patterns or strategies? In other words, does the child build his/her phonological inventory around certain sounds? If so, do these sounds represent a child's preference for a particular sound or set of sounds? Ferguson and Farwell (1975) referred to conditions like these as **salience** and **avoidance** factors. They imply that the child will acquire words that contain sounds within his/her phonological inventory. Words containing sounds which are important or remarkable (salient) to the child will actively be selected for early word productions. Words which do not contain sounds within their inventory will be avoided. (This principle seems to apply only to the production of words, comprehension has not been similarly organized (see Hoek, Ingram, and Gibson, 1986).) Productional selection and avoidance have often been observed; for example, Schwartz and Leonard (1982) add experimental support to this claim.

Individual strategies employed may include preferences for certain sounds, certain syllable structures and/or sound classes or sound features. Yet, we must never forget that all children will be acquiring somewhat different vocabularies in accordance with their varying environments. Individual preference can also refer to those objects and contexts which the child enjoys more than others. The child's preference in this respect will most certainly have an effect on which words are acquired as well and, as a consequence, which phonetic inventory is utilized during the production of the first 50 words.

SUPRASEGMENTAL DEVELOPMENT

Another important means of communication during the first 50 word stage is prosodic variation. Examples of children's speech during this time have included pitch variations to indicate differences in meaning, such as [nanæ] indicating "banana" versus [nanɔ] which was used consistently for the child's stuffed animal. Also suprasegmentals are used to indicate differences in syntactical function. Bruner (1975) describes these prosodic units as "place-holders." A demand or question, for example, is often established using prosody first, words are then later added. The most widely held view is that these prosodic units provide a social function. They are seen as a means to signal joint participation in an activity shared by the child and the caregiver. Dore (1975) suggests that prosodic features provide evidence for developing speech acts. A word with a specific intonation pattern might signal, for example, requesting, calling, or demanding.

Intonational changes seem to develop prior to stress. While they appear prior to the first meaningful words, contrastive stress is initially evidenced only at the beginning of the two word stage or at approximately 1;6. During the first 50 words, the observed pitch variations can be said to represent directional sequences (rising versus falling, for example) or range patterns (high versus low within the child's pitch range). For a more detailed analysis of early intonational development see Crystal (1986).

ACROSS LINGUISTIC BOUNDARIES/UNIVERSALS

As was previously discussed, Jakobson (1941/1968) believed that there is a universal sequence of sound acquisition for children in at least this early stage of development. While not dismissing this view, the individual variations reported in several studies do not really substantiate the claim. To adjust for these disparities, Ingram (1988, 1992) proposes a Neo-Jakobsonian theory of acquisition. It relates back to Jakobson's theory in that it states that there are general patterns of phonological acquisition across all languages. Also, according to this view, children begin phonological processing at the time of the first words, and word acquisition is accomplished through the acquisition of distinctive features. This natural phonology plus generative phonology model is termed "Neo" because of the addition of more recent findings and—on the basis of that—an elaboration on the old theory. (For more information the reader is referred to Ingram, 1988.) The revival of universal aspects of language and, especially, sound acquisition, should provide interesting discussion material for the future.

Two other concepts have also played a role in our quest for language universals: the maturational theory and the refinement-attunement theory. The maturational theory proposes that all children have certain biological constraints that impose limitations on the developing child.

The linguistic environment, therefore, should not have an effect on the child's language acquisition until after the first 50 word stage. The refinement-attunement theory states, on the other hand, that the native language background does play a role in the development of early language skills. Through the interaction of perceiving and producing within this language, the child fine tunes these skills more and more. Only through longitudinal studies of children acquiring languages with phonological systems quite different from English could we examine these largely opposing viewpoints.

An interesting study which addresses this issue has been reported by Pye, Ingram, and List (1987). The authors analyzed the early speech of Quiché children. Quiché is a Mayan language which has a phonological inventory unlike English. If the first 50 words of these children are analyzed and compared to children learning English the following inventories are established:

English children	Quiché children
[m] [n]	[m] [n]
[b] [d] [g]	
[p] [t] [k]	[p] [t] [k] [ʔ]
[f] [s] [h]	[x]
[w]	[w]
	[l]
	[ʧ]

Although similarities can be found, for example, the use of bilabial and dental stops and nasals, clear dissimilarities exist. The use of [ʧ] and [l], for instance, were among the most frequent sounds used by the Quiché children. However, these sounds were not seen in the early inventory of the English children. On the other hand, the English children utilized [f] and [s] to some degree, sounds which were not found in the Quiché inventory. Ingram concluded that such differences must have language-based reasons. Ingram also explores the concept of **functional load** in this respect. Functional load is measured by the number of oppositions or minimal pairs which occur with that sound in a given language. By using this method Ingram discovered that the functional load for [ʧ] and [l] are high in Quiché; relatively more minimal pairs occur with [ʧ] and [l] initially.

Although these results are by no means conclusive, they do open up new avenues in an attempt to answer the question of language universals. However, if we analyze the information presently available, results like this are still not convincing enough to disregard any of the other viable theories.

CONCLUSIONS

This section examined phonological characteristics of the first 50 word stage. Although certain trends can be detected in children such as the use of [a] vowels and bilabial and dental nasals and stops, these findings are not the entire picture by any means. Individual variation is an important factor in this phase of development. Also, as noted throughout this discussion, other features begin more and more to play a role in the phonological development: word preferences, sound preferences, perceptual and cognitive development are only a few of the variables which will influence the parameters of a specific child's phonological acquisition.

PRESCHOOL CHILD

This section stresses information on the developing phonology of the child from 18 months, the approximate end of the 50 word stage, to the beginning of the sixth year. It is during this time that the largest growth within the phonological system takes place, but let us first look at some other gains the child typically makes during this time span.

Around 18 months of age the child is seen to have a productive vocabulary of about 50 words, although the receptively available vocabulary typically amounts to about 200 words. The transition from one-word utterances to two-word sentences, a large linguistic step, occurs also around this 18-month marker. With the production of two-word sentences the child has entered the period of expressing specific semantic relationships—the beginning of syntactical development. It is around this time as well that the child's vocabulary increases substantially.

By the end of this time period, around the fifth birthday, the child's vocabulary has expanded to approximately 8000 words. Also, almost all of the basic grammatical forms of the language are now present, such as questions, negative statements, dependent clauses, and compound sentences. More importantly the child knows now how to use language to communicate in a really effective manner. Children talk differently to babies than they do to their friends, for example. They also know how to tell jokes and riddles and they are quite able to handle the linguistic subtleties of being polite and being rude.

Phonologically children start with a rather limited inventory of speech sounds and phonotactic possibilities. However, by the time they are 2-years old preliminary phonological analyses are beginning to take place. At this time perception seems to precede production somewhat, children can now identify single segment differences between words. By the end of this period, around the child's fifth birthday, an almost complete phonological system has emerged.

All these changes occur in less than 4 years. Although this section focuses on phonological development, such a discussion must always remain within the context of the large expansions in morphosyntax, semantics, and pragmatics which occur during this time.

SEGMENTAL DEVELOPMENT—CONSONANTS

It appears that no chapter on phonological development can be complete without looking at the large sample studies which began in the 1930s (Wellman, Case, Mengert, and Bradbury, 1931) and have continued periodically since. However, it seems necessary to preface such a discussion with the problems inherent in these studies.

Large sample studies were initiated to look at many children in order to find out which sounds were mastered at which age levels. To this end they evaluated most of the speech sounds within a given native language. With a few exceptions (Irwin and Wong, 1983; Olmsted, 1971; Stoel-Gammon, 1985) these studies have used methods similar to articulation tests to acquire their data, i.e., the child was asked to name pictures and certain sounds were then judged as being productionally "correct" or "incorrect."

In this type of procedure general as well as specific problems arise. First, the fact that the child produces the sound correctly in a one-word response does not mean that he/she can produce that sound in natural speech conditions. Practitioners have always been aware of the often large articulatory discrepancies between one-word responses and the same sounds produced in conversation. Second, the choice of pictures/words will certainly affect the production of the individual sounds within the word. Not only does the child's familiarity with the word play a role but so do factors such as the length of the word, its structure, the stressed or unstressed position of the sound within the word, and the phonetic context the sound occurs in. These factors help or hinder standard production. Therefore, strictly speaking, all we can conclude from cross-sectional studies is that the children could or could not produce that particular sound in that specific word. Let's say the [j] was "correct" in the word "yellow." No problem here. It is when this result is generalized to include all [j] sounds in all words that the problem begins.

The third point is a theoretical issue. As stated at the beginning, there has been an adoption of certain new concepts and terminology within the field of speech-language pathology. This chapter, for example, is called developing phonology and not developing speech sounds. With the inclusion of the terms phonology, phonological development, and phonological disorders we have decided to accept certain conceptual changes which are simply part of the definition of phonology. These cross-sectional studies are perhaps indicative of a specific inventory of speech sounds a child possesses but they are not in any way indicative of a particular child's phonological system.

Some specific problems with cross-sectional studies are also not to be ignored. These include the criteria used to determine whether or not the child has "mastered" a particular sound. Although this has been elaborated upon in several articles and books (e.g., Smit, 1986; Vihman, 1988b) it is worth mentioning again. Table 3.4 provides a comparison between several of the larger cross-sectional studies.

Looking at age comparisons on this chart, a difference in reported mastery of 3 years or more can be noted for specific sounds. For example, this is true when the [s] sound is compared in the more recent Prather, Hedrick, and Kern (1975) study to the older Poole (1934) study. The Poole investigation has a mastery age of 7½ years while the Prather, et al., investigation shows an age level of 3 years. Also, a 3 year difference can be found for [z] acquisition when the Prather, et al., data are compared to the Templin (1957) results. Again Prather, et al., assigns a much earlier level of mastery. One question often asked in this context is: Does that mean children are now producing sounds "correctly" at an earlier age? Many of these differences are a consequence of the way "mastery" was defined. Poole, for instance, stated that 100% of the children must use the sound correctly in each of the positions tested. Prather, et al., and Templin, on the other hand, set this level at 75%. In addition, rather than using the 75% cut-off level for all three positions (initial, medial, and final) as Templin had done, Prather, et al., used only two positions (initial and final) for their calculations. This clearly changes the ages to which mastery can be assigned. Obviously, the shift to earlier acquisition noted in the Prather study could be accounted for by these methodological changes. Also, as Smit (1986) points out, the Prather results are based on incomplete data sets, especially at the younger age groupings. Although Prather began with 21 subjects in each age group, several of these children did not respond to many of the words. At times only 8–12 subjects were used to calculate the norms. The children who did not respond to some words may have been avoiding them because they felt that they could not say them correctly. This, too, would alter the age norms. Table 3.5 (Smit, 1986) compensates for the incomplete data sets of Prather and uses the two-position norms from Templin (1957).

TABLE 3.4. Age Levels for Phoneme Development According to Six Studies

	Wellman (1931)	Poole (1934)	Templin (1957)	Sander (1972)	Prather (1975)	Arlt (1976)
m	3	3½	3	before 2	2	3
n	3	4½	3	before 2	2	3
h	3	3½	3	before 2	2	3
p	4	3½	3	before 2	2	3
f	3	5½	3	3	2–4	3
w	3	3½	3	before 2	2–8	3
b	3	3½	4	before 2	2–8	3
ŋ		4½	3	2	2	3
j	4	4½	3½	3	2–4	
k	4	4½	4	2	2–4	3
g	4	4½	4	2	2–4	3
l	4	6½	6	3	3–4	4
d	5	4½	4	2	2–4	3
t	5	4½	6	2	2–8	3
s	5	7½	4½	3	3	4
r	5	7½	4	3	3–4	5
ʧ	5		4½	4	3–8	4
v	5	6½	6	4	4	3½
z	5	7½	7	4	4	4
ʒ	6	6½	7	6	4	4
θ		7½	6	5	4	5
ʤ			7	4	4	4
ʃ		6½	4½	4	3–8	4½
ð		6½	7	5	4	5

With these adjustments the Templin and Prather data suddenly look very similar. There are even instances where the Templin acquisition norms show younger ages than those reported by Prather, et al. If we realign the information in such a way we see clearly that, when compared to older studies, children are by no means mastering the sounds earlier now.

Ingram (1989, p. 366) points out additional problems related to the Templin study and sums them up with the following words of wisdom:

> Templin's study provides useful descriptive overview of English phonological acquisition. . . . Here, however, we will conclude with a caution about using large sample data such as these for anything more than the most general of purposes, setting out a series of problems with Templin's study in particular and large sample studies in general. The limitations of such studies need to be emphasized since their results may be inappropriately used both for theoretical and practical purposes, the latter including cases where a child might be misidentified as being speech-delayed because of his performance of a Templin-style articulation test.

TABLE 3.5. Ages of Acquisition of Specific Sounds as Provided by Prather, Hedrick, and Kern (1975) and by Templin (1957)*

Sound	Prather, Hedrick, and Kern (1975) Two-position Norms (I,F)			Templin (1957)	
	All Data Sets	Complete Data Sets	Sets with Data from at Least 14 Ss	Two-position Norms (I,F)	Three-position Norms (I,M,F)
m	≤2;0	4;0	2;4	≤3;0	≤3;0
n	≤2;0	3;8	2;4	≤3;0	≤3;0
h[a]	≤2;0	>4;0	2;8	≤3;0	≤3;0
p	≤2;0	>4;0	2;4	≤3;0	≤3;0
ŋ[a]	≤2;0	4;0	2;4	≤3;0	≤3;0
f	2;4	4;0	2;4	≤3;0	≤3;0
j[a]	≤2;0	>4;0	3;0	3;6	3;6
k	2;4	4;0	2;4	4;0	4;0
d	2;4[b]	3;8	2;4[b]	4;0	4;0
w[a]	≤2;0[b]	4;0	2;8	≤3;0	≤3;0
b	2;8	4;0	2;8	4;0[b]	4;0[b]
t	2;8	3;8	2;8	≤3;0[b]	6;0
g	2;4[b]	4;0	2;4[b]	4;0[b]	4;0[b]
s	3;0[b]	3;8	3;0[b]	4;6	4;6[b]
r	3;4[b]	>4;0	3;4[b]	4;0	4;0
l	3;4[b]	4;0	3;4[b]	6;0	6;0
ʃ	3;8	3;8	3;8	4;0	4;6[b]
ʧ	3;8	3;8	3;8	4;6	4;6
ð	>4;0	>4;0	>4;0	7;0	7;0
ʒ[a]	4;0	>4;0	4;0	7;0	7;0
ʤ	3;4[b]	>4;0	3;4[b]	7;0	7;0
θ	>4;0	>4;0	>4;0	6;0	6;0
v	>4;0	>4;0	>4;0	6;0	6;0
z	>4;0	>4;0	>4;0	7;0	7;0
hw[a]	>4;0	>4;0	>4;0	>8;0	>8;0

Note: The age of acquisition in each case is the earliest age at which at least 75% of children produced the designated sound correctly in each indicated word position
[a]Sound does not occur in all word positions in English
[b]A reversal occurs in older age groups

What then is the alternative? Several investigators (e.g., Irwin and Wong, 1983; Stoel-Gammon, 1985) have attempted to improve upon the situation by using spontaneous speech and/or longitudinal investigations. While this is in some respects better than the picture naming tasks, several problems remain. The use of spontaneous speech, for instance, can also give us a biased sample. We actually probe only a minute portion of the child's conversation and then generalize assuming this is representative of the child's overall performance. Also, factors outside of our control determine which words and sounds the child does produce and which ones not. As a result the sample obtained will probably not contain all the sounds in that particular child's phonetic inventory.

On the other hand, longitudinal data can give us a real insight into the individual acquisition process, an important aspect missing in all cross-sectional studies. Several longitudinal studies exist (e.g., Leopold, 1947; Menn, 1971; Vihman, et al., 1985) but they either report on a single child or a small group of children. Therefore, the data cannot be readily generalized. One longitudinal investigation which utilizes spontaneous speech and looks at a sizable number of children is that presented by Stoel-Gammon (1985).

Thirty-four children between 15–24 months of age participated in this study. All children were evaluated at 15, 18, 21, and 24 months of age. The investigation was constructed to look at meaningful speech only. Thus, the number of subjects in each of these groups varied according to the age at which the child began to achieve meaningful speech. The children had been assessed as having normal cognitive and motor development based on the Bayley Scales of Infant Development (Bayley, 1969). An interesting point is that at 15 months only nine of the 34 subjects had true words (produced 10 different word types) while at 24 months there was still one child who had failed to reach the meaningful speech stage. As can be seen, the individual age variation for onset of this stage is considerable.

In Tables 3.6 and 3.7 the data are analyzed according to the inventory of the initial word position, final word position, and the age of onset of the meaningful word stage. Group A began this stage at 15 months, Group B at 18 months, and Group C at 21 months.

To summarize:

1. Early inventories contain stops, nasals, and glides. Fricatives and liquids do not appear until later.

TABLE 3.6.   Initial Position: Inventory Size and Phones in 50% of Inventories Organized by Group (*n*) and Age at Onset of Meaningful Speech

Group (*n*) by Age	Inventory Size: Mean (Range)	Phones in Inventories of 50% of Subjects
Group A (7)		
15 mos.	3.4(2–5)	b^{a}d^{a}h
18	7.9(5–10)	b^{a}td^{a}kgmnhw
21	10.1(5–13)	pb^{a}td^{a}kgm^{a}nhwf
24	11.6(9–16)	btd^{a}k^{a}gm^{a}nhwjfs
Group B (12)		
18 mos.	5.3(2–9)	b^{a}d^{a}mnh
21	7.4(3–11)	b^{a}td^{a}mnh^{a}w
24	9.3(5–12)	b^{a}t^{a}d^{a}kmnh^{a}wfs
Group C (13)		
21 mos.	4.2(2–8)	bd
24	8.5(4–12)	btd^{a}gmnhs

^{a}Indicates phone occurred in 90% of the inventories

TABLE 3.7. Final Position: Inventory Size and Phones in 50% of Inventories Organized by Group (*n*) and Age at Onset of Meaningful Speech

Group (*n*) by Age	Inventory Size: Mean (Range)	Phones in Inventories of 50% of Subjects
Group A (7)		
15 mos.	0.6(0–2)	(none)
18	4.0(0–6)	tk
21	5.7(4–7)	pt^{a}kn^{a}r
24	8.1(5–11)	pt^{a}k^{a}nŋr^{a}s
Group B (12)		
18 mos.	2.2(0–5)	t
21	4.7(1–7)	ptkn
24	6.1(4–8)	pt^{a}kmn^{a}rs
Group C (13)		
21 mos.	1.5(0–4)	(none)
24	4.5(1–8)	pt^{a}kn

^{a}Indicates phone occurred in 90% of the inventories

2. More anteriorly produced sounds precede posteriorly produced ones.
3. There was always a larger inventory of sounds used in the initial when compared to the final word position.
4. Differences existed in the inventories of initial versus final word productions. Initial inventories contained voiced stops prior to voiceless ones while the reverse was true for final word productions.
5. The liquid [r] nearly always appeared first in word-final position.
6. If the mean percentage of standard consonant productions was calculated (Shriberg and Kwiatkowski, 1982) 70% accuracy was achieved. While there is a large difference in the inventory produced by the 2-year-olds and adults, this accuracy level suggests that children are primarily attempting words that contain sounds within their articulatory abilities.

Vihman and Greenlee (1987) also used a longitudinal methodology to examine the phonological development of ten 3-year-old children. Only the substitutions of [θ] and [ð] by other consonants, such as stops and other fricatives, were regularly used by all subjects. Over half of the subjects also substituted [r] and [l] sounds (gliding) and employed palatal fronting where a palatal sound is replaced by an alveolar ([ʃ] becomes [s]). Vihman and Greenlee point to the differences in the error pattern of two of the children. Based on the information gathered, it appeared to them that these children had their own particular "style" of phonological acquisition. This is an important concept. It stresses again individual variation which has also been documented in other areas of language acquisition (e.g., Bloom, Lightbown, and Hood, 1975; Bretherton, McNew, Snyder, and Bates, 1983; Nelson, 1973).

Vihman and Greenlee also looked at the intelligibility of these children. All of them were understood at least half of the time. On the average 73% of their utterances were judged intelligible by three raters unfamiliar with the children. However, the range of intelligibility was broad, extending from 54%–80%. As to be expected, children with fewer errors were more intelligible than those with multiple errors. However, another factor also played a role. The children who used more complex sentences tended to be more difficult to understand.

This finding is significant. It documents the complex interaction between phonological development and the acquisition of the language system as a whole. The simultaneous acquisition of complex morphosyntactic and semantic relationships could well have a momentary impact on the growth of the phonological system. What has been labeled **phonological idioms** (Moskowitz, 1971) or **regression** (Leopold, 1947) might be the result of such a burden. Both terms refer to accurate sound productions which are later replaced by inaccurate ones. Thus, the child's previously correct articulations appear to be lost, replaced by nonstandard pronunciation. It has been hypothesized that these regressions are occurring as the child attempts to master other complexities of language. In view of all the other linguistic properties to be learned at the same time, such regressions are really not surprising.

SEGMENTAL DEVELOPMENT—VOWELS

One area of acquisition which has been widely neglected in most discussions of phonological development is the acquisition of vowels. This neglect has at least partially been justified, for example by Templin (1957), with the statement that children have acquired all the vowels within the English inventory by the age of 3. Little information is available on the development of vowels. This final section of the segmental phonological development will utilize the data presented by Irwin and Wong (1983). Although several methodological problems with this investigation have been pointed out (see Smit, 1986), it does examine the vowel productions in spontaneous conversations of children from 18 to 72 months of age.

If the criterion is set at 70% accuracy, the children show acquisition of [ɑ], [ʊ], [i], [ɪ], and [ʌ] at 18 months. For the individual subjects at this age level, the correct production of vowels ranged from 23%–71%. The group mean of correct vowel production was 59%. By 24 months the only vowels which did not reach 70% group accuracy were [ɝ] and [ɚ]. At 24 months the group mean accuracy percentage rose to 91% (range 77%–96%). By the age of 3 all the vowels were accounted for with virtually no production errors. Interestingly enough, though, at 4 years the accuracy for [ɚ], [u], and [ə] dropped again to less than 90%.

These findings generally support Templin's claim that vowels are mastered at age 3. As the drop in accuracy at age 4 indicates, it may be that the younger children simply avoided those difficult vowels before.

Another view of vowel acquisition is offered by diary studies. Velten's data (1943) show that prior to the age of 21 months her daughter utilized the [a] vowel. After a surge in vocabulary at 21 months the vowel [u] was added. When comparing this child to Irwin and Wong's data large discrepancies between the two become obvious. Again, the previously discussed concepts of salience and avoidance may apply to the described differences. Some children possibly select, for the most part, words that consist of sounds within their repertoire, avoiding those sounds that are not. Salience and avoidance in conjunction with individual phonetic preference could skew the investigative results.

Far more information is needed in the area of vowel acquisition. From the limited amount of data presently available it appears that vowels are, indeed, generally mastered by the age of

3. Whether individual variation plays a large role in this process still needs to be documented. This is an interesting area of research especially in light of the deviant vowel systems which are often noted in children with phonological disorders.

SUPRASEGMENTAL DEVELOPMENT

At the time when children begin to use two-word utterances a further development in the usage of suprasegmentals occurs: **contrastive stress**. This term indicates that one syllable within an utterance becomes prominent. The acquisition process seems to proceed in the following order. First, within the child's two-word utterance a single prosodic pattern is maintained. The two words have a pause between them which becomes shorter and shorter. The next step appears to be the prosodic integration of the two words into one **tone-unit**. A tone-unit, or what is often called a **sense-group**, is an organizational unit imposed upon prosodic data. A tone-unit conveys meaning beyond that which is implied by only the verbal production. When the two words become one tone-unit (i.e., without the pause between them and with one intonational contour) one of these words becomes more prominent than the other, usually louder associated with an identifiable pitch movement (Crystal, 1986). Now there exists a unifying rhythmic relationship between the two items, thus, pauses become less likely. The following developmental pattern could be observed:

Daddy :: eat
Daddy : eat
'Daddy 'eat (no pause, both stressed)
'Daddy eat (first word stressed)

This development is important because the use of contrastive stress in the two-word stage signals semantic relationships (Brown, 1973). It is assumed that the meaning of the combined one-tone utterance is different than the meaning of the two words in sequence. Later we see that this contrastive stress is used to signal differences in meaning with similar words. Thus, "'Daddy eat" could indicate that "Daddy is eating," while "Daddy 'eat" could indicate, perhaps, that "Daddy should sit down and eat."

The relatively few existing studies of suprasegmental development agree that the acquisition of intonation and stress begin at an early age. Adult-like intonational patterns are noted prior to the appearance of the first word, while the onset of stress patterns seems to occur clearly before the age of 2. However, true mastery of the whole suprasegmental system does not seem to take place until children are at least 12-years old. Thus, while the acquisition of the suprasegmentals begins early, it represents a long process which may extend well beyond the acquisition of the child's segmental phonological system.

ACROSS LINGUISTIC BOUNDARIES/UNIVERSALS

The concept that there is a universal acquisition of phoneme contrasts was first authentically presented by Roman Jakobson (1941/1968). He stated that children initially acquire [a], then [i] and [u]. These vowels represent extreme corners of the vowel quadrilateral. Only later are the intermediate vowels acquired, making the distance between them smaller and smaller.

With respect to consonants, Jakobson suggested two principles. First, the place of articulation tends to be acquired from the front of the mouth to the back. Labials, therefore, are generally produced before dentals and alveolars, whereas dentals and alveolars appear before palatals and velars. The second principle pertains to the manner of articulation. On the whole, consonants are acquired in this order: stops, nasals, fricatives, affricates, and liquids. The interaction of both of these principles predicts that /p, b, m/ will precede /t/. Also, according to this principle we would expect /t, d/ before /n/ and /n/ before /s/ and /z/. How much does this theory of universal acquisition mirror actual research findings?

Stoel-Gammon (1985, p. 511) notes in her data set (see Tables 3.6 and 3.7 earlier in this chapter) that "The findings reported here are in close agreement with Jakobson's statements (1941/1968) regarding the universal patterns of phonemic acquisition." How do these principles survive, however, if they are scrutinized cross-linguistically?

Locke (1983) provides cross-linguistic sequences of phonological mastery for English, German, Japanese, Russian, Italian, Arabic, Slovenian, Swedish, Norwegian, and Czech. Some of the information is based on cross-sectional data while others come from detailed diary studies. Although differences can be found, it appears that consonants produced more anteriorly are acquired earlier than posterior consonants. Also, stops seem universally to be appear before fricatives. Very early sounds are traditionally bilabial stops and nasals, followed by dental and alveolar stops. On the other hand, the affricates and liquids are often among the later sounds to appear and be mastered.

This theory of universal acquisition has often been criticized. However, it seems less and less wise to disregard it completely. At the same time, the amount of individual variation in the course of phonological development will probably not allow too strict an adherence to these principles.

CONCLUSIONS

In this section an attempt has been made to point out some of the problems inherent in the large cross-sectional studies which continue to dominate the field of developmental phonology. Although these normed findings can be used as broad, general guidelines, or rough points of orientation, great caution must be exercised if they are applied to the diagnosis of speech/language deficient children. Discrepancies in "mastery" ages of particular sounds reflecting various investigative methodologies are misleading. Also, the basic premise that the results of a picture naming task can be generalized to indicate overall phonological competency is very weak. In contrast, longitudinal studies have been presented to allow some insight into actual developmental processes of individual children. The impact of individual variation should not be reduced to averaged norms. That does not contradict the finding that certain universal principles of acquisition apply as well.

SCHOOL-AGE CHILD

By the time children enter school their phonological development has progressed considerably. At age 5;0 most of them can converse freely with everyone and make themselves understood clearly to peers and adults alike. However, their pronunciation is still recognizably different from the adult norm. Phonologically they have yet a lot to learn. While their phonological inventory is nearly complete, this system must now be adapted to many more and different contexts, words, and situations. Other phonological features are obviously not mastered at all at this time. Certain sounds are still frequently misarticulated and specific aspects of suprasegmental development are only beginning.

Most of the research in child phonology has centered around the development of phonological skills in the first 5 years of life. However, recent interest in later phonological acquisition has evolved due to the established relationship between learning to speak and learning to read. Not only does the school-age child still have a lot to learn to complete his/her phonological system, but so do we in the field of child phonology, especially about later development and its relation to other language skills such as reading and writing. New insights will be gained when more about the relationship between phonological development and emerging literacy becomes known.

SEGMENTAL DEVELOPMENT

The mastery of a child's phonological system includes both perceptual and productional maturation. While it is not the focus of this chapter to discuss perception, it should be emphasized that the school-age child's perceptual skills are still very much in the process of growing. The gradual establishment of phonemic categorization skills, for example, continues well beyond 5-years of age and it may be as late as age 14 when children can reliably give categorical responses to certain types of synthetic stimuli (Fourcin, 1978). Tallal, Stark, Kallman, and Mellits (1980) reported that the perceptual constancy of children's phonemic categorizations still changes between 5- and 9-years of age. Also, the recognition of isolated words under quiet and noisy environmental conditions appears to be improving until at least age 10 (Elliott, Connors, Kille, Levin, Ball, and Katz, 1979). The processing ability of specific continuous speech samples is measurably slower for fifth graders than for adults (Cole and Perfetti, 1980), and the ability to understand specifically structured sentences under difficult listening conditions continues to develop until the age of 15 (Elliott, 1979). Perceptually children are still fine-tuning, certainly during the beginning school years and in some respects far beyond.

Information on the productional development of the phonological system comes from quite different methodological backgrounds. Most of the information available is based on the results of articulation tests, i.e., on responses to picture naming. If we look at these investigations (e.g., Lowe, 1986; Templin, 1957) we find that acceptable pronunciation of certain sounds is not achieved until between 4;6 and 6;0. The most common later sounds are [θ], [ð], [ʒ] (Sander, 1972). Other findings (Ingram, Christensen, Veach, and Webster, 1980) include one or more of these sounds: [r], [z], [v]. Based on single item pronunciation, most investigators agree that children complete their phonemic inventory by the age of 6;0 or at the latest 7;0. Table 3.8 indicates the later developing sounds found in large cross-sectional studies.

One must keep in mind that most of these results are responses to single word tasks. To assume, based on this type of task, that these sounds are now "learned" does not take into account the complexity of their use in naturalistic contexts, in new words and in conversational situations.

Consonant clusters also prove difficult for the school-age child. The acquisition of clusters usually takes place anywhere from about age 3;6 to 5;6. During this time the child may demonstrate consonant cluster reduction, lengthening of certain elements of the cluster, for example

TABLE 3.8.   Age Levels of Sound ''Mastery'' in School-Age Children

Sound	Age of Mastery	Source
[d]	5	Wellman (1931)
[t]	5	Wellman (1931)
[s]	5: 7½	Wellman (1931): Poole (1934)
[z]	5: 7½: 7	Wellman (1931): Poole (1934): Templin (1957)
[r]	5: 7½	Wellman (1931): Poole (1934)
[v]	5: 6½: 6	Wellman (1931): Poole (1934): Templin (1957)
[ʃ]	6½	Poole (1934)
[ʒ]	6: 6½: 7	Wellman (1931): Poole (1934): Templin (1957)
[θ]	7½: 6: 5	Poole (1934): Templin (1957): Sander (1972)
[ð]	6½: 7: 5	Poole (1934): Templin (1957): Sander (1972)
[tʃ]	5	Wellman (1931)
[ʤ]	7	Templin (1957)

[s:no] or epenthesis. In epenthesis the child inserts a schwa vowel between two consonantal elements of a cluster ([səno], for example).

The timing of the sounds within consonant clusters is also not yet comparable to adult performance (Gilbert and Purves, 1977; Hawkins, 1979). When the temporal relationships between the elements of a cluster were compared for children and adults, it was found that differences, particularly in voice onset time, were still present at 8;0 years of age.

While this information indicates that phonological development extends past the age of 7, we continue to focus on the phonological inventory or on the phonotactic development. Unfortunately, other features of the phonological system are still relatively uncharted territory. For example, the development of allophonic variation in older children should also be addressed. How do children learn the acceptable range of phonetic variation in different contexts within their speech community? Local (1983) followed this process exemplified by the acquisition of one vowel produced by a boy between the ages of 4;5 and 5;6. The variability of sound production and the learning of its acceptable allophonic limitations are decisively important tasks for the developing school-age child.

The intricate interrelation of normal phonological development with other areas of language growth, which has been previously emphasized, demands attention at this point in the child's development as well. The acquisition of vocabulary, for example, is a monumental task to be accomplished in a relatively short time. When children begin kindergarten they are said to have a vocabulary of approximately 8000 words. Obviously, the phonological rules valid for the analysis of previously used words often will not suffice any longer. New sound sequences occurring in words which will now be attained require not only an increased oral-motor control and improved timing skills, they also necessitate the internalization of new phonological rules. For instance, the conditions under which voiceless stops in English need to be aspirated or not might now become a new achievement.

The acquisition of morphology is also related to phonological growth. The learning of specific morphological structures implies the learning of phonological rules. The child has to understand under which conditions the plural suffix -s is voiced or voiceless, for example. This interconnection between morphology and phonology (morphophonology) refers to the study of the different allomorphs of the morpheme and the rules governing their use. Thus, the child's production of [əz] to indicate the plural form for ''glass'' versus [s] as the plural of ''boat'' falls within the study of morphophonology as well as the rules which govern the productional changes from divide/division, explode/explosion. Research findings in this area (e.g., Atkinson-King, 1973; Ivimey, 1975; Myerson, 1978) substantiate that children as old as 17 are still acquiring certain morphophonological patterns. The complex interrelationship between the phonological system and other components of language continues into the later school years of the child.

One other important aspect which needs to be addressed in this section pertains to the parallel between learning to speak and learning to read. Although a general concensus has not been reached as to which variables are indispensable for acquiring reading, there does seem to be a close relationship between early speech and emerging literacy. Thus, a strong correlation between the phonological development, especially segmentation skills, and later reading achievement has been found (e.g., Lundberg, Olofsson, and Wall, 1980). Moreover, early language development, specifically the perceptual processing of sounds, has been found to be one of the strongest predictors of later reading acquisition (Lundberg, 1988). Some of these skills develop during the early school years.

Metaphonological skills are also related to reading. A subcategory of metalinguistics, metaphonology involves the child's conscious awareness of the sounds within that particular language. It includes how those sounds are combined to form words. Metaphonological skills pertain to the child's ability to discern how many sounds are in a word or which sound constitutes its beginning or end. Certain metaphonological abilities seem to be related to the child's acquisition of reading. Although it is not yet clear whether the metaphonological skills are precursors of emerging literacy or a result of the developing reading skills (Hakes, 1982; Liberman, Shankweiler, Liberman, Fowler, and Fisher, 1977; Read, 1978), two factors remain: (a) metaphonology is related to reading performance and (b) these skills develop at the time when most children start to read, i.e., within the age range of 5–6 years. Research (e.g., Brady, 1986; Brady and Fowler, 1988; Liberman and Shankweiler, 1985) examining the phonological abilities of school children with poor reading skills has confirmed the following metaphonological difficulties:

- *Phonological awareness.* Poor readers have difficulty analyzing words into syllables and sounds.
- *Memory storage of phonetic coding.* Poor readers are less efficient at creating and maintaining the necessary phonological code for storing verbal information. They can recall fewer items from lists of material. This may contribute to poor phonological awareness tasks.
- *Phonetic perception in recreating a phonological code.* On repetition tasks poor readers exhibit clearly greater difficulties if background noise is introduced or if the words to be read are somewhat longer or less familiar. Although this affects good readers as well, the group differences established are remarkable.

Investigations relating reading and phonological skills have been primarily correlational in nature. Therefore, they do not allow us to say that the previous skills are precursors of reading ability. However, the degree of phonological skills, both productional and perceptual, seems to be one of the basic units in emerging literacy.

SUPRASEGMENTAL DEVELOPMENT

Very little documented research is available on the suprasegmental acquisition of the school-age child. This lack of information is not restricted to our knowledge about prosodic progress during this later developmental period. It pertains to the evolution of suprasegmentals in children in general. Several reasons could account for this gap: (*a*) the linguistic meaning of the suprasegmentals is somewhat elusive (Grunwell, 1986); (*b*) what actually has to be identified is obscured by different methods and analytical frames of reference (Wode, 1980); and (*c*) the acquisition of suprasegmentals is often held to be essentially completed by around age 2 (Crystal, 1986). While the suprasegmentals in their variation of pitch, loudness, and duration can be used to signal attitudes and emotions, they can also assume grammatical function. For example, specific intonation patterns have to be employed to differentiate between statements and certain questions in English ("He is coming." versus "He is coming?"). Contrasting stress realizations might signal different word classes ('construct versus con'struct). On the sentence level the combined effects of higher pitch and increased loudness usually convey communicatively important modifications of basic meaning ("This is a *pen*." versus "*This* is a pen."). This section looks at the grammatical function of the suprasegmentals in school-age children and their relationship to phonological development.

As previously noted, the child begins to use intonational patterns towards the end of the first year of life. As the child's grammatical abilities develop, new uses of intonation emerge. For example, the contrast between rising and falling pitch differentiates the two grammatical functions of a tag question in English ("asking" as in "We're ready, aren't we?" and "telling" as in "We're ready, aren't we!"). Differences in intonation patterns like these appear to be learned during the child's third year (Crystal, 1987). However, the learning of intonation goes on for a very long time. Studies (Cruttenden, 1985; Ianucci and Dodd, 1980) report that children as old as 12-years were still acquiring some of the fundamental functions of English intonation, especially those for signaling grammatical contrasts. As reported by Crystal (1987) even teenagers have been shown to have difficulty understanding sentences where intonation and pausing are used to differentiate meanings. His example: "She dressed, and fed the baby." (indicating she dressed herself and then fed the baby) versus "She dressed and fed the baby." (indicating she dressed as well as fed the baby). Thus, while certain intonational features seem to be among the earliest phonological acquisitions, others may be some of the last.

Several studies (e.g., Atkinson-King, 1973; Chomsky, 1971; Hornby and Hass, 1970; Myers and Myers, 1983) have examined the use of contrastive stress both on the word level ('record versus re'cord) and on the sentence level (differentiating between whom Mary hit in the following sentences: "John hit Bill and then *Mary* hit him" versus "John hit Bill and then Mary hit *him*."). Although the ages differ depending on the type and design of the research, results suggest that children are still learning certain aspects of contrastive stress up until the age of 13.

The acquisition of the suprasegmentals is a gradual process which in some respects extends into the teens. It is closely connected to the new phonological, morphosyntactic, semantic, and pragmatic demands which are placed upon the developing child. As the complexity of the linguistic environment and the child's interaction with that environment increase, so do the subtle intricacies of each of these language levels.

Across Linguistic Boundaries/Universals

It has been reported in other sections of this chapter that certain universals do seem to exist. For example, a relatively small repertoire of sounds noted in infants' babbling appeared to be common to infants from many different language backgrounds. As the child developed, other universals were mentioned. For example, regardless of the language in question, stops seem to be acquired before fricatives. Do universal trends also exist in the production of phonological systems in the school years?

To answer this question a cross-linguistic comparison must be made of the phonological abilities of older children. Table 3.9 is based on information provided by Locke (1983) and, for German, Bauman-Waengler and Waengler (1990).

As can be seen, fricatives (especially sibilants), affricates, and consonant clusters appear to dominate the articulatory difficulties encountered by older children. The "r" problems mentioned are rather incomparable due to the language dependent articulatory differences in pronunciation. The flapped "r" of Italian cannot be compared to the uvular trilled "r" of German. Both are phonetically incomparable to typical American-English "r" productions. In spite of these differences a trend can be seen.

However, this concentrates once more on the phonetic inventory of the children. Although the available phonetic inventory is one important component of the phonological system in its totality, it is by no means the only, or even most important, one. A far more detailed examination of the condition under which phonological features were verified would be necessary before any definite statements could be attempted. For example, the German children (Bauman-Waengler and Waengler, 1990) substituted or omitted certain sounds only in unstressed syllables. Also, the frequent devoicing of normally voiced stops could be the result of an overgeneralization of the phonological principle in German that all word final stops are devoiced. A more in-depth analysis of children's speech in many different contexts and situations taking phonological features other than just pronunciation into account would need to be available before universal claims can be made.

Conclusions

This section has addressed the phonological development of school-age children, here defined as those who are 5;0 years old or older. As is generally known, these children are still demonstrating difficulty with certain sounds and sound combinations.

TABLE 3.9. Cross-Linguistic Comparison of Later Acquired Sounds

Language	Sounds	Age	Source
English	[l,r,ʃ,ʒ,v,z,ʤ,θ,ð]	4+	Locke (1973)
German	[ʃ,s,z,ʀ]	6;7–7;0	Bauman-Waengler and Waengler (1990)
Japanese	[dz,ts,s,r]	4;6–5;11	Umebayashi and Takagi (1965) cited in Yasuda (1970)
Arabic	[ʃ, ʒ, ç, ř, q]	4;0–6;6	Omar (1973)
Czech	[r, ř]	500 word stage	Pačesova (1968)

It is not, however, just that certain sounds are not yet quite accurate in their phonetic realization. School-age children still must master a considerable amount of phonological detail. If they do not, they might suffer consequences in the continuous growth of other language skills and/or their total language development. In addition, problems with further phonological analyses can also translate into reading and writing deficiencies. The importance of continued phonological development during these ''later'' years should not be underestimated.

REFERENCES

Atkinson-King K. Children's acquisition of phonological stress contrasts. UCLA Working Papers in Phonetics 1973; 25:184–191.

Atkinson K, MacWhinney B, Stoel C. An experiment on the recognition of babbling. In Language behavior research laboratory working paper # 14. Berkeley: University of California, 1968.

Bauer HR. The ethologic model of phonetic development: I. clinical linguistics and phonetics 1988;2:347–380.

Bauer HR, Robb MP. Phonetic development between infancy and toddlerhood: the phonetic product estimator. Paper presented at the Annual ASHA Convention, St. Louis,1989.

Bauman-Waengler JA, Waengler H-H. Speech sound acquisition and phonological analysis of three groups of German children age 6;7 to 7;0. Beiträge zur Phonetik und Linguistik. Neue Tendenzen in der Angewandten Phonetik III 1990;62:7–58.

Bayley N. Bayley Scales of Infant Development. New York: Academic Press, 1969.

Bloom L, Lightbown P, Hood L. Structure and variation in child language. Society for Research in Child Development Monographs 1975;40:119–318.

Bonvillian J, Raeburn V, Horan E. Talking to children—the effect of rate, intonation and length on children's sentence imitation. Journal of Child Language 1979;6:459–467.

Brady S. Short-term memory, phonological processing and reading ability. Annals of Dyslexia 1986;36:138–153.

Brady SA, Fowler AE. Phonological precursors to reading acquisition. In Masland RL, Masland MW, eds. Prevention of reading failure. Parkton, MD: York Press, 1988.

Bretherton I, McNew S, Snyder L, Bates E. Individual differences at 20 months: analytic and holistic strategies in language acquisition. Journal of Child Language 1983;10:293–320.

Brown R. Words and things. Glencoe: Free Press, 1958.

Brown R. A first language: the early stages. London: Allen and Unwin, 1973.

Bruner J. The ontogenesis of speech acts. Journal of Child Language 1975;2:1–21.

Camp B, Burgess D, Morgan L, Zerbe G. A longitudinal study of infant vocalizations in the first year. Journal of Pediatric Psychology 1987;12:321–331.

Chomsky C. Linguistic Development in Children from 6 to 10. U.S. Office of Education: Final Report. Washington, DC: 1971.

Cole RA, Perfetti CA. Listening for mispronunciations in a children's story: the use of context by children and adults. Journal of Verbal Learning and Verbal Behavior 1980:19:297–315.

Cruttenden A. A phonetic study of babbling. British Journal of Communication 1970:5:110–117.

Cruttenden A. Item-learning and system-learning. Journal of Psycholinguistic Research 1981:10:79–88.

Cruttenden A. Intonation comprehension in 10-year-olds. Journal of Child Language 1985;12:643–661.

Crystal D. Prosodic development. In Fletcher P, Garman M, eds. Language acquisition. Cambridge: Cambridge University Press, 1986.

Crystal D. The Cambridge encyclopedia of language. Cambridge: Cambridge University Press, 1987.

de Boysson-Bardies B, Halle P, Sagart L, Durand, C. A cross-linguistic investigation of vowel formants in babbling. Journal of Child Language 1989;16:1–17.

de Boysson-Bardies B, Sagart L, Bacri N. Phonetic analysis of late babbling: a case study of a French child. Journal of Child Language 1981;8:511–524.

Dore J. Holophrases, speech acts and language universals. Journal of Child Language 1975;3:22–39.

Dore J, Franklin MB, Miller RT, Ramer ALH. Transitional phenomena in early language acquisition. Journal of Child Language 1976;3:13–29.

Dyson A, Paden E. Some phonological acquisition strategies used by two-year-olds. Journal of Childhood Communication Disorders 1983;7:6–18.

Edwards ML, Shriberg LD. Phonology: applications in communicative disorders. San Diego: College-Hill, 1983.

Elbers L. Operating principles in repetitive babbling: a cognitive approach. Cognition 1982;12:45–63.

Elliott LL. Performance of children aged 9–17 years on a test of speech intelligibility in noise using sentence material with controlled word predictability. Journal of the Acoustic Society of America 1979;66:651–653.

Elliott LL, Connors S, Kille E, Levin S, Ball K, Katz D. Children's understanding of monosyllabic nouns in quiet and in noise. Journal of the Acoustic Society of America 1979;66:12–21.

Farwell CB. Some strategies in the early production of fricatives. Papers and reports on child language development 1976;12:97–104.

Ferguson CA. Learning to pronounce: the earliest stages of phonological development in the child. In Minifie FD, Floyd LL, eds. Communicative and cognitive abilities: early behavioral assessment. Baltimore, MD: University Park Press, 1978.

Ferguson CA. Phonological processes. In Greenberg JH, ed. Universals of language. Vol. 2: Phonology. Stanford: Stanford University Press, 1978.

Ferguson CA, Farwell C. Words and sounds in early language acquisition: English initial consonants in the first fifty words. Language 1975;51:419–439.

Ferguson CA, Garnica O. Theories of phonological development. In Lenneberg E, Lenneberg E, eds. Foundation of language development. New York: Academic Press, 1975.

Fernald A, Simon T. Expanded intonation contours in mother's speech to newborns. Developmental Psychology 1984; 20:104–113.

Fernald A, Taeschner T, Dunn J, Papousek M, de Boysson-Bardies B, Fukui I. A cross- language study of prosodic modification in mother's and father's speech to preverbal infants. Journal of Child Language 1989;16:477–503.

Fisichelli RM. An experimental study of the prelinguistic speech development of institutionalized infants [unpublished Doctoral Dissertation]. New York: Fordham University, 1950.

Fourcin AJ. Acoustic patterns and speech acquisition. In Waterson N, Snow C, eds. Development of communication. New York: John Wiley and Sons, 1978.

French A. The systematic acquisition of word forms by a child during the first-fifty-word stage. Journal of Child Language 1989;16:69–90.

Fry DB. The development of the phonological system in the normal and deaf child. In: Smith F, Miller GA, eds. The genesis of language. Cambridge, MA: MIT Press, 1966.

Gesell A, Thompson H. Infant behavior: its genesis and growth. New York: McGraw Hill, 1934.

Gilbert JHV, Purves BA. Temporal constraints on consonant clusters in child speech production. Journal of Child Language 1977;4:417–432.

Grunwell P. Aspects of phonological development in later childhood. In Durkin K, ed. Language development in the school years. London: Croom Helm Ltd., 1986.

Haelsig P, Madison C. A study of phonological processes by 3-, 4- and 5-year-old children. Language, Speech, and Hearing Services in Schools 1986;17:107–114.

Hakes DT. The development of metalinguistic abilities: what develops. In Kuczaj S, ed. Language development, Vol. II. Hillsdale, NJ: Lawrence Erlbaum, 1982.

Hawkins S. Temporal coordination of consonants in the speech of children: further data. Journal of Phonetics 1979;13: 235–267.

Hoek D, Ingram D, Gibson D. Some possible causes of children's early word extensions. Journal of Child Language 1986;13:477–494.

Holmgren K, Lindblom B, Aurelius G, Jalling B, Zetterstrom R. On the phonetics of infant vocalization. In Lindblom B, Zetterstrom R, eds. Precursors of early speech. New York: Stockton Press, 1986.

Hornby PA, Hass WA. Use of contrastive stress by pre-school children. Journal of Speech and Hearing Research 1970; 13:395–399.

Ianucci D, Dodd D. The development of some aspects of quantifier negation. Papers and Reports on Child Language Development 1980;19:88–94.

Ingram D. Phonological rules in young children. Journal of Child Language 1974;1:49–64.

Ingram D. Phonological disability in children. London: Edward Arnold, 1976a.

Ingram D. Phonological analysis of a child. Glossa 1976b;10:3–27.

Ingram D. Procedures for the phonological analysis of children's language. Austin: Pro-Ed, 1981.

Ingram D. Phonological development: production. In Fletcher P, Garman M, eds. Language acquisition. Cambridge: Cambridge University Press, 1986.

Ingram D. The acquisition of word initial [v]. Language and Speech 1988;31:77–85.

Ingram D. First language acquisition. Cambridge: Cambridge University Press, 1989.

Ingram D. Early phonological acquisition, a cross-linguistic perspective. In Ferguson CA, Menn L, Stoel-Gammon C, eds. Phonological development: models, research, implications. Timonium, MD: York Press, 1992.

Ingram D, Christensen L, Veach S, Webster B. The acquisition of word-initial fricatives and affricates in English by children between 2 and 6 years. In Yeni-Komshian GH, Kavanagh JF, Ferguson CA, eds. Child phonology. Vol. I: Production. New York: Academic Press, 1980.

Irwin OC. Infant speech: consonantal sounds according to place of articulation. Journal of Speech and Hearing Disorders 1947a;12:397–401.

Irwin OC. Infant speech: consonant sounds according to manner of articulation. Journal of Speech and Hearing Disorders 1947b;12:402–404.

Irwin OC. Infant speech: development of vowel sounds. Journal of Speech and Hearing Disorders 1948;13:31–34.

Irwin OC, Chen HP. Infant speech: vowel and consonant frequency. Journal of Speech and Hearing Disorders 1946;11: 123–125.

Irwin JV, Wong SP. Phonological development in children 18 to 72 months. Carbondale: Southern Illinois University Press, 1983.

Ivimey GP. The development of English morphology: an acquisition model. Language and Speech 1975;18:120–144.

Jacobson J, Boersma D, Fields R, Olson K. Prelinguistic features of adult speech to infants and small children. Child Development 1983;54:436–442.

Jakobson R. Kindersprache, Aphasie und allgemeine Lautgesetze. Uppsala: Almquist and Wiksell, 1941.

Jakobson R. Child language, aphasia and phonological universals. The Hague: Mouton, 1968.

Jakobson R, Halle M. Fundamentals of language. The Hague: Mouton, 1956.

Jensen TS, Boggild-Andersen B, Schmidt B, Ankerkus J, Hansen E. Prenatal risk factors and first-year vocalizations: influence on preschool language and motor performance. Developmental Medicine and Child Neurology 1988;30: 153–161.

Jusczyk PW. Developing phonological categories for the speech signal. In Ferguson CA, Menn L, Stoel-Gammon C, eds. Phonological development: models, research, implications. Parkton, MD: York Press, 1992.

Kagan J. Change and continuity in infancy. New York: John Wiley and Sons, 1971.

Kent RD. The psychobiology of speech development: co-emergence of language and movement system. American Journal of Physiology 1984;R 888–R 894.

Kent RD, Bauer HR. Vocalizations of one-year-olds. Journal of Child Language 1985;13:491–526.

Kiparsky P, Menn L. On the acquisition of phonology. In Macnamara J, ed. Language learning and thought. New York: Academic Press, 1977.

Labov W, Labov T. The phonetics of "cat" and "mama." Language, 1978;57:816–852.

Lenneberg EH. Biological foundations of language. New York: John Wiley and Sons, 1967.

Leonhard L, Newhoff M, Mesalam L. Individual differences in early childhood phonology. Applied Psycholinguistics 1980;1:7–30.

Leopold WF. Speech development of a bilingual child. Evanston: Northwestern University Press, 1947.

Liberman IY, Shankweiler D. Phonology and the problems of learning to read and write. Topical Issues: Remedial and Special Education 1985;6:8–17.

Liberman IY, Shankweiler D, Liberman AM, Fowler C, Fischer FW. Phonetic segmentation and recording in the beginning reader. In Reber AS, Scarborough H, eds. Toward a psychology of reading. Hillsdale, NJ: Lawrence Erlbaum, 1977.

Local J. How many vowels in a vowel? Journal of Child Language 1983;10:449–453.

Locke JL. Mechanisms of phonological development in children: maintenance, learning, and loss. Papers from the Sixteenth Regional Meeting of the Chicago Linguistic Society. Chicago: Chicago Linguistic Society, 1980.

Locke JL. Phonological acquisition and change. New York: Academic Press, 1983.

Locke JL. Speech perception and emergent lexicon. In Fletcher P, Garman M, eds. Language acquisition. Cambridge: Cambridge University Press, 1986.

Lowe R. Assessment link between phonology and articulation: ALPHA. Moline, IL: LinguiSystems, Inc., 1986.

Lundberg I. Preschool prevention of reading failure: does training in phonology work? In Masland RL, Masland MW, eds. Prevention of reading failure. Parkton, MD: York Press, 1988.

Lundberg I, Olofsson A, Wall S. Reading and spelling skills in the first school years predicted from phonemic skills in kindergarten. Scandinavian Journal of Psychology 1980;21:159–173.

Macken MA. Phonological development: a crosslinguistic perspective. In Fletcher P, Garman M, eds. Language acquisition. Cambridge: Cambridge University Press, 1986.

Macken M, Barton D. The acquisition of the voicing contrast in English: a study of voice onset time in word-initial stop consonants. Journal of Child Language 1980;7:41–74.

Mehler J. Language acquisition: models and methods. In Huxley R, Ingram D, eds. Comments at a conference held in 1969. New York: Academic Press, 1971.

Menn L. Phonotactic rules in beginning speech. Lingua 1971;26:225–251.

Menn L. Evidence for an interactionist discovery theory of child phonology. Stanford Papers and Reports on Child Language Development, 1975:12.

Menn L. Pattern, control and contrast in beginning speech: a case study in the development of word form and word function. Bloomington, IN: Indiana University Linguistics Club, 1978.

Menn L. Phonological theory and child phonology. In Yeni-Komshian G, Kavanagh J, Ferguson CA, eds. Child phonology. Vol. I: Production. New York: Academic Press, 1980.

Menyuk P, Liebergott J, Schultz M. Predicting phonological development. In Lindblom B, Zetterstrom R, eds. Precursors of early speech. New York: Stockton Press, 1986.

Menyuk P, Menn L. Early strategies for the perception and production of words and sounds. In Fletcher P, Garman M, eds. Language acquisition. Cambridge: Cambridge University Press, 1979.

Minifie FD, Lloyd LL, eds. Communicative and cognitive abilities, early behavior assessment. Baltimore, MD: University Park Press, 1978.

Mitchell PR, Kent R. Phonetic variation in multisyllable babbling. Journal of Child Language 1990;17:247–265.

Moskowitz A. Acquisition of phonology [Doctoral Dissertation]. Berkeley: University of California, 1971.

Myers FL, Myers RW. Perception of stress contrasts in semantic and non-semantic contexts by children. Journal of Psycholinguistic Research 1983;12:327–338.

Myerson RF. Children's knowledge of selected aspects of sound pattern of English. In Campbell RN, Smith PT, eds. Recent advances in the psychology of language. New York: Plenum Press, 1978.

Nelson K. Structure and strategy in learning to talk. Monographs of the Society of Research in Child Development 1973;38(149).

Oller DK. The emergence of the sounds of speech in infancy. In Yeni-Komshian G, Kavanagh J, Ferguson CA, eds. Child phonology. Vol. I: Production. New York: Academic Press, 1980.

Oller DK, Eilers R. Similarity of babbling in Spanish- and English-learning babies. Journal of Child Language 1982;9: 565–577.

Oller DK, Weiman LA, Doyle WJ, Ross C. Infant babbling and speech. Journal of Child Language 1976;3:1–11.

Olmsted D. Out of the mouth of babes. The Hague: Mouton, 1971.

Olney RL, Scholnick EK. Adult judgements of age and linguistic differences in infant vocalization. Journal of Child Language 1976;3:145–155.

Omar MK. The acquisition of Egyptian arabic as a native language. The Hague: Mouton, 1973.

Pačesova J. The development of vocabulary in the child. Brno: Universita J.E. Purkyne, 1968.

Piaget J. The origins of intelligence in children. New York: International University Press, 1952.

Pierce JR, Hanna IV. The development of a phonological system in English speaking American children. Portland: HaPi Press, 1974.

Pike KL. Phonetics. Ann Arbor: University of Michigan Press, 1941.

Poole E. Genetic development of articulation of consonant sounds in speech. Elementary English Review 1934;11:159–161.

Prather ED, Hedrick C, Kern C. Articulation development in children aged two to four years. Journal of Speech and Hearing Disorders 1975;40:179–191.

Preisser DA, Hodson BW, Paden EP. Developmental phonology: 18–29 months. Journal of Speech and Hearing Disorders 1988;53:125–130.

Pye C, Ingram D, List H. A comparison of initial consonant acquisition in English and Quiché. In Nelson KE, van Kleek A, eds. Children's language, Vol. 6. Hillsdale, NJ: Lawrence Erlbaum, 1987.

Read C. Children's awareness of sounds, with emphasis on sound systems. In Sinclair A, Jarvella RJ, Leveit WJM, eds. The child's conception of language. Berlin: Springer Verlag, 1978.

Roe KV. Amount of infant vocalization as a function of age: some cognitive implications. Child Development 1975; 46:936–941.

Roe KV. Relationship between infant vocalizations and preschool cognitive functioning. Paper presented at the Annual Meeting of the Washington Psychological Association, Seattle, WA, 1977.

Sander EK. When are speech sounds learned? Journal of Speech and Hearing Research 1972;37:55–63.

Schwartz R, Leonard LB. Do children pick and choose? An examination of phonological selection and avoidance in early lexical acquisition. Journal of Child Language 1982;9:319–336.

Schwartz R, Leonard L, Wilcox J, Folger M. Again and again: reduplication in child phonology. Journal of Child Language 1980;7:75–87.

Shriberg L, Kwiatkowski J. Natural process analysis (NPA). New York: John Wiley and Sons, 1980.

Shriberg L, Kwiatkowski J. Phonological disorders III: a procedure for assessing severity of involvement. Journal of Speech and Hearing Disorders 1982;47:242–256.

Shvachkin NK. The development of phonemic speech perception in early childhood. In Ferguson CA, Slobin DI, eds. Studies of child language development. New York: Holt, Rinehart and Winston, 1973.

Smith BL, Brown-Sweeney S, Stoel-Gammon C. A quantitative analysis of reduplicated and variegated babbling. First Language 1989;9:175–190.

Smit A. Ages of speech sound acquisition: comparisons and critiques of several normative studies. Language, Speech, and Hearing Services in Schools 1986;17:175–186.

Stark R. Features of infant sounds: the emergence of cooing. Journal of Child Language 1978;5:379–390.

Stark R. Prespeech segmental feature development. In Fletcher P, Garman M, eds. Language acquisition. Cambridge: Cambridge University Press, 1979.

Stark R. Stages of speech development in the first year of life. In Yeni-Komshian G, Kavanagh J, Ferguson CA, eds. Child phonology. Vol. I: Production. New York: Academic Press, 1980.

Stern D, Spieker S, Barnett R, MacKain K. The prosody of maternal speech: infant age and context related changes. Journal of Child Language 1983;10:1–15.

Stern D, Wasserman G. Maternal language to infants. Paper presented at a meeting of the Society for Research in Child Development, 1979.

Stockman I, Woods D, Tishman A. Listener agreement on phonetic segments in early childhood vocalizations. Journal of Psycholinguistic Research 1981;10:593–617.

Stoel-Gammon C. Phonetic inventories, 15–24 months: a longitudinal study. Journal of Speech and Hearing Research 1985;28:505–512.

Stoel-Gammon C, Cooper JA. Patterns of early lexical and phonological development. Journal of Child Language 1984; 11:247–271.

Stoel-Gammon C, Dunn C. Normal and disordered phonology in children. Baltimore, MD: University Park Press, 1985.

Stoel-Gammon C, Otomo K. Babbling development of hearing-impaired and normally hearing subjects. Journal of Speech and Hearing Disorders 1986;51:33–41.

Tallal P, Stark RE, Kallman C, Mellits D. Perceptual constancy for phonemic categories: a developmental study with normal and language-impaired children. Journal of Applied Linguistics 1980;1:49–64.

Templin M. Certain language skills in children: their development and interrelationships (Institute of Child Welfare Monograph 26). Minneapolis: The University of Minnesota Press, 1957.

Trubetzkoy NS. Grundzüge der Phonologie. Prague: TCLP, 1939(4).

Trubetzkoy NS. Principles of phonology. Berkeley: University of California Press, 1969.

Velten H. The growth of phonemic and lexical patterns in infant language. Language 1943;19:281–292.

Vihman MM. Sound change and child language. In Traugott EC, Labrum R, Shepherd S, eds. Papers from the Fourth International Congress on Historical Linguistics. Amsterdam: John Benjamins, 1980.

Vihman MM. Words and babble at the threshold of language acquisition. In Smith MD, Locke JL, eds. Emerging lexicon in the child's development of a linguistic vocabulary. New York: Academic Press, 1988a.

Vihman MM. Early phonological development. In Bernthal JE, Bankson NW, eds. Articulation and phonological disorders. Englewood Cliffs: Prentice Hall, 1988b.

Vihman MM. Early syllables and the construction of phonology. In Ferguson CA, Menn L, Stoel-Gammon C, eds. Phonological development: models, research, implications. Timonium, MD: York Press, 1992.

Vihman MM, Ferguson CA, Elbert M. Phonological development from babbling to speech: common tendencies and individual differences. Applied Psycholinguistics 1986;7:3–40.

Vihman MM, Greenlee M. Individual differences in phonological development: ages one to three years. Journal of Speech and Hearing Research 1987;30:503–521.

Vihman MM, Macken MA, Miller R, Simmons H, Miller J. From babbling to speech: a reassessment of the continuity issue. Language 1985;61:395–443.

Waterson N. Child phonology: a prosodic view. Journal of Linguistics, 1971;7:179–211.

Waterson N. Prosodic phonology: the theory and its application to language acquisition and speech processing. Newcastle upon Tyne: Grevatt and Grevatt, 1987.

Weir R. Some questions on the learning of phonology. In Smith F, Miller GA, eds. The genesis of language. Cambridge, MA: MIT Press, 1966.

Wellman BL, Case IM, Mengert EG, Bradbury DE. Speech sounds of young children. University of Iowa Studies in Child Welfare, 5. Iowa City: University of Iowa Press, 1931.

Whalen DH, Levitt AG, Wang Q. Intonational differences between reduplicative babbling of French- and English-learning infants. Journal of Child Language 1991;18:501–516.

Wode H. Grammatical intonation in child language. In Yeni-Komshian G, Kavanagh J, Ferguson CA, eds. Child phonology. Vol. I: Production. New York: Academic Press, 1980.

Yasuda A. Articulatory skills in three-year-old children. Studia Phonologica 1970;5:52–71.

Yeni-Komshian G, Kavanagh J, Ferguson CA, eds. Child phonology. Vol. I: Production. New York: Academic Press, 1980.

Distinctive Features and Phonological Rules

Chapter 4

Robert J. Lowe

Dɪꜱᴛɪɴᴄᴛɪᴠᴇ ꜰᴇᴀᴛᴜʀᴇ theory and analysis as practiced in the United States has its roots in the work of Roman Jakobson. Jakobson, Fant, and Halle (1952) and Jakobson and Halle (1956) developed the first complete theory of distinctive features. Their goal was to establish a set of subphonemic properties that could be used in the description of any known language. These properties were called distinctive features.

DISTINCTIVE FEATURES

Berko and Brown (1960, pp. 525–526) define distinctive features as "those aspects of the process of articulation and their acoustic consequences that serve to contrast one phoneme from another." Jakobson, Fant, and Halle viewed features as a set of properties that occurred at the same time for the production of a given sound. They could be compared to musical notes that when played together make a chord. Distinctive features are considered the smallest indivisible units that make up phonemes and most are described in terms of acoustic or articulatory characteristics. Particular sets or bundles of these characteristics (features) are used to define phonemes (see Table 4.1).

In their development of distinctive feature theory, Jakobson, et al., were concerned about language in general, and thus did not develop their distinctive feature system based on any one particular language. It was their goal to develop a set of features that could be applied universally. As a result, each of the features would not necessarily apply to every language. Only nine of the features, for example, applied to English.

Schane (1973, p. 25) describes features as fulfilling three functions. First, they can be used in the description of systematic phonetics, which refers to the phonetic descriptions typically used in narrow transcription. Second, features can be used to differentiate lexical items—a

TABLE 4.1. Chomsky and Halle Distinctive Feature Matrix for English Consonants*

	Voc	**Con**	**Son**	Hi	Bck	Rnd	Ant	Cor	Voi	Cnt	Del	Nas	Str
p	−	+	−	−	−	−	+	−	−	−	−	−	−
b	−	+	−	−	−	−	+	−	+	−	−	−	−
t	−	+	−	−	−	−	+	+	−	−	−	−	−
d	−	+	−	−	−	−	+	+	+	−	−	−	−
k	−	+	−	+	+	−	−	−	−	−	−	−	−
g	−	+	−	+	+	−	−	−	+	−	−	−	−
f	−	+	−	−	−	−	+	−	−	+	−	−	+
v	−	+	−	−	−	−	+	−	+	+	−	−	+
θ	−	+	−	−	−	−	+	+	−	+	−	−	−
ð	−	+	−	−	−	−	+	+	+	+	−	−	−
s	−	+	−	−	−	−	+	+	−	+	−	−	+
z	−	+	−	−	−	−	+	+	+	+	−	−	+
ʃ	−	+	−	+	−	−	−	+	−	+	−	−	+
tʃ	−	+	−	+	−	−	−	+	−	−	+	−	+
dʒ	−	+	−	+	−	−	−	+	+	−	+	−	+
j	−	−	+	+	−	−	−	−	+	+	−	−	−
r	+	+	+	−	−	−	−	+	+	+	−	−	−
l	+	+	+	−	−	−	+	+	+	+	−	−	−
w	−	−	+	+	+	+	−	−	+	+	−	−	−
m	−	+	+	−	−	−	+	−	+	−	−	+	−
n	−	+	+	−	−	−	+	+	+	−	−	+	−
ŋ	−	+	+	−	+	−	−	−	+	−	−	+	−
h	−	−	−	−	−	−	−	−	−	+	−	−	−

*Major class features are in bold face.

phonemic function. In other words, the distinctive features differentiate among phonemes. For example, /t/ and /d/ contrast in the voicing feature. Third, distinctive features can define natural classes—those segments that as a group undergo similar sound changes.

Features can be distinctive or nondistinctive depending upon the language they are describing. Distinctive features are those properties which differentiate between phonemes in a language. Nondistinctive features are properties that describe the phoneme but do not contrast it with other phonemes. For example, the feature of voicing differentiates the /t/ and /d/ and is thus distinctive in English. The feature of aspiration, however, does not distinguish between English phonemes but does describe a phonetic feature. Contrast this with the Hindi language in which aspiration is distinctive as it differentiates between voiceless stops to change word meaning.

The feature system as developed by Jakobson, et al., did not live up to its proposed purpose. Contrasts, for example, existed in various languages which the 12 feature system could not handle (Sommerstein, 1977). As a result, the distinctive feature theory and the features themselves have been revised time and time again.

One of the more influential revisions was by Chomsky and Halle (1968) and published in *The Sound Patterns of English*. The Chomsky and Halle distinctive feature system is based on binary values. If the feature is present it is given a "+" value or a "1," and if not present a "−" or "0" is assigned. Their system also differs from earlier systems by placing more emphasis on articulatory features and less on acoustic. They list 36 features which they describe as representing the phonetic capabilities of man. Later in this section are some of the features of the Chomsky and Halle system which pertain to English speech sounds. For ease of reference, Table 4.1 provides a matrix of the features pertaining to English consonants. The following are definitions of selected features from the Chomsky and Halle system.

CHOMSKY AND HALLE DISTINCTIVE FEATURES

1. Vocalic. Two conditions are necessary for a sound to be labeled vocalic: the constriction in the oral cavity cannot be greater than that required for the /i/ and /u/, and the vocal cords must be positioned to allow spontaneous voicing. In producing nonvocalic sounds one or both of these conditions are not satisfied. Vocalic sounds include the liquids and the vowels. (Negative: nonvocalic.)
2. Consonantal. Consonantal sounds are made with a narrow constriction in the midsagittal region of the vocal tract as in the production of fricative consonants. All liquids, nasal consonants, and nonnasal consonants have this feature. Glides and vowels do not. (Negative: nonconsonantal)
3. Sonorant. Sonorant sounds are produced with the vocal tract cavity in a configuration that allows spontaneous voicing. Nonsonorant sounds (obstruents) are produced with a cavity configuration that makes spontaneous voicing impossible. Sonorants include all vowels, glides, liquids, and nasals. (Negative: nonsonorant).
4. Rounded. Rounded sounds have a narrowing of the lip orifice during production. Rounded consonants are sometimes called labialized consonants. (Negative: nonround.)
5. Tense. Tense sounds are produced with a deliberate, distinct articulatory gesture with considerable effort by supraglottal musculature. The articulatory organs maintain their configurations for a relatively long period. The tense feature applies to vowels. (Negative: nontense.)
6. Nasal. When the velum is lowered to allow the air to be directed through the nose during sound production, the nasal feature is present. The sounds with this feature include the /m/, /n/, /ŋ/. (Negative: nonnasal.)
7. Continuant. Continuant sounds are produced with a partial obstruction to the air flow but not a total blockage. Continuants include liquids and fricatives. (Negative: noncontinuant or stops).
8. Delayed Release. The delayed release consonants are the affricates. During their production, turbulence is created in the vocal tract so that the release of the affricate is very similar to the homorganic fricative. The delayed release consonants are /ʤ/, and /ʧ/. (Negative: Instantaneous release.)
9. Voiced. During production of voiced sounds the vocal cords are vibrating. (Negative: nonvoiced.)
10. Strident. The main characteristic of a strident sound is its acoustic noisiness. Strident sounds have greater noisiness that results when air is passed over a rough surface. The

phonemes /f/, /v/, /s/, /z/, /ʃ/, /ʒ/, /ʧ/, and /ʤ/ have the strident feature. (Negative: nonstrident.)

11. Coronal. Coronal sounds are made with the blade of the tongue raised from the neutral position and is associated only with consonants. (Negative: noncoronal.)

12. High. The high feature describes the body of the tongue as raised above the neutral position. (Negative: nonhigh.)

13. Low. The low feature describes the body of the tongue as being lowered below the neutral position. (Negative: nonlow.)

14. Back. This feature means the body of the tongue is retracted from the neutral position. (Negative: nonback.)

15. Anterior. The anterior feature is present when a sound is produced in the front of the mouth anterior to the palato-alveolar region where the /ʧ/ is produced. (Negative: nonanterior.)

Table 4.1 displays the Chomsky and Halle distinctive features in matrix form. Note that each speech sound can be described by the bundle of features listed beneath it. These feature bundles can be compared to determine how similar or dissimilar two sounds are in terms of features. The less features two sounds have in common the more dissimilar they are considered. This feature counting is used in the analysis of misarticulations using distinctive features.

Three of the Chomsky and Halle features are considered major class features as they differentiate among the major sound classes. These are consonantal, sonorant, and vocalic. The sonorant category differentiates between ''true'' consonants and vowels or vowel-like consonants (vowels, liquids, glides, and nasals). The consonantal feature differentiates between sounds made with obstruction in the vocal tract (stops, fricatives, affricates, nasals, and liquids) and those with little or no obstruction (vowels, glides, and also /h/). The vocalic feature is also based on degree of obstruction. Those with plus vocalic are made with no more obstruction than is associated with production of /i/. In addition, the folds must be positioned so that there is the possibility of spontaneous voicing (Edwards and Shriberg, 1983). Most of the plus vocalic sounds are vowels though liquids are also considered plus vocalic. The other features are considered nonmajor features. Gierut (1992) summarizes current research evaluating use of major versus nonmajor features in programming intervention (see Chapter 7).

McReynolds and Engmann (1975) describe Chomsky and Halle's features as operating on two levels: classificatory and phonetic. At the classificatory level the features are binary, ''they specify whether the segment (the consonant or vowel in an utterance) is within a feature category. Thus a segment may be classified as a member of a feature category, or as not a member of a feature category'' (p. 8).

At the phonetic level they describe features as functioning as properties or characteristics. McReynolds and Engmann state:

> In their phonetic function, features receive a physical interpretation. Instead of a binary specification, the description is multivalued on a physical and acoustical continuum. In particular, the degree to which a segment is characterized by the feature is specified. For example, a sound may be described as ''noncontinuant'' and ''moderately aspirated'' on the phonetic feature level. At this level, contextual variables are taken into account. (p. 80.)

The two levels are connected by phonological rules. These rules specify how the phono-logical representation will be produced at the phonetic level. Phonological rules will be discussed later in this chapter.

SINGH AND POLEN DISTINCTIVE FEATURE SYSTEM

Singh and Polen (1972) developed a simpler distinctive feature system that is more closely related to speech production and perception. Their system has only seven features and focuses on consonants. These features are also given a binary value but using numbers "1" and "0" rather than plus and minus.

1. Front/back. Front (0) consonants are those that are articulated on or in front of the alveolar ridge. Back (1) consonants are articulated posterior to the ridge. Front (0) consonants include /p/, /b/, /t/, /d/, /f/, /v/, /θ/, /ð/, /s/, /z/, /l/, /m/, and /n/.
2. Nonlabial/labial. Labial consonants are produced with the lips as the main place of artic-ulation. Nonlabial consonants are articulated without the lips. Labial (1) consonants include /p/, /b/, /m/, /f/, /v/, and /w/.
3. Nonsonorant/sonorant. The sonorant consonants are those that are articulated with an unrestricted airflow and spontaneous voicing. They include the liquids, glides, and nasals. Sonorant (1) consonants are /l/, /r/, /j/, /w/, /m/, /n/, and /ŋ/.
4. Nonnasal/nasal. Nasal consonants are those that are produced with nasal resonance. Nasal (1) consonants include /m/, /n/, and /ŋ/.
5. Stop/continuant. Stop consonants are those which are produced with an abrupt termi-nation of airflow while continuants have an airflow that is sustained. The continuants are the fricatives and approximants. The continuant (1) sounds are /f/, /v/, /θ/, /ð/, /s/, /z/, /ʃ/, /ʒ/, /h/, /j/, /r/, /l/, /w/, /m/, /n/, and /ŋ/.
6. Nonsibilant/sibilant. Sibilant sounds are those whose airflow creates high-frequency tur-bulence. Included in sibilant (1) sounds are /s/, /z/, /ʃ/, /tʃ/ and /dʒ/.
7. Voiceless/voiced. These features refer to the presence or absence of voicing during sound production. The voiced (1) sounds include /b/, /d/, /g/, /v/, /ð/, /z/, /ʒ/, /dʒ/, /m/, /n/, /ŋ/, /l/, /r/, /j/, and /w/.

Table 4.2 is a listing of the distinctive features in chart form from Singh and Polen (1972). Note that some of the feature values are in parentheses. This indicates that the feature is redundant for the consonant (e.g., all labial consonants must also be front consonants). The Singh and Polen system has been used in the analysis of misarticulations (Costello, 1975). It is a convenient system as it has few features and focuses on the consonants; however, one drawback of the system is that it does not distinguish between some sound classes (e.g., glides and liquids). Singh and Singh (1976) developed a revised feature system based on the same features but with finer definitions which successfully differentiate between glides and liquids. In this system /r/ is considered to have the labial feature which allows it to be differentiated from the /j/.

It should be noted that the features describe phonemes which means that the actual produc-tions may or may not include all of the features associated with any given speech sound. For example, a voiced stop in word-final position may be produced without voicing. Thus the feature associated with the stop at the phonological level is [+voice] but at the phonetic level the pro-duction is [−voice]. In distinctive feature analysis the examiner will want to compare the intended production with what is actually said to determine how they differ in features.

TABLE 4.2. Singh and Polen Distinctive Feature Matrix

0 / 1	Front / Back	Nonlabial / Labial	Nonsonorant / Sonorant	Nonnasal / Nasal	Stop / Continuant	Nonsibilant / Sibilant	Voiceless / Voiced
p	0	1	(0)	(0)	0	(0)	0
b	0	1	0	0	0	(0)	1
t	0	0	(0)	(0)	0	(0)	0
d	0	0	0	0	0	(0)	1
k	1	(0)	(0)	(0)	0	(0)	0
g	1	(0)	0	0	0	(0)	1
f	0	1	(0)	(0)	1	0	0
v	0	1	0	0	1	0	1
θ	0	0	(0)	(0)	1	0	0
ð	0	0	0	0	1	0	1
s	0	0	(0)	(0)	1	1	0
z	0	0	0	0	1	1	1
ʃ	1	(0)	(0)	(0)	1	1	0
tʃ	1	(0)	(0)	(0)	0	1	0
ʤ	1	(0)	0	0	0	1	1
j	1	(0)	1	0	(1)	(0)	(1)
r	1	(0)	1	0	(1)	(0)	(1)
l	0	0	1	0	(1)	(0)	(1)
w	1	1	1	0	(1)	(0)	(1)
m	0	1	1	1	(1)	(0)	(1)
n	0	(0)	1	1	(1)	(0)	(1)
h	1	(0)	(0)	(0)	1	0	(0)

NATURAL CLASSES

One of the values of distinctive features is their utility in identifying natural classes. Naturalness in phonology is discussed in Chapter 1. Here natural class refers to "a class of segment types which, in the feature system that is being used, can be defined with fewer features than any of its members" (Sommerstein, 1977, p. 97). For example, the three nasal consonants can be defined by one feature, [+nasal]. To identify any of the nasals separately would require more features. The /m/ would require [+labial, +nasal], /n/ would require [+coronal, +nasal] and / ŋ/ requires [−front, +nasal].

This descriptive ability of features is important as natural classes of sounds frequently undergo similar changes or act together in phonological processes (Schane, 1973, p. 33). Thus, with the help of distinctive features it may be possible to capture some generalities that occur in sound changes that would be otherwise missed. Features have also been used to differentiate phonetic inventories of phonologically disordered children into five characteristic types which may have future application in assessment and intervention (Dinnsen, Chin, Elbert, and Powell, 1990; see Chapter 6).

Some of the common natural classes using the Chomsky and Halle system include:

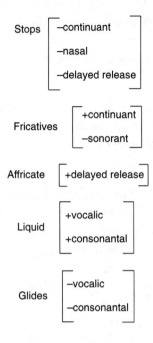

Stops
−continuant
−nasal
−delayed release

Fricatives
+continuant
−sonorant

Affricate
+delayed release

Liquid
+vocalic
+consonantal

Glides
−vocalic
−consonantal

DISTINCTIVE FEATURES AND STAGES OF DEVELOPMENT

Blache (1982) outlines six stages of distinctive feature acquisition. The work is based on Jakobson's model for phonological acquisition, developmental sound studies, and psychoacoustic research. At each stage, as more features are mastered, the child develops new phonemic contrasts. This follows Jakobson's principle of maximal contrast whereby "the grossest phonemic contrasts are learned before the more refined, more difficult tasks" (Blache, p. 114). Although no universal order of sound acquisition has been found, acquisition does follow a general trend. Blache identifies the following six stages of acquisition: (*a*) primitive, (*b*) vocalic, (*c*) stop-nasal, (*d*) semivowel, (*e*) continuant, and (*f*) the sibilant stage.

Primitive System

Between the end of the prelinguistic stage and 3 years of age, the child develops control of the nasal/non-nasal and the labial/lingual features. "At this stage, the child produces utterances of four types: a nasal, labial utterance (usually in the form of [m]), a nasal, lingual utterance (usually in the form of [n]), a non-nasal, labial utterance (usually in the form of [p]), and a non-nasal, lingual utterance (usually in the form of [t])" (Blache, 1982, p. 82).

Vocalic System

The development of the vowel system is completed by the end of the child's third year of life. The child initially learns to produce distinctions among high-front, low-front, high-back and low-back vowel utterances. Finer distinctions between the vowels are learned later.

Stop-Nasal System

The stop-nasal system is learned by 4 years of age. This stage results in finer distinctions of the nasal/nonnasal and the labial/lingual features. The stops and nasals are now distinguished by three places of articulation (lip, front of tongue, and back of tongue) and an additional manner (voiced versus voiceless). The result is a nine category consonantal system.

Semivowel System

Near the end of the fourth year the child will establish production of consonants with vowel-like characteristics. Like the stops and nasals, these semivowels are organized into a three-point place of articulation scheme (Blache, 1982).

Continuant System

The continuant system is based on control of duration. The child begins controlling this feature in his/her fifth year. The introduction of this feature greatly expands the child's sound system and presents a difficult task for the child. Whereas before there were only nine consonants (stop/nasal system), the child must now acquire sounds with the continuant feature that are also distinguished by voicing and place features.

Sibilant System

The sibilant system is developed when the child learns the strident/mellow feature. It is a refinement of the continuancy feature with strident sounds being continuants that are made with an unobstructed airflow striking the teeth. Mellow sounds are made with the airflow against the teeth being obstructed. The mellow sounds are the [θ] and [ð] and are established after 6 years of age. See Appendix 4.1, Exercise 4.1.

PHONOLOGICAL RULES

Phonological rules are used to describe sound changes. As descriptors they state three things. First, the rule specifies what segments are affected or changed. This represents the input for the rule. In child phonology, the input is often assumed to be the adult representation. Second, the rule tells us how the segment changes, what the child actually produces. Third, the rule describes the conditions under which the change occurs. Use of phonological rules provides the practitioner with a shorthand for describing sound changes that occur in speech. Edwards and Shriberg (1983) provide an excellent resource for rule writing as does Schane (1973). Some of the general aspects of rule writing follow.

Rules are written following the general form presented below:

$$A \rightarrow B \: / \: X \underline{\quad} Y$$

Using this format, (A) represents the adult form, which serves as input to the rule. The arrow means "changes to" or "becomes" and (B) indicates what is actually produced (surface form), the output of the rule. The (/) means "in the environment of" and the phonetic context is represented by the (X) and (Y). The blank (____) indicates where the segment that changes is located.

Word boundaries are indicated by using the (#) symbol or generic vowel symbols (V). A sound that changes word-initially, is indicated by #____. A word-final position is shown by ____# and intervocalic by V____V. Sometimes the context involves more than one word position. The following rule states that /s/ is changed to [t] in both word-initial and final positions.

$$s \rightarrow t \; / \; \#\rule{1cm}{0.4pt}$$
$$\rule{1cm}{0.4pt}\#$$

When a consonant is involved it is represented by a capital (C) or by a particular phone. Sometimes the consonants or vowels that make up the phonetic context represent a class of related segments. In such a case, features that define the class of segments are listed below the consonant or vowel symbol. An example from Schane (1973, p. 64) is a rule in French where a vowel is nasalized when it precedes a nasal consonant that ends a word.

$$V \longrightarrow [+ \text{nasal}] \; / \rule{1cm}{0.4pt} \begin{bmatrix} C \\ + \text{nasal} \end{bmatrix} \#$$

Segments that are optional are usually enclosed in parentheses. The following rule states that two or three member clusters are reduced to one member when in word-initial position.

$$CC(C) \rightarrow C \; / \; \#\rule{1cm}{0.4pt}$$

The rule points out that there must be at least two consonants as input but that there could be as many as three which are replaced by just one consonant. Some systems use subscripts and superscripts to indicate optional segments. The subscript is used to represent the minimum number of segments in the rule and the superscript the maximum. The rule above rewritten using this notation would be:

$$C^3 \rightarrow C \; / \; \#\rule{1cm}{0.4pt}$$

Brackets are used when two or more rules are collapsed to write a more general rule. Edwards and Shriberg (1983, p. 292) provide the following examples of two rules:

(a) l $\longrightarrow$ ø/ ____ # (b) r $\longrightarrow$ ø/ ____ C

These rules can be rewritten using brackets as one rule:

$$\begin{bmatrix} l \\ r \end{bmatrix} \longrightarrow ø/ \rule{1cm}{0.4pt} \begin{bmatrix} \# \\ C \end{bmatrix}$$

In using brackets the segments must be matched horizontally so that the context condition matches the sound change. In the above example it would be inappropriate for the (C) and (#) to be flip flopped as that would indicate that /r/ was deleted in word-final position and /l/ deleted when preceding a consonant (C).

Braces are used when the same sound change occurs but in different environments. For example, if /s/ is deleted in word final position or when preceding a consonant, the rule could be written as:

$$s \longrightarrow \emptyset / \underline{\quad} \left\{ \begin{matrix} \# \\ C \end{matrix} \right\}$$

DEGREES OF FORMALITY

Rules can be written with different degrees of formality. Informal notation typically uses phones (segments). Sometimes the segments are written with the input in slant brackets (/ /) and the output in square brackets ([ ]). This notation assumes that the input is the phoneme (phonological or underlying representation) and the child's output is the phonetic form (surface representation). For example, a rule that describes the /r/ changing to a [w] in word initial position would be written as:

$$/r/ \rightarrow [w] / \# \underline{\quad}$$

Formal notation in rule writing typically makes use of distinctive features. The input lists the relevant features to identify the segment(s) that changes. Features that are not relevant to whether the rule applies are omitted from the input. Features that are noted in the input but not the output have remained the same, thus the output lists only the feature(s) that change. The advantage of using features is that classes of sounds can be designated without having to list each of the individual sounds. This option is particularly important in describing child phonology, because rules typically apply to classes of sounds rather than to unrelated or individual segments. The following rule from Schane (1973, p. 63) demonstrates this advantage. It states that all obstruents are voiced in intervocalic position:

$$[-sonorant] \rightarrow [+voiced] / V \underline{\quad} V$$

Clinicians unfamiliar with distinctive features may prefer to use the abbreviated feature system of place-manner-voicing. The above rule using the abbreviated system would be written as:

$$\begin{bmatrix} \text{stops} \\ \text{fricatives} \\ \text{affricates} \end{bmatrix} \longrightarrow [+ \text{voice}] / \quad V \underline{\quad} V$$

CONTEXT SENSITIVE VERSUS CONTEXT FREE

Sometimes a phonetic condition statement in the rule is not necessary. It would depend upon whether the sound changes are context sensitive or context free. If a sound change occurs without regard to the phonetic context it is said to be context free. Context free phonological rules do not require a statement of the conditions under which the sound change occurs (as it always occurs). Thus the right half of the rule need not be written. As an example, for a child who substitutes [t] for /s/ in all phonetic environments, the rule would be written as:

$$/s/ \rightarrow [t] \text{ or } s \rightarrow t$$

When a sound change occurs only under specific phonetic conditions it is context sensitive. The context that triggers the sound change could be word position, place, manner or voicing characteristics of neighboring phones (vowels or consonants), or the influence of sounds in adjacent words. The following rule states that the sound change only occurs when the /s/ is in word-initial position and followed by a stop consonant.

$$/s/ \longrightarrow [t] \ / \ \# \ \underline{\hspace{1cm}} \begin{bmatrix} C \\ -\text{continuant} \end{bmatrix}$$

Context sensitive sound changes must include a condition statement describing the phonetic context in which the sound changes occur. Sometimes these sound changes do not occur with 100% consistency. Rules that describe sound changes that occur with less than 100% consistency are called optional rules. Rules that describe sound changes that occur with 100% consistency are called obligatory rules.

STATIC VERSUS DYNAMIC RULES

Another means of classifying rules is to divide them into static and dynamic categories. **Static** rules are those which describe sounds and sound sequences allowable in a phonological system and are sometimes referred to as phonotactic constraints. Elbert and Gierut (1986) describe three types of phonotactic constraints: positional, inventory, and sequential.

Static Rules

Positional. This type of constraint refers to sounds that function as phonemes but only in certain positions. Positional constraints limit where production occurs, thus they are context sensitive. For example, if fricatives occurred only in word-final position in a child's inventory, this would be a positional constraint.

Inventory. If a child has an inventory constraint it means that certain sounds never occur in the child's phonemic or phonetic inventories. Inventory constraints are context free meaning that the sounds do not occur in any phonetic environment. For example, a child who produces no lingual fricatives in any context would have an inventory constraint for lingual fricatives.

Sequential. Sequence constraints refer to the sequence of sounds that can occur in a child's phonological system. Elbert and Gierut (1986) give the example of a child who produces only singleton consonants. Such a child would have a sequence constraint that does not allow production of consonant clusters. Sequence constraints are similar to co-occurrence restrictions as described by Bleile (1991). Bleile describes these as restrictions that specify which combinations of units are permitted by the child's phonology. As an example he notes a common restriction in child phonology in which both consonants of a word must be made at the same place of articulation.

Dynamic Rules

The second category of phonological rules are called **dynamic** as they function to alter production by adding, deleting, or changing sounds. As described by Elbert and Gierut the dynamic rules function differently from static rules. "Dynamic rules make changes in the production of sounds in contrast to static rules that act as filters accepting or rejecting sounds or sound combinations" (p. 57).

Dynamic rules include rules that describe allophonic variations (sound changes that do not effect meaning) and neutralization rules. For the clinician the neutralization rules are of more interest as they may be useful in describing articulation errors. Neutralization rules occur when a child has knowledge of two different phonemes but loses this contrast in specific environments. For example, the child that contrasts stops and fricatives in word-final position but only uses stops in word-medial position. For such a child a contrast present in one context (stops versus fricatives) is lost in another position (stops used in place of fricatives in word-medial position). The contrast is said to have been neutralized in the medial context. Chapter 6 describes criteria for neutralization rules in more detail with respect to identifying phonological processes.

RULE ORDERING AND UNDERLYING REPRESENTATION

It is possible for more than one rule to apply to a sound change. In such cases the rules may be ordered, meaning that they must follow a set sequence for the output to occur. As described by Schane (1973, p. 86), "A crucial property of ordered rules is that they apply or fail to apply to the most recent representation—that is, the output of one rule becomes the input to the next rule."

To understand rule ordering, surface forms must be considered in conjunction with the rules. In the following we have two rules, (a) and (b). Rule (a) states that fricatives become stops when followed by stops. Rule (b) states that stops are deleted in word-final position.

Rule (a)

[+ continuant] ⟶ [−continuant] / # ___ [−continuant]
e.g., seat [ti]; see [si]

Rule (b)

[−continuant] ⟶ ø/ ___#
e.g., boat [bo]; gate [ge]

In this example Rule (a) must be applied prior to Rule (b). If Rule (b) had been applied first, the word-final stops would be deleted and there would be no context for fricatives to be changed to stops. Thus the following derivation for the word "seat."

Derivation with Rule (b) first:

/sit/	Underlying representation
si	Deletion of final stop—Rule (b)
[si]	Surface representation—Rule (a) not applied

Derivation with Rule (a) first:

/sit/	Underlying representation
tit	Fricative changes to stop
ti	Final stop is deleted
[ti]	Surface representation

Only by ordering the rules can the derivation explain the surface forms in the two examples. In this case, the surface form for "seat" is [ti] with one ordering and [si] for the other. The rule ordering has a definite impact upon the derivation.

The derived surface form is dependent on the rule ordering but what happens when the underlying representation does not match the adult form? For instance, if in the above example the child's underlying representation for "seat" had been /si/, how would this effect the phonological rules?

/si/	Underlying representation for "seat"
ti	Fricative changes to stop when followed by stop
[ti]	Surface representation

Again we see that the phonological rules required for the derivation have changed. In this case there was need for only one rule to account for the derivation. The point to be made is that the clinician must not only consider rule ordering but also the assumptions being made about the underlying representation. If those assumptions are in error then the derivational rules will also be wrong. As the underlying representation may be difficult or impossible to determine, many clinicians use rules only as descriptors of sound changes rather than as explanations of any mental operations used to derive the surface form. As a result, they make the assumption that the underlying representation is the same as the adult form and that may or may not be the case.

References

Berko J, Brown R. Psycholinguistic research methods. In Mussen PH, ed. Handbook of research methods in child development. New York: John Wiley and Sons, 1960.

Blache S. Minimal word-pairs and distinctive feature training. In Crary M, ed. Phonological intervention: concepts and procedures. San Diego: College-Hill Press, 1982:61–96.

Bleile K. Child phonology: a book of exercises for students. San Diego: Singular Publishing Group, 1991.

Chomsky N, Halle M. The sound pattern of English. New York: Harper and Row, 1968.

Costello J. Articulation instruction based on distinctive features theory. Language, Speech, and Hearing Services in Schools 1975;6(2):61–71.

Dinnsen D, Chin S, Elbert M, Powell T. Some constraints on functionally disordered phonologies: phonetic inventories and phonotactics. Journal of Speech and Hearing Research 1990;33:28–37.

Edwards ML, Shriberg LD. Phonology: applications in communicative disorders. San Diego: College-Hill Press, 1983.

Elbert M, Gierut J. Handbook of clinical phonology: approaches to assessment and treatment. Boston: College-Hill Publication, 1986.

Gierut J. The conditions and course of clinically induced phonological change. Journal of Speech and Hearing Research 1992;35:1049–1063.

Jakobson R, Fant G, Halle M. Preliminaries to speech analysis. Cambridge, MA: MIT Press, 1952.

Jakobson R, Halle M. Fundamentals of language. The Hague: Mouton, 1956.

McReynolds L, Engmann D. Distinctive feature analysis of misarticulations. Baltimore: University Park Press, 1975.

Schane S. Generative phonology. Englewood Cliffs, NJ: Prentice-Hall, 1973.

Singh S, Polen S. Use of a distinctive feature model in speech pathology. Acta Symbolica 1972;3:17–25.

Singh S, Singh K. Distinctive features: principles and practices. Baltimore: University Park Press, 1976.

Sommerstein A. Modern phonology. Baltimore: University Park Press, 1977.

Identifying Distinctive Features—
Exercises and Answers

EXERCISE 4.1

Vocalic (Voc)	Consonantal (Con)	Continuant (Cnt)
Sonorant (Son)	Nasal (Nas)	Delayed Release (Del)
Voiced (Voi)	Strident (Str)	Anterior (Ant)
Round (Rnd)	Coronal (Cor)	

Underline the positive Chomsky and Halle features associated with the following speech sounds.

Sound	Features										
1. [t]	Voc	Son	Con	Voi	Nas	Str	Cnt	Del	Cor	Rnd	Ant
2. [s]	Voc	Son	Con	Voi	Nas	Str	Cnt	Del	Cor	Rnd	Ant
3. [j]	Voc	Son	Con	Voi	Nas	Str	Cnt	Del	Cor	Rnd	Ant
4. [ʃ]	Voc	Son	Con	Voi	Nas	Str	Cnt	Del	Cor	Rnd	Ant
5. [m]	Voc	Son	Con	Voi	Nas	Str	Cnt	Del	Cor	Rnd	Ant
6. [tʃ]	Voc	Son	Con	Voi	Nas	Str	Cnt	Del	Cor	Rnd	Ant
7. [θ]	Voc	Son	Con	Voi	Nas	Str	Cnt	Del	Cor	Rnd	Ant
8. [l]	Voc	Son	Con	Voi	Nas	Str	Cnt	Del	Cor	Rnd	Ant
9. [z]	Voc	Son	Con	Voi	Nas	Str	Cnt	Del	Cor	Rnd	Ant
10. [b]	Voc	Son	Con	Voi	Nas	Str	Cnt	Del	Cor	Rnd	Ant
11. [dʒ]	Voc	Son	Con	Voi	Nas	Str	Cnt	Del	Cor	Rnd	Ant
12. [r]	Voc	Son	Con	Voi	Nas	Str	Cnt	Del	Cor	Rnd	Ant
13. [d]	Voc	Son	Con	Voi	Nas	Str	Cnt	Del	Cor	Rnd	Ant
14. [n]	Voc	Son	Con	Voi	Nas	Str	Cnt	Del	Cor	Rnd	Ant
15. [g]	Voc	Son	Con	Voi	Nas	Str	Cnt	Del	Cor	Rnd	Ant

EXERCISE 4.2

Vocalic (Voc)	Consonantal (Con)	Continuant (Cnt)
Sonorant (Son)	Nasal (Nas)	Delayed Release (Del)
Voiced (Voi)	Strident (Str)	Anterior (Ant)
Round (Rnd)	Coronal (Cor)	

The following are common substitutions seen in child phonology. Identify what features distinguish between the sounds.

Substitution	Different Features
1. t/s	
2. f/θ	
3. w/l	
4. d/g	
5. t/tʃ	
6. p/f	

EXERCISE 4.3

Vocalic (Voc)	Consonantal (Con)	Continuant (Cnt)
Sonorant (Son)	Nasal (Nas)	Delayed Release (Del)
Voiced (Voi)	Strident (Str)	Anterior (Ant)
Round (Rnd)	Coronal (Cor)	

The following are common substitutions seen in child phonology. Identify what features distinguish between the sounds.

Substitution	Different Features
1. d/ʤ	
2. v/θ	
3. w/r	
4. t/k	
5. f/s	
6. b/v	

ANSWERS TO EXERCISE 4.1

Vocalic (Voc)	Consonantal (Con)	Continuant (Cnt)
Sonorant (Son)	Nasal (Nas)	Delayed Release (Del)
Voiced (Voi)	Strident (Str)	Anterior (Ant)
Round (Rnd)	Coronal (Cor)	

Underline the positive Chomsky and Halle features associated with the following speech sounds.

Sound	Features						
1. [t]	Con	Cor	Ant				
2. [s]	Con	Str	Cnt	Cor	Ant		
3. [j]	Son	Voi	Cnt				
4. [ʃ]	Con	Str	Cnt	Cor			
5. [m]	Son	Con	Voi	Nas	Ant		
6. [ʧ]	Con	Str	Del	Cor			
7. [θ]	Con	Cnt	Cor	Ant			
8. [l]	Voc	Son	Con	Voi	Cnt	Cor	Ant
9. [z]	Con	Voi	Str	Cnt	Cor	Ant	
10. [b]	Con	Voi	Ant				
11. [ʤ]	Con	Voi	Str	Del	Cor		
12. [r]	Voc	Son	Con	Voi	Cnt	Cor	
13. [d]	Con	Voi	Cor	Ant			
14. [n]	Son	Con	Cor	Voi	Nas	Ant	
15. [g]	Con	Voi					

ANSWERS TO EXERCISE 4.2

Vocalic (Voc)	Consonantal (Con)	Continuant (Cnt)
Sonorant (Son)	Nasal (Nas)	Delayed Release (Del)
Voiced (Voi)	Strident (Str)	Anterior (Ant)
Round (Rnd)	Coronal (Cor)	

The following are common substitutions seen in child phonology. Identify what features distinguish between the sounds.

Substitution	Different Features
1. t/s	Continuant, Strident
2. f/θ	Coronal, Strident
3. w/l	Vocalic, Consonantal, Back, Round, Anterior, Coronal
4. d/g	Back, Anterior, Coronal
5. t/ʧ	Anterior, Delayed Release, Strident
6. p/f	Continuant, Strident

ANSWERS TO EXERCISE 4.3

Vocalic (Voc)	Consonantal (Con)	Continuant (Cnt)
Sonorant (Son)	Nasal (Nas)	Delayed Release (Del)
Voiced (Voi)	Strident (Str)	Anterior (Ant)
Round (Rnd)	Coronal (Cor)	

The following are common substitutions seen in child phonology. Identify what features distinguish between the sounds.

Substitution	Different Features
1. d/ʤ	Anterior, Delayed Release, Strident
2. v/θ	Coronal, Voice, Strident
3. w/r	Vocalic, Consonantal, Back, Round, Coronal
4. t/k	Back, Anterior, Coronal
5. f/s	Back, Coronal
6. b/v	Continuant, Strident

Writing Phonological Rules—
Exercises and Answers

EXERCISE 4.4

Using segments, write informal rules for the following sound changes.

1. t/s in word-initial position.

2. d/z in all word positions.

3. t/d and k/g in word-final position.

4. Deletion of /s/ in word-initial position.

5. w/r in word-initial clusters.

6. t/s in intervocalic position.

7. Clusters simplified to one member in all positions.

8. t/s in word-initial position preceding a stop consonant.

EXERCISE 4.5

Using features (Chomsky and Halle) write formal rules for the following sound changes.

1. d/z in word-final position.

2. f/θ in all positions.

3. p/f in word-initial singletons.

4. t/z in word-initial and final positions.

5. t/k in all positions.

ANSWERS TO EXERCISE 4.4

Using segments, write informal rules for the following sound changes.

1. t/s in word-initial position.
   /s/ → [t] / # _____
2. d/z in all word positions.
   /z/ → [d]
3. t/d and k/g in word-final position.

$$\begin{bmatrix} d \\ g \end{bmatrix} \rightarrow \begin{bmatrix} t \\ k \end{bmatrix} / \underline{} \#$$

4. Deletion of /s/ in word-initial position.
   /s/ → ø / # _____
5. w/r in word-initial clusters.
   /r/ → [w] / CC(C)_____
6. t/s in intervocalic position.
   /s/ → [t] / V___V
7. Clusters simplified to one member in all positions.
   C(C)(C) → C
8. t/s in word-initial position preceding a stop consonant.

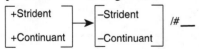

$$/s/ \rightarrow t / \# \underline{} \begin{bmatrix} C \\ Stop \end{bmatrix}$$

ANSWERS TO EXERCISE 4.5

Using features (Chomsky and Halle) write formal rules for the following sound changes.

1. d/z in word-final position.

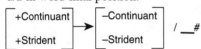

$$\begin{bmatrix} +Continuant \\ +Strident \end{bmatrix} \rightarrow \begin{bmatrix} -Continuant \\ -Strident \end{bmatrix} / \underline{}\#$$

2. f/θ in all positions.

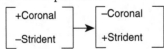

$$\begin{bmatrix} +Coronal \\ -Strident \end{bmatrix} \rightarrow \begin{bmatrix} -Coronal \\ +Strident \end{bmatrix}$$

3. p/f in word-initial singletons.

$$\begin{bmatrix} +Strident \\ +Continuant \end{bmatrix} \rightarrow \begin{bmatrix} -Strident \\ -Continuant \end{bmatrix} /\# \underline{}$$

4. t/z in word-initial and final positions.

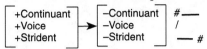

5. t/k in all positions.

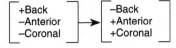

Phonological Processes

Chapter **5**

Robert J. Lowe

F<small>ROM A HISTORICAL</small> viewpoint, the study of speech sound development and sound errors has undergone a number of changes in emphasis, beginning with an interest in isolated segments and gradually changing to the current focus on how sounds function within a language. Several systems of analysis have been utilized, including error to target substitutions, place-manner-voicing descriptions, distinctive features, and phonological processes. Of these, phonological processes has surfaced as the preferred method for analyzing and describing patterns of sound errors.

Phonological processes, as described in Chapter 1, are systematic sound changes that affect a class of sounds or a sound sequence (Edwards and Shriberg, 1983). As defined by Hodson and Paden (1983, p. 102), they are a ''regularly occurring deviation from standard adult speech patterns; may occur across a class of sounds, a syllable shape, or syllable sequence.'' In short, processes are descriptions of regularly occurring patterns observed in child speech which operate to simplify adult targets.

How phonological processes are used depends largely on the user's background. Theorists when referring to a child using processes generally assume that the phonological level of representation is the same as the adult target form and that the processes are being applied to result in the observed surface form. Clinicians, however, tend to use phonological processes in a descriptive sense. As noted by Bernthal and Bankson (1988, p. 115), ''references to 'phonological processes' are generally a descriptive convenience rather than an attempt to reflect the child's mental activity.'' In other words, the processes are used to describe patterns of sound change.

As we will discover in Chapters 6 and 7, the underlying representation may be very important and probably should be taken into consideration when evaluating a phonological system and planning intervention. Elbert and Gierut (1986), for example, argue that the extent of phonological knowledge may influence target selection and programming for the remediation of phonological disorders. Gierut and Dinnsen (1986) present evidence that children having similar surface patterns may have very different productive knowledge of the sounds in error, which will have implications for intervention. Before the issue of underlying representation is tackled, however, the reader must have a clear understanding of phonological processes. This chapter will provide a detailed description of phonological processes observed in both normal and phonologically disabled children.

CRITERIA FOR PROCESSES

The identification of processes is not a straightforward procedure. Different criteria have been suggested but no uniform guidelines adopted by the profession. McReynolds and Elbert (1981) demonstrated the effects of applying different criteria, noting that the application of criteria significantly changes what sound patterns qualify as processes. In their report they suggested that a particular sound change should have a possibility of occurring four times and be used at least 20% of the time to qualify as a process. Most other studies only stipulate that a particular sound change occur and make no demands on its frequency.

Test instruments such as the ALPHA (Lowe, 1986) rely on normative data to determine if a process should be targeted for intervention but, other than meeting the pattern of sound change described by the process description, no quantitative criteria are used. Thus, if a particular sound change occurs even once, a phonological process is identified.

Some minimal criteria should be set for the identification of phonological processes. Returning to our earlier definition, we said that a process was a sound change that affected a class of sounds or a sound sequence. One criteria that should be considered then is the number of sounds affected. The definition indicates that a class of sounds is affected. What constitutes a class? If a child only has isolated errors (residual errors) would they qualify as processes? For example, a child who consistently uses a [t] for the /s/ phoneme might be described as having a stopping process. Yet if the /s/ were the only fricative that changed, the sound change would not represent a class of sounds. Is it a process or not?

The answer depends on the definition of class. A class can be defined as a natural grouping of sounds that share a common dimension. All fricatives, for example, represent a class of sounds. The grouping could be narrowed by adding qualifiers. For example, all voiced fricatives would represent a smaller grouping than the class of all fricatives. Distinctive features have been used for determining natural classes, those that share common features. Generally, it will take more features to describe a smaller class. It is suggested that sound changes affect classes of sounds rather than individual segments or unrelated segments because the rules required to affect isolated sounds would involve more features and thus be more complex (Sloat, Taylor, and Hoard, 1978). In any case the smallest grouping possible would have two members that share some dimension. Given this criteria, the identification of a phonological process would require that at least two sounds (having a common dimension) be changed in a similar manner.

The second half of the process definition stipulates changes in sound sequences. A sound sequence refers to the arrangement of consonants and vowels within syllable and word shapes. Examples would include deletions of initial or final consonants, additions of sounds (epenthesis), or rearrangements of sounds (metathesis). Although this part of the process definition appears clear, we are again left with the question of how often must a particular sound change occur before it qualifies as a phonological process? If the change in sequence occurs one time is it a process? Perhaps the answer lies in the idea that processes are used to describe sound change patterns. Patterns are regularly occurring events. If a sound sequence change only occurs one time this would hardly qualify as a pattern. A minimal criteria then for changes in sound sequences would be at least two occurrences of the particular sound change before it could qualify as a process.

COMMON PHONOLOGICAL PROCESSES

Although more than 40 different processes have been identified as occurring in child phonology, only a handful occur with any frequency. Those processes that commonly occur developmentally in normal children across languages are called natural processes. Processes that never occur, or occur only rarely, in normal child phonology are called unusual or idiosyncratic processes (Stoel-Gammon and Dunn, 1985).

Phonological processes are categorized into three groupings: syllable structure, substitution, and assimilatory. Later in this section is a summary of definitions and some developmental information. The common processes are also summarized in Table 5.1. Much of the developmental information for the descriptions comes from Ingram (1989) and two studies, Prater and Swift (1982) and Haelsig and Madison (1986). The Prater and Swift study divided 60 children between the ages of 21 and 48 months into six MLU groups to examine the use of various phonological processes across MLU. Haelsig and Madison studied the phonological processes exhibited by 3-, 4-, and 5-year-old children (10 in each group).

Syllable Structure Processes

Syllable structure processes describe sound changes that affect the syllable structure of the child's production of an adult target word. These processes are most frequently seen in younger children with MLUs between 1 and 4 morphemes (Prater and Swift, 1982).

Deletion of Final Consonant (DFC)

As with most processes, the name describes the sound change. Deletion of final consonants involves the deletion of a final consonant or final consonant cluster so the final form of the word ends with a vowel. It is common in children between the ages of 1;6 and 3;0 but rare beyond 3 years of age (Ingram, 1989). Examples:

$$gate \rightarrow [ge]$$
$$most \rightarrow [mo]$$

Cluster Reduction (CR)

Cluster reduction can be subdivided into Total, Partial, and Substitution. Total Cluster Reduction (TCR) involves the deletion of all members of the cluster. Partial Cluster Reduction (PCR) occurs when some of the cluster members are deleted but others remain. Cluster Substitution (CS) occurs when there is a substitution of a cluster member. Cluster substitution is sometimes treated as a form of partial cluster reduction. The member that is typically deleted or substituted tends to be the marked member of the cluster. Unmarked cluster members can be deleted or substituted but this is rare. Examples:

Target	Form	Cluster Reduction
tree	[i]	TCR
tree	[ti]	PCR
tree	[twi]	CS

Dyson and Paden (1983) report that in normally developing children, cluster reduction is most common for clusters containing /s/ and /z/, liquid segments, or strident segments. Haelsig and Madison (1986) report 7% occurrence of cluster reduction in the total responses of ten 5-year-old children. Applying the 20% criteria, the process of cluster reduction is not likely to occur beyond 4 years of age, but in comparison to most natural processes it is suppressed late in phonological development.

Clusters tend to develop following four stages. Using information from the work of Greenlee (1974), Ingram (1989) reports these stages using the target word "play":

TABLE 5.1. Definitions of Some Common Phonological Processes

Process	Description	Example
Consonant Deletion	Deletion of singleton consonant in word-initial or -final position	boat → [ot] or [bo]
Cluster Reduction	Consonant clusters are reduced by one or more members	street → [trit], [tit], or [it]
Syllable Deletion	A polysyllabic word is reduced by one or more syllables; typically the weak syllable is deleted	potato → [tedo]
Stopping	A fricative or affricate is replaced by a stop; some classification systems also include glides and liquids being replaced by stops	soap → [top]
Stridency Deletion	The deletion of a strident consonant either through consonant deletion or substitution of a nonstrident consonant	sew → [o] or [to]
Fronting	A palatal or velar is replaced with a front consonant (typically an alveolar)	goat → [dot]
Gliding	A liquid is replaced with a glide	rake → [wek]
Alveolarization	A labial or interdental is replaced by an alveolar consonant	thief → [sif]
Labialization	A labial consonant substitutes for an alveolar or interdental consonant; some classifications include all lingual consonants	they → [ve]
Deaffrication	A fricative replaces an affricate; some classifications include stops replacing the affricate as well	cheese → [siz]
Vocalization	A liquid is replaced by a vowel; this typically occurs in postvocalic position	beater → [bido]
Prevocalic Voicing	Voiceless singletons in prevocalic position are replaced with a voiced consonant	cake → [gek], [det]
Postvocalic Devoicing	Voiced consonants in postvocalic positions are replaced with voiceless consonant	made → [met] or [mep]

Stage 1   Deletion of entire cluster [ey]
Stage 2   Reduction of cluster to one member [pey]
Stage 3   Use of cluster with substitution for one of the members [pwey]
Stage 4   Correct articulation [pley]

Weak Syllable Deletion (WSD)

This process, also called unstressed syllable deletion or just syllable reduction, describes the deletion of one or more syllables from a polysyllabic word. Typically the syllable with the least stress is deleted in the production. The process seldom occurs in children with normally developing sound systems after age 3. Haelsig and Madison (1986) did observe its occurrence in the speech of 4½- and 5-year-old children, but if a criterion of 20% occurrence were applied the sound changes would not qualify as processes. Examples:

telephone → *[tɛfon]*
tomato → *[medo]*

Reduplication (Rd)

Reduplication (also called Doubling) occurs when a child repeats a syllable of a word making it into a polysyllabic form. Most classification systems categorize reduplication as a syllable structure process, but some consider it an assimilatory process. Reduplication may be total or partial. Total reduplication occurs when all of a syllable is repeated. Partial reduplication occurs when only part of the syllable is repeated. Examples:

bottle → *[ba ba]*
bottle → *[ba da]*

A special form of partial reduplication is the diminutive in which the final vowel is produced as an [i]. Stoel-Gammon and Dunn (1985) give this sound change status as a separate process called Diminutization and describe it as the addition of [i], or sometimes [Ci] to a target form. Examples:

blanket → *[babi]*
egg → *[ɛgi]*

Ingram (1989) describes reduplication as an early process of acquisition associated with the first 50 words. However, Lleo (1990) reports that reduplication may disappear after the 50 word stage but reappear when the child begins production of trisyllables at or about 3 years of age. As the child passes from bisyllable production to trisyllables he/she will reduplicate one of the syllables so a three syllable pattern is produced. At this point the child appears more concerned about producing the three syllables than about the correctness of the segments. Lleo suggests that use of reduplication simplifies the mental representation and storage so more complex patterns (trisyllables) can be produced.

Epenthesis (Epn)

Khan (1985) describes epenthesis as a process that results in the insertion of a schwa between two consonants. She also points out that epenthesis might involve insertion of a consonant but the most common occurrence is a vowel between two consonants. Leonard (1985) categorizes the addition of consonants to adult forms as an unusual or idiosyncratic process. Examples:

spoon → [səpun]
plate → [pəlet]

Khan notes that the insertion of a vowel between two consonants functions to simplify the cluster but does not include the process under cluster reduction as all members of the cluster are retained. Shriberg and Kwiatkowski (1980) state that vowel insertion occurs during stage 3 of cluster development at or about 2½ years of age when it will alternate with correct articulation of the cluster.

Stoel-Gammon and Dunn (1985) note that vowels also can be added in word-final position and that this seems to occur as the first stage of a voicing contrast between stops in that position. They describe the progression of the word bead; "*bead* may first be pronounced [bit], then [bi:t] with vowel lengthening, then [bi:də], and finally [bi:d]" (p. 39).

SUBSTITUTION PROCESSES

Substitution processes involve sound changes whereby one sound class replaces another class of sounds. The names of these processes typically reflect the replacing sound class. Thus, in stopping we find sounds are replaced with stops, and in fronting we find that the replacing sounds are made more anterior than the adult target.

Stopping (St)

One of the most common substitution processes is that of stopping. Perhaps the hardest choice to be made concerning stopping is what definition to use. Ingram (1989) describes stopping as the replacement of fricatives or affricates with stop consonants. Dyson and Paden (1983) define stopping as the replacement of a continuant phoneme by a stop, affricate, or nasal, and/or the replacement of an affricate by a stop or nasal. Their definition reflects the identification of stops, affricates, and nasals as noncontinuant by Chomsky and Halle (1968). Hodson and Paden (1983) describe stopping as primarily affecting fricatives, but also note that sonorants (nasals, liquids, and glides) can be stopped. Stoel-Gammon and Dunn (1985) would list glides being stopped as an idiosyncratic process.

The most frequently seen form of stopping is the replacement of fricatives and affricates with stops and is the preferred definition for this text. Other forms of stopping (those affecting glides, liquids, and nasals) will be considered as special cases of stopping and treated separately.

Stopping is more often seen on prevocalic consonants than postvocalic (Dyson and Paden, 1983). It appears to operate most effectively in normally developing children with MLUs between 1 and 4.99 (Prater and Swift, 1982). The replacing stops are typically homorganic to the sounds substituted though this is not always the case. Examples:

soap → [top]
jeep → [dip]

Stridency Deletion (StD)

A process that is closely associated with stopping is stridency deletion. This process occurs when a strident sound [f, v, s, z, ʃ, ʒ, tʃ, ʤ] is either deleted or replaced with a nonstrident sound. An easy manner in which to remember which sounds are strident is the following—strident sounds are all affricates and fricatives except "th." The "th" represents the /θ/, /ð/ and the /h/.

Stridency deletion typically occurs through stopping though it is possible for stopping to occur without stridency deletion (e.g., stop replacing /θ/). Both stopping and stridency deletion are very common in the speech patterns of phonologically disordered children. Hodson and Paden (1983) note that the most unintelligible children omit the strident sound while children with less severe problems use nonstrident substitutes. Examples:

soap → [op] or [top]

Deaffrication (DeA)

This process involves the substitution of a fricative for an affricate. The fricative may or may not be homorganic (same place) to the affricate. There appears to be some confusion concerning the status of deaffrication. Some authors list it as a common process and others as an idiosyncratic process. Roberts, Burchinal, and Footo (1990) indicate that deaffrication occurs more frequently than some common processes, so for this text it will be considered a common phonological process. Deaffrication is usually suppressed prior to 4 years of age. Example:

jeep → [zip]
cheese → [ʃiz]

Fronting (Fr)

Two forms of fronting have been identified in the research literature: velar and palatal. Velar fronting involves the replacement of a velar consonant [k, g, ŋ] by a more anterior consonant (typically alveolar). Palatal fronting (sometimes called depalatalization) is the replacement of a palatal by a sound made farther forward in the mouth (Lowe, Knutson, and Monson, 1985). Grunwell (1987) indicates that occasionally children will replace velars with palatals, and that this, too, is a form of fronting. Fronting occurs more often in word-initial position than in word-final position.

Stoel-Gammon and Dunn (1985) stipulate that depalatalization is the substitution of an alveolar fricative for a palatal fricative or an alveolar affricate for a palatal affricate. Khan (1985) makes a similar distinction for palatal fronting, indicating that this results in the forward production of palatal consonants. The examples given do not list [t] or [d] as possible substitutions. The replacement of a palatal affricate or fricative with an alveolar stop is called stopping in their systems. For this text the more general of the definitions will be used. Palatal fronting will include sound changes to stops as long as they are made anterior to the palatals.

Lowe, Knutson, and Monson (1986) screened 1048 children between the ages of 31 and 54 months for the presence of fronting. They observed fronting in 6% of the preschoolers, with velar fronting occurring more frequently than palatal fronting. Fronting rarely occurred after the age of 42 months. Examples:

cake→ [tek]
shoe → [su]

Gliding (Gl)

The replacement of liquids by glides is called gliding. Gliding is most commonly seen in 3- and 3½-year old children. Haelsig and Madison (1986) observed gliding in older children (4½- and 5-year-olds) but not at a frequency high enough to qualify as a process. There is a greater incidence of gliding for prevocalic /r/ than for /l/ (Dyson and Paden, 1983). Stoel-Gammon and Dunn (1985) indicate that substitution patterns for the /l/ may sometimes be controlled by the following vowel. The /l/ is substituted by [j] before front vowels and by [w] elsewhere. The most common substitute for /r/ is the [w].

Gliding is a common process in the speech of phonologically disordered children. Hodson and Paden (1981) list it as one of the most common processes observed in the speech of unintelligible children. The /l/ appears to develop first followed by suppression of gliding for the /r/. Examples:

red → [wɛd]
leaf → [jif] or [wif]

Vocalization (Vc)

Vocalization or vowelization affects syllabic consonants. In vocalization a full vowel is substituted for syllabic liquids or nasals. The typical vowel substitutions are [o], [ʊ] and [ə]. Stoel-Gammon and Dunn (1985) note that vocalization can also affect nonsyllabic consonants and list rhotic diphthongs as examples.

Vocalization was the most frequently occurring substitution process in the Prater and Swift (1982) study of process development. They noted that the process was used very actively when MLU was less than five morphemes, but some use of vocalization was still observed in Group 6 which had an upper MLU of 6.99 morphemes. Examples:

paper → [pepə]
bottle → [bado]

ASSIMILATORY PROCESSES

Assimilation is the process in which a sound becomes similar to (or is influenced by) another sound in the word (Ingram, 1989, p. 34). Assimilation can be total or partial. Total assimilation means that after the sound change, the sound that changes and the sound that influenced the change are the same. A partial assimilation occurs when the sound change results in the two sounds being more similar but not the same. Assimilation can be to voicing, place, manner, or a combination of these features, but usually affects the place of articulation. Assimilation can be between consonants or between a consonant and a vowel.

Assimilation can also be categorized as contiguous or noncontiguous. Contiguous means that the sound that changes and the one that influences the change are adjacent to one another. Noncontiguous assimilation occurs when there is at least one segment separating the sound that changes and the influencing segment. Noncontiguous consonant assimilation is sometimes given the special name of consonant harmony and Bernthal and Bankson (1989) equate it with partial reduplication.

Another dimension of assimilation is direction. Assimilation can be progressive (affected segment follows the one that influences it) or regressive (affected segment precedes the one that influences it). In English, most assimilation is regressive.

Grunwell (1986, p. 215) notes that the assimilation process causes a structural simplification in that (a) it results in a phonetically simpler sequence of consonants and (b) the harmonized target consonants are usually found to occur in other contexts. In other words, if it were not for the presence of the influencing segment, the sound change may not have occurred and the sound probably does occur correctly in other contexts.

Vihman (1978) comments that consonant harmony is common in child phonology. She suggests that consonant harmony functions to (a) provide a source of substitutions for sounds the child cannot pronounce and (b) allow the child to focus on new segments or extra syllables by reducing the overall complexity of the word. In support of this Leonard, Miller, and Brown (1980) reported on the speech patterns of eight language disordered children noting that assimilation typically affected consonants not in the children's productive repertoires.

Velar Assimilation (VeA)

Velar assimilation (back assimilation) results when an alveolar sound changes to become more like a velar consonant. Most velar assimilation is noncontiguous and regressive. The example below shows potential velar assimilation. To verify assimilation, evidence is required to indicate that the sound change occurs only in the presence of a velar consonant (e.g., correct production of /t/ in a word lacking the velar: tea → [ti]). The same condition of context as specified here holds for the other forms of assimilation. Example:

take → [kek]

Labial Assimilation (LbA)

Labial assimilation occurs when a nonlabial consonant is replaced by a labial consonant in a context containing a labial consonant. The most common form occurs when alveolars change to labials. This assimilation also is typically noncontiguous and regressive, though progressive forms have been observed. Labial assimilation requires the presence of a labial consonant in the adult form. Typically a noncontiguous alveolar consonant changes to become more like a following labial consonant. This process was observed to occur in all six MLU groups in the Prater and Swift (1982) study. This would reflect an age range from 1–4 years. Examples:

knife → [maɪp]
bone → [bom]

Nasal Assimilation (NsA)

Stoel-Gammon and Dunn (1985, p. 41) describe this process as the "assimilation of a nonnasal to a nasal consonant; place of articulation of the affected consonant may also be assimilated." Examples:

gun → *[nʌn]*
candy → *[næni]*

Prevocalic Voicing (PrV)

Ingram (1981) describes this process as the change of a voiceless obstruent (fricative, affricate, or stop) into a voiced one when preceding a vowel within the same syllable. Prater and Swift (1982) report that prevocalic voicing was used primarily by subjects with MLUs of less than four morphemes (under 3 years of age). Examples:

take → *[dek]*
pen → *[bɛn]*

Final Consonant Devoicing (DeV)

This process, also called devoicing, involves the devoicing of a voiced obstruent when it occurs at the end of a syllable. Ingram (1989) indicates that the assimilation is to the silence following the end of the word. The devoicing, however, is as likely due to the complex of aerodynamic conditions that exist in the production of word-final obstruents. Examples:

made → *[met]*
dad → *[dæt]*

Ingram (1989) adapted data from Velten (1943) to derive the following stages for the suppression or final consonant devoicing:

Stage 1   Devoicing of final consonant.
Stage 2   Lengthening of vowel before voiced consonants and devoicing of those voiced consonants.
Stage 3   Loss of the process of final consonant devoicing.

CO-OCCURRENCE OF PROCESSES

It is possible for more than one process to occur in a child's production. The processes may be applied to different positions in the same word or to the same sound change. This co-occurrence is very probable in cases of stopping and stridency deletion and in fronting of palatals as seen in these examples:

Target Form	Potential Processes
1. same → [dem]	stopping, stridency deletion, prevocalic voicing
2. shoe → [to]	stopping, fronting, stridency deletion

In some instances processes may be applied in an ordered sequence (as are phonological rules). Following is a derivation of the word ''soap'' as influenced by the processes of labial assimilation and deletion of final consonant.

Derivation A: Labial assimilation precedes final consonant deletion.

/sop/	Underlying representation
pop	Labial assimilation
po	Final consonant deletion
[po]	Surface form

Derivation B: Final consonant deletion precedes labial assimilation.

/sop/   Underlying representation
so   Final consonant deletion
[so]   Surface form

Note that two different forms result depending on the order of process application. Rule ordering should always be considered when the clinician comes across patterns that are inconsistent.

OVERVIEW OF COMMON PROCESSES AND DEVELOPMENT

In general, the research on the normal use and suppression of phonological processes indicates that most children, regardless of the language being learned, use the common processes early in their development of the sound system. The rate at which processes are suppressed varies between children but the greatest rate of process suppression occurs between 2½ and 4 years of age. Roberts, Burchinal, and Footo (1990) note that the most commonly occurring processes (children between 2½- and 4-years-old) are deletion of final consonants, cluster reduction, fronting, stopping, and liquid gliding.

Dyson and Paden (1983) studied five processes in 40 normally developing 2-year-olds over a 7 month period. They noted that gliding was most frequently used, followed by cluster reduction, fronting, stopping, and final consonant deletion. Gliding was more common on /r/ than on the /l/, and fronting of palatals more frequent than that of velars. Stopping of liquids occurred almost as frequently as stopping of stridents, and final consonant deletion was most apt to occur with nasals and stridents.

In children between 4 and 5 years of age, Hodson and Paden (1981) noted little use of phonological processes that have a significant effect on intelligibility. They observed devoicing of final obstruents, production of anterior strident phonemes to replace nonstrident interdentals, liquid deviations, tongue protrusions, depalatalization, nasal assimilation, labial assimilation, velar assimilation, and metathesis.

Norms from the ALPHA (Lowe, 1986) indicate that sound changes associated with stridency deletion, stopping, gliding, vocalization, and cluster reduction still occur in some children between 6 and 7 years of age. In this sampling, one instance of a sound change constituted a process. Grunwell (1987) provides a useful profile for phonological development in Table 5.2. See Exercises 5.1–5.4 in Appendix 5.1.

IDENTIFYING ASSIMILATION PROCESSES

Assimilation processes occur when one sound changes to become more like another sound in the same word. It is easy to confuse assimilation processes with other common processes. For example, if fronting occurs in the word "gate" the resulting surface form would be [det]. This might also be identified as assimilation to word final /t/, an alveolar assimilation. (Remember assimilation can be to place, manner, voicing, or a combination of these.) To ascertain whether the sound change is due to assimilation or to fronting, other sound changes in the child's speech sample must be examined.

TABLE 5.2. Profile of Phonological Development

Stage	Consonant inventory	Phonological processes	
Stage I (0;9–1;6)	LABIAL LINGUAL NASAL PLOSIVE FRICATIVE APPROXIMANT	*First Words* tend to show: —individual variation in consonants used; —phonetic variability in pronunciations; —all simplifying processes applicable.	
Stage II (1;6–2;0)	m n p b t d w	Reduplication Consonant Harmony FINAL CONSONANT DELETION CLUSTER REDUCTION	FRONTING of velars STOPPING GLIDING /r/ → [w] CONTEXT SENSITIVE VOICING
Stage III (2;0–2;6)	m n (ŋ) p b t d (k g) w h	Final Consonant Deletion CLUSTER REDUCTION	(FRONTING of velars) STOPPING GLIDING /r/ → [w] CONTEXT SENSITIVE VOICING
Stage IV (2;6–3;0)	m n ŋ p b t d k g	Final Consonant Deletion CLUSTER REDUCTION	STOPPING /v ð z tʃ dʒ/ /θ/ → [f] FRONTING /ʃ/ → [s] GLIDING /r/ → [w] Context Sensitive Voicing
Stage V (3;0–3;6)	f s j h w (l)	Clusters appear: obs. + approx. used; /s/ clusters may occur	STOPPING /v ð/ (/z/) /θ/ → [f] FRONTING of /tʃ dʒ ʃ/ GLIDING /r/ → [w]
Stage VI (4;0–4;6) (3;6–4;0)	ŋ m t d tʃ dʒ k g p b s z ʃ h f v l (r) j w	Clusters established: obs. + approx.: approx. 'immature' /s/ clusters: /s/ → FRICATIVE obs. + approx. acceptable /s/ clusters: /s/ → type FRICATIVE	/θ/ → [f] /ð/ → [d] or [v] (PALATALISATION of /tʃ dʒ ʃ/) GLIDING /r/ → [w]
Stage VII (4;6 <)	m n ʲ ŋ p b t d tʃ dʒ k g f v θ ð s z ʃ ʒ h w l r j	(/θ/ → [f]) (/ð/ → [d] or [v]) (/r/ → [w] or [ʊ])	

Assimilation is present if the sound change occurs only in environments where there is an influencing sound. In the previous example, we would examine the child's speech sample for other cases of fronting. If we find that fronting occurs regardless of the phonetic context of the words then the sound change probably reflects the fronting process. However, if the sound change only occurs in the presence of alveolar or anterior consonants then the process is probably a form of assimilation.

Comparing minimal pair words where one changes and the other doesn't provides evidence that the segment that distinguishes the pair has an influence on the sound change. Try Exercise 5.5 in Appendix 5.2.

IDIOSYNCRATIC/UNUSUAL PROCESSES

There has been some question about the appropriateness of the label of natural processes (Fey, 1985). Many of the processes described in the speech of children with phonological disorders do not qualify as ''natural.'' Stoel-Gammon and Dunn (1985, pp. 116–117) refer to these unusual processes as idiosyncratic processes and define them as error patterns that have never been documented in normal children or that occur infrequently in the normal population. Examples of idiosyncratic processes are backing, where a velar consonant substitutes for a more anterior consonant, and deletion of initial consonant.

How uncommon are the idiosyncratic processes? Little is known about frequency of occurrence, but by definition it is thought that these processes occur only rarely. Roberts, Burchinal, and Footo (1990), however, point out that for some of their normally developing subjects (145 subjects between the ages of 2½ and 8 years), the unusual processes (e.g., deletion of medial consonant and deaffrication) were more common than some of the processes labeled common (reduplication and syllable deletion). Part of the confusion may be in the categorizing of the processes. For example, Roberts, Burchinal, and Footo (1990) categorize deaffrication as an unusual process, but Dodd and Iacano (1989) list it as a developmental process. Judging from the Roberts, Burchinal, and Footo (1990) study, categorization as a developmental process may be more appropriate.

Leonard (1985, p. 4) describes some of the characteristics of unusual sound changes:

> Including (a) cases where a presumably later-developing sound replaces a presumably earlier-developing sound, (b) cases where the child's production constitutes an addition to the adult surface form, (c) cases where the child shows systematic use of a sound not present in the ambient language or use of a suprasegmental feature in a manner not seen in that language, and (d) cases where the child shows systematic use of a sound not seen in any natural language.

To these characteristics we can add the counterfeature to what defines a natural process or sound change, namely, cases where the sound change is rarely seen in any natural language.

Edwards (1992) points out there may be some clinical value to differentiating between normal and idiosyncratic processes. Some evidence for this clinical application is found in the research literature. Dodd, Hambly, and Leahy (1989) compared groups of children with only developmental processes with children who used both unusual and developmental processes. The results showed that the groups varied in two ways. (*a*) The group having only developmental processes pronounced words in the same way in imitation, picture naming, and spontaneous naming tasks. The group with unusual patterns made the fewest errors in imitation, more with picture naming, and the most errors occurred in spontaneous speech. (*b*) When given a forced-choice task of choosing phonologically legal nonsense words (e.g., thripi) or illegal words (thlipi) as names for animals, the group using unusual processes showed no preference. The group using only developmental processes preferred the phonologically legal names. This suggests a difference in the underlying phonological knowledge of the two groups.

Another difference between children who use developmental processes versus those using unusual or idiosyncratic processes is that children showing unusual processes may be more resistant to change. Leonard (1973) suggested that the speech of children using deviant processes may be more resistant to change without direct intervention. Leahy and Dodd (1987) observed that while the phonological systems of normal children improve steadily over time, systems of disordered children who exhibit unusual processes show little change in the number and types of errors made. A list of unusual processes and their definitions is provided in Table 5.3.

TABLE 5.3.   Unusual/Idiosyncratic Phonological Processes

Process	Definition
[1]Atypical Cluster Reduction ACR	Deletion of the member that is usually retained Example: play → [le]
[2]Initial Consonant Deletion ICD	The deletion of word-initial consonant or cluster so that the initial sound is a vowel Example: shoe → [u], star → [ar]
[2]Medial Consonant Deletion MCD	The deletion of intervocalic consonants Example: beetle → [bio]
[2]Backing of Stops BkS	The replacement of front consonants by phonemes made posterior to the target phonemes (typically velars) Example: toe → [ko]
[3]Apicalization Apl	A labial is replaced by an apical (tongue tip) consonant Example: bow → [do]
[1]Glottal Replacement Glt	Substitution of a glottal stop for a consonant usually in medial or final position Example: bat → [bæʔ]
[2]Backing of Fricatives BkF	The replacement of fricatives with fricatives that are made in a more posterior position Example: suit → [ʃut]
[2]Medial Consonant Substitutions MCS	The replacement of intervocalic consonants with one or more phonemes Example: butter → [bʌja]
[2]Denasalization DeN	The substitution of nasal consonants by a homorganic, nonnasal Example: no → [do]
[2]Devoicing of Stops DeVl	Replacement of a voiced stop with a voiceless phoneme (usually a stop) in word-initial position Example: daddy → [tædi]
[1]Fricatives Replacing Stops FRS	Substitution of a fricative consonant for a stop consonant Example: bat → [bæs]
[1]Stops Replacing Glides SRG	Substitution of a stop consonant for a glide Example: yellow → [dɛlo]
[3]Metathesis Met	The reversal of position of two sounds; the sounds may or may not be adjacent Example: most → [mots]
[4]Migration Mgr	The movement of a sound from one position in a word to another position Example: soap → [ops]
[2]Sound Preference Substitutions SPS	The replacement of groups of consonants by one or two particular consonants Example: /s/, /z/, /ʃ/, /tʃ/, /dʒ/ → [t]

[1]From Stoel-Gammon C, Dunn C. Normal and disordered phonology in children. Baltimore: University Park Press, 1985. Copyright 1985 by University Park Press.
[2]Dodd R, Iacano T. Phonological disorders in children: changes in phonological process use during treatment. British Journal of Disorders of Communication 1989; 24:342.
[3]Roberts J, Burchinal M, Footo M. Phonological process decline from 2½ to 8 years. Journal of Communication Disorders 1990; 23:205–217.
[4]Leonard L, McGregor K. Unusual phonological patterns and their underlying representations: a case study. Journal of Child Lanugage 1991; 18:261–271.

Leonard, Schwartz, Swanson, and Loeb (1987) investigated some conditions that appear to promote unusual phonological behavior. They suggested three conditions in which unusual patterns might occur:

1. The child uses the sound appearing in the adult surface form, but in contexts that may be problematic, an unusual pattern is adopted.
2. In most contexts the child uses a substitution for the sound appearing in the adult surface form. For the remaining contexts the child adopts an unusual pattern.
3. The child never uses the sound appearing in the adult surface form and does not use a substitution for them (omission with no substitution). The words requiring these sounds do not lend themselves to the child's usual sound changes (substitutions). As a result, an unusual pattern is adopted.

Using nonsense words as stimuli, Leonard, et al., simulated the three conditions described above. They predicted that normally developing children would tend to use unusual patterns or sound changes more often when the stimuli approximated Condition 3. The results were true to predictions; however, there were a greater number of unusual sound changes associated with Conditions 1 and 2 than expected.

A second study used children with specific language impairments (SLI) as subjects. This group demonstrated a significantly larger percentage of unusual sound patterns showing a mean percentage of 47.47% compared to only 27.67% for the normally developing children. The SLI children showed about the same number of errors for each of the conditions. The type of condition did not have an apparent influence on the production of unusual sound errors.

Leonard, et al. (1987, p. 32) interpreted the SLI results as indicating limited ''ability to identify phonetic regularities among words and to adopt production patterns that take advantage of these regularities.'' This finding supports findings of the Dodd, Hambly, and Leahy (1989) study, reported earlier, in which children using unusual processes showed no preference between phonologically legal and illegal nonsense words. The researchers suggest that the task tapped into the children's unconscious awareness of the ways in which phonemes are combined. Again, this suggests a limited ability to abstract phonological patterns. See Exercises 5.6–5.7 in Appendix 5.2.

PROCESSES COMMON TO PHONOLOGICAL DISORDERS

Hodson and Paden (1981) evaluated the speech errors of 60 normally developing children (ages between 4 and 5 years) in comparison to 60 unintelligible children (ages 3–8 years). The processes most prevalent in the unintelligible children's speech included cluster reduction, stridency deletion, stopping, liquid deviations (gliding and vocalization), and assimilation (labial and nasal). Secondary to these processes were velar fronting or omission, backing, final consonant deletion, syllable reduction, prevocalic voicing, and glottal replacement.

The normally developing children did not exhibit processes that interfered significantly with intelligibility. Hodson and Paden noted that while all of the unintelligible children showed processes of cluster reduction, stridency deletion, and stopping, these processes were evident in fewer than five of the intelligible children. The processes also differed in impact on intelligibility. The unintelligible children tended to use processes that crossed manner. For example, the ''th'' targets were replaced with stops. For the same sounds, the intelligible children tended to substitute other fricatives (maintaining manner). The two groups also differed in frequency of use with the unintelligible children using processes much more frequently.

The reader should note that the two groups differed to some extent in the types of processes used. However, keep in mind that the intelligible group were between 4 and 5 years of age which is beyond the age at which they would be expected to have suppressed use of processes. The processes used by the unintelligible children have all been reported as occurring in normally developing children at younger ages.

Stoel-Gammon and Dunn (1985) compared error patterns from eight studies (not including Hodson and Paden, 1981) on phonologically disordered children. The most frequently occurring processes they noted were:

Deletion of Final Consonant	Cluster Reduction
Weak Syllable Deletion	Stopping
Velar and Palatal Fronting	Gliding
Vocalization	Assimilation (nasal, labial, velar)
Prevocalic Voicing	Final Consonant Devoicing

In comparison, Stoel-Gammon and Dunn identified most of the processes observed by Hodson and Paden (1981), including cluster reduction, stopping, gliding, vocalization, assimilation, velar fronting, consonant deletion, weak syllable deletion, and prevocalic voicing. Both studies note that other processes occur, but less frequently. Cluster reduction was the only process that occurred in all of the children. Stoel-Gammon and Dunn make the point that though children use some of the same processes, they may use them variably. In other words, for one child fronting may be an infrequently used process while another child may use it heavily.

DIFFERENCES IN USE OF PROCESSES

Grunwell (1987) observes that many of the processes used in phonological disabilities are also used in normally developing children. The difference between the groups however, appears to be in the use of those processes. She classifies these differences as

Persisting Normal Processes
Chronological Mismatch
Unusual/Idiosyncratic Processes
Variable Use of Processes
Systematic Sound Preference

The descriptions of these classifications are from Grunwell (1988, p. 252).

Persisting Normal Processes

Persisting Normal Processes are those normal phonological processes which remain in the child's pronunciation patterns long after the age at which they would be expected to have been "suppressed." If the processes evidenced in a data sample are all "normal" and are homogeneous in terms of their chronology, then it is clear that a child's phonological development is delayed to a greater or lesser extent, depending upon his/her age, or is "arrested" at a particular stage of development.

Chronological Mismatch

Chronological Mismatch is the co-occurrence of some of the earliest normal simplifying processes with some patterns of pronunciation characteristic of later stages in phonological development. Such "uneven" progress by comparison with the normal chronology of development is clearly suggestive of disrupted or disordered development.

Unusual/Idiosyncratic Processes

Unusual/Idiosyncratic Processes are simplifying patterns which have been rarely attested in normal speech development, or which appear to be different from normal developmental processes and which may therefore be idiosyncratic. Leonard (1985) classifies these unusual phonological behaviors into two categories: (a) salient sound changes with readily detectable systematicity, for example early sounds replaced by late sounds, additions to adult surface forms, use of sounds absent from the target language or from natural languages; and (b) salient sound changes with less readily detectable systematicity, for example context-based speech patterns such as harmony/assimilation, dissimilation, metathesis.

Variable Use of Processes

Variable Use of Processes occurs where more than one simplifying process routinely operates with the same target type of structure, so that the child's realizations of these target types are variable and unpredictable. This variability is abnormal when there are no indications that one of the variable pronunciations is potentially progressive, that is, entails the possible development of a new contrast.

Grunwell (1987) describes two types of variable use. The first is variability between the presence and absence of a process in which sometimes the target sound is produced correctly and at other times a process is used. The second type of variability occurs when two different processes affect the same sound. For example, fronting of a /k/ on one occasion and deletion of the /k/ on another.

Systematic Sound Preference

Systematic Sound Preference occurs when one type of consonant phone is used for a large range of different target types. Often several different processes can be identified as resulting in a massive reduction of the phonological contrasts in the child's system. The processes "conspire" to "collapse" the adult system of contrasts to the one phone the child prefers to use in his pronunciation patterns—a "favorite articulation." The massive lack of contrasts is clearly indicative of a severe phonological learning disability, given the communicative inadequacies of the child's pronunciation patterns which must ensue.

BETWEEN-WORD PROCESSES

The emphasis of phonological process descriptions has traditionally been on sound changes at the word level. However, multiword productions should also pose problems for the child acquiring the sound system. Stemberger (1988, p. 40) suggests that "the extra complexity of multiword utterances would prove difficult in certain ways and lead to the rise of phonological processes that involve two or more words." Stemberger refers to these as between-word processes.

Most of the research on between-word processes has focused on the operating of consonant harmony across words (Donahue, 1986; Matthei 1989). Stemberger (1988) describes several additional between-word processes that occurred in his daughter's speech, including vowel deletions, doubling of /l/, nasal assimilation, and word-initial deletion.

Between-word processes obviously operate in disordered phonologies as well as those that are normally developing. If these processes are to be recognized, assessment will have to include connected speech samples in addition to the standard isolated word instruments.

PHONOLOGICAL STRATEGIES

An interesting behavior observed in the speech patterns of children is that of strategies. Stoel-Gammon and Dunn (1985, p. 50) note that while "there is no consensus on the exact definition of the term 'strategy,' it is generally agreed that phonological strategies allow children to organize and simplify the complex phonological system being acquired." The use of strategies appears to help the young language learner cope temporarily with the growing complexity of the phonological system. The strategies operate to simplify the child's underlying representations and storage of a rapidly growing lexicon. Four strategies will be discussed here: fronting, syllable-maintaining, syllable-reducing, and homonomy. (Another strategy commonly identified is sound preference substitution or systematic sound preference. This strategy was discussed earlier in this chapter under Differences in Use of Processes.)

FRONTING

Fronting as a strategy differs from fronting as a process. Recall that the process of fronting involved the substitution of anterior consonants (typically alveolars) for velar or palatal consonants. Ingram (1974) describes the strategy of fronting as an ordering of the sounds in a child's production so sounds produced toward the beginning of a word form are made more anterior to sounds that follow in the same word form. He proposes that back consonants are less marked in syllable-final position than in syllable-initial position, and the reverse for anterior consonants.

Ingram describes two subjects—one English and one French—evidencing the fronting strategy. In the strategy, the word forms are produced so the initial consonants are made at the same or a more anterior position than following consonants. He notes that the children use different processes in their speech patterns to achieve the anterior-posterior relationship in their word forms. Some of the processes used included metathesis, assimilation, reduplication, and syllable deletion.

SYLLABLE-MAINTAINING AND SYLLABLE-REDUCING

Klein (1981) published a very comprehensive paper on syllable-maintaining and syllable-reducing strategies based on her doctoral dissertation. These strategies make use of various phonological processes to allow the child's production to retain the number of syllables present in the adult target form. Klein identifies several processes that operate to maintain or reduce the number of syllables and notes that children appear to rely on particular processes. For example, one of her subjects relied mainly on neutralization to maintain syllables, while another relied more heavily on reduplication.

Syllable-Maintaining

Klein considered the following processes as helping to maintain the number of syllables in the child's production: consonant assimilation, reduplication, diminutive, metathesis, and neutralization. All of these processes function to simplify production so the child can still maintain the number of syllables that are present in the adult target. Of these, only neutralization has not been discussed previously. Neutralization occurs when two sounds that are contrastive in one environment are represented by the same segment in another environment. Thus, their contrastiveness has been neutralized. Schane (1973, p. 59) uses the example of /t/ versus /d/ in German. The two sounds contrast in initial and medial word position, but only the /t/ appears word finally. Thus, the contrast is neutralized in word-final position (only one representation).

Syllable-Reducing

These processes operate to "minimize the number of phonemic and/or syllable units in a lexical item" (Klein, 1981, p. 24). As defined in her study, if the processes resulted in the loss of at least one syllable it was considered syllable-reducing. Included in these processes are weak syllable deletion, accented syllable, bisyllabic retention, and coalescence.

Three of these terms need clarification. Accented syllable refers to syllable reduction where only one syllable is retained. This differs from weak syllable deletion where only the weak syllable is lost. Bisyllable retention refers to the retaining of two syllables of a polysyllabic word. It differs from weak syllable deletion because the syllable that is deleted may be stressed. Coalescence is a process in which segments that are present in two syllables are combined into one. An example of coalescence from Klein is the word pacifier being produced as [pæf] where the [p] is retained from the first syllable and the [f] from the third.

HOMONYMY

Vihman (1981) describes homonymy as a strategy used by children who are "seeking to combine adult word-patterns to limit their output repertoire" (p. 239). As a result of homonymy one child form is used to represent several adult forms. As an example, Ingram (1989) describes the speech of a language delayed child (Aaron) as having the form [dado] representing the words, butter, ladder, letter, spider, water, and whistle. Lleo (1990) investigated use of homonymy by her daughter over a 1 year period (ages 1;7 to 2;7). She compared the number of lexical types (i.e., adult words as used by the child) with an articulation score based on the total number of word-initial and final consonants occurring in relation to the number of words in the child's lexicon.

Lleo noted that, between 1;7 and 2;11, as her child's lexicon and articulation score increased, her use of homonyms decreased. This trend was reversed between ages 1;11 and 2;3 when her daughter's use of homonyms increased significantly. Use of homonyms continued to increase until the emergence of trisyllabic words after which use of homonyms decreased markedly.

As explanation, Lleo looks to the syllable structure of her child's lexicon. Between the ages of 1;11 and 2;3 her daughter's lexicon is growing rapidly but the relative numbers of one, two, and three syllable words remains about the same. During this time Lleo suggests that her child adopted homonymy to simplify the lexicon which had grown so fast. The homonyms are mostly bisyllabic forms representing trisyllabic adult targets. When her daughter increases her use of trisyllabic words, the homonyms do not appear to be needed and their use declines.

This analysis would seem to agree with Stoel-Gammon and Cooper (1981), as cited in Stoel-Gammon and Dunn (1985), who interpreted the presence of many homonymous forms as allowing the child to produce many adult words using only a few articulatory patterns.

VOWEL PATTERNS IN CHILD PHONOLOGY

Although the emphasis of research on phonological development and disorders has been placed on consonants, some recent studies have focused on the development of the vowel system (Pollock and Keiser, 1990; Stoel-Gammon and Herrington, 1990; and Reynolds, 1990). Linguists have long been aware of processes that affect vowels. Schane (1973) describes vowel epenthesis, vowel deletion, vowel harmony, and vowel coalescence. He also covers vowel shift and vowel neutralization. The following are some vowel errors observed in phonologically disordered children.

Pollock and Keiser (1990) evaluated 15 phonologically disordered children for the presence of vowel errors. They posited that the errors would fall into one of three subtypes: (*a*) feature changes in which a vowel feature (height, frontness, roundness) changes it value, (*b*) complexity changes which involve changes in the diphthongal nature of vowels, and (*c*) vowel harmony in which a vowel changes to become more like another vowel in the same word (p. 169). They noted that most errors were feature changes followed by complexity changes. Harmony processes were rare. Some of the more common vowel processes are described next. Most of the vowel patterns noted, along with examples, are taken from the Pollock and Keiser article.

FEATURE CHANGING PROCESSES

Vowel Backing. This feature changing process results in a vowel being replaced with a more posterior vowel. Example: /æ/ → [a].

Vowel Lowering. This sound change occurs when a vowel is replaced with a vowel made with lower tongue height. Pollock and Keiser observed /ɪ/ changing to [ɛ] in several of their subjects.

Centralization. This process is the replacement of a vowel with a more central vowel, typically the schwa or its stressed form. Example: /e/ → [ʌ]

Vowel Unrounding. In this sound change a vowel that is normally rounded is produced without the rounding. Example: /ɔ/ → [a]

Other forms of feature changing processes include vowel fronting, raising, tensing, laxing, and raising. In the Pollock and Keiser study these occurred with less frequency than those previously described more fully.

COMPLEXITY CHANGES

Diphthongization. A monophthong vowel is produced as a diphthong. Diphthongization is common in the speech of deaf children (MacKay, 1987). Example: /a/ → [aɪ]

Diphthong Reduction. A vowel that is normally produced as a diphthong is reduced to a monophthong. Example: /aɪ/ → [a]

Vowel Harmony

Complete Vowel Harmony. In this sound change one vowel is changed so that both vowels in the word are the same. Example: /ɔfɪs/ → [ɔfɔs]

Tenseness Harmony. Pollock and Keiser (1990) give the example of a lax vowel becoming tense when there is another tense vowel in the same word. Example: /kʊki/ → kuki]

Height Vowel Harmony. This sound change occurs when a vowel is replaced with a vowel that is closer in production to the height of another vowel in the same word. Example: /himæn/ → [himɪn]

Consonant Vowel Harmony. Some vowels change due to the presence of a neighboring consonant. Reynolds (1990) describes a tendency for vowels to be replaced with a more open vowel when preceding nasals and of vowel lowering and backing preceding the dark /l/.

Other forms of vowel harmony suggested by Pollock and Keiser include frontness vowel harmony and rounding vowel harmony. These were not observed in the subjects of their study.

References

Bernthal J, Bankson N. Articulation and phonological disorders. 2nd ed. Englewood Cliffs: Prentice-Hall, 1988.

Chomsky N, Halle M. The sound pattern of English. New York: Harper and Row, 1968.

Dodd B, Hambly G, Leahy J. Phonological disorders in children: underlying cognitive deficits. British Journal of Developmental Psychology 1989;7:55–71.

Dodd B, Iacano T. Phonological disorders in children: changes in phonological process use during treatment. British Journal of Disorders of Communication 1989;24:333–351.

Donahue M. Phonological constraints on the emergence of two-word utterances. Journal of Child Language 1986;13:209–218.

Dyson A, Paden E. Some phonological acquisition strategies used by two-year-olds. Journal of Childhood Communication Disorders 1983;7(1):26–18.

Edwards M. Phonological assessment and treatment in support of phonological processes. Language, Speech, and Hearing Services in Schools 1992;23:233–240.

Edwards M, Shriberg L. Phonology: applications in communicative disorders. San Diego: College-Hill Press, Inc., 1983.

Elbert M, Gierut J. Handbook of clinical phonology: approaches to assessment and treatment. Boston: College-Hill Publication, 1986.

Fey M. Articulation and phonology: inextricable constructs in speech pathology. Human Communication 1985;9:7–16.

Gierut J, Dinnsen D. On word-initial voicing: converging sources of evidence in phonologically disordered speech. Language and Speech 1986;29(Part 2):97–114.

Greenlee M. Interacting processes in the child's acquisition of stop-liquid clusters. Papers and Reports on Child Language Development 1974;6:97–106.

Grunwell P. Clinical phonology. 2nd ed. Baltimore: Williams and Wilkins, 1987.

Grunwell P. Phonological assessment, evaluation and explanation of speech disorders in children. Clinical Linguistics and Phonetics 1988;2(3):221–252.

Haelsig P, Madison C. A study of phonological processes exhibited by 3-, 4-, and 5-year-old children. Language, Speech, and Hearing Services in Schools 1986;17(April):107–114.

Hodson B, Paden E. Phonological processes which characterize unintelligible and intelligible speech in early childhood. Journal of Speech and Hearing Disorders 1981;46:369–373.

Hodson B, Paden E. Targeting intelligible speech. San Diego: College-Hill Press, 1983.

Ingram D. Fronting in child phonology. Journal of Child Language, 1974;1:233–241.

Ingram D. Procedures for the phonological analysis of children's language. Baltimore: University Park Press, 1981.

Ingram D. Phonological disability in children. 2nd ed. London: Whurr Publishers, 1989.

Khan L. Basics of phonological analysis: a programmed learning text. San Diego: College-Hill Press, 1985.

Klein H. Productive strategies for the pronunciation of early polysyllabic lexical items. Journal of Speech and Hearing Research 1981;24:389–405.

Leahy J, Dodd B. The development of disordered phonology: a case study. Language and Cognitive Processes 1987;2:115–132.

Leonard L. The nature of deviant articulation. Journal of Speech and Hearing Disorders 1973;38:151–161.

Leonard L. Unusual and subtle phonological behavior in the speech of phonologically disordered children. Journal of Speech and Hearing Disorders 1985;50:4–13.

Leonard L, McGregor K. Unusual phonological patterns and their underlying representations: a case study. Journal of Child Language 1991;18:261–271.

Leonard L, Miller J, Brown H. Consonant and syllable harmony in the speech of language disordered children. Paper presented at the First Wisconsin Symposium on Research in Child Language Disorders, June 6–7, University of Wisconsin-Madison, 1980.

Leonard L, Schwartz R, Swanson L, Loeb D. Some conditions that promote unusual phonological behavior in children. Clinical Linguistics and Phonetics 1987;1(1):23–34.

Lleo C. Homonymy and reduplication: on the extended availability of two strategies in phonological acquisition. Journal of Child Language 1990;17:267–278.

Lowe R. Assessment link between phonology and articulation (ALPHA). Moline, IL: LinguiSystems, Inc., 1986

Lowe R, Knutson P, Monson M. Incidence of fronting in preschool children. Language, Speech, and Hearing Services in Schools 1985;16(2):119–123.

Mackay I. Phonetics: the science of speech production. Boston: College-Hill Publications, 1987.

Matthei E. Crossing boundaries: more evidence for phonological constraints on early multi-word utterances. Journal of Child Language 1989;16:41–54.

McReynolds L, Elbert M. Criteria for phonological process analysis. Journal of Speech and Hearing Disorders 1981; 46:197–204.

Norris M, Harden J. Natural processes in the phonologies of four error-rate groups. Journal of Communication Disorders 1981;14:195–213.

Pollock K, Keiser N. An examination of vowel errors in phonologically disordered children. Clinical Linguistics and Phonetics 1990;4(2):161–178.

Prater R, Swift J. Phonological process development with MLU-referenced guidelines. Journal of Communication Disorders 1982;15:395–410.

Reynolds J. Abnormal vowel patterns in phonological disorder: some data and a hypothesis. British Journal of Disorders of Communication 1990;25:115–148.

Roberts J, Burchinal M, Foote M. Phonological process decline from 2½ to 8 years. Journal of Communication Disorders 1990;23:205–217.

Schane S. Generative phonology. Englewood Cliffs: Prentice-Hall, 1973.

Shriberg L, Kwiatkowski J. Natural process analysis (NPA). New York: John Wiley and Sons, 1980.

Sloat C, Taylor S, Hoard J. Introduction to phonology. Englewood Cliffs: Prentice-Hall, 1978.

Stemberger J. Between-word processes in child phonology. Journal of Child Language 1988;15:39–61.

Stoel-Gammon C, Cooper J. Individual differences in early phonological and lexical development. Paper presented at the Second International Congress for the Study of Child Language, August 9–14, Vancouver, BC, 1981.

Stoel-Gammon C, Dunn C. Normal and disordered phonology in children. Baltimore: University Park Press, 1985.

Stoel-Gammon C, Herrington P. Vowel systems of normally developing and phonologically disordered children. Clinical Linguistics and Phonetics 1990;4(2):145–160.

Velten H. The growth of phonemic and lexical patterns in infant language. Language 1943;19:281–292.

Vihman M. Consonant harmony: its scope and function in child language. In Greenberg J, Ferguson C, Moravcsik E, eds. Universals of Human Language, Vol. 2. Stanford University Press, Stanford, CA, 1978:281–334.

Vihman M. Phonology and the development of the lexicon: evidence from children's errors. Journal of Child Language 1981;8:239–264.

Identification of Common Phonological Processes— Exercises and Answers

EXERCISE 5.1

Stopping (St)	Deletion of Final Consonant (DFC)	Final Consonant Devoicing (DeV)
Fronting (Fr)	Weak Syllable Deletion (WSD)	Velar Assimilation (VeA)
Gliding (Gl)	Vocalization (Vc)	Labial Assimilation (LbA)
Stridency Del (StD)	Prevocalic Voicing (PrV)	Nasal Assimilation (NsA)
Epenthesis (Epn)	Cluster Reduction (CR)	

For the following, first indicate the sound change and then underline the abbreviation of the process or processes that might be occurring.

Target	Form	Snd Change	Potential Processes
1. shoot	[sut]	→ s	St Fr Gl StD Epn DFC WSD Vc PrV CR DeV VeA LbA NsA
2. star	[tar]	_____	St Fr Gl StD Epn DFC WSD Vc PrV CR DeV VeA LbA NsA
3. booth	[but]	_____	St Fr Gl StD Epn DFC WSD Vc PrV CR DeV VeA LbA NsA
4. rain	[we]	_____	St Fr Gl StD Epn DFC WSD Vc PrV CR DeV VeA LbA NsA
5. knees	[nis]	_____	St Fr Gl StD Epn DFC WSD Vc PrV CR DeV VeA LbA NsA
6. gate	[det]	_____	St Fr Gl StD Epn DFC WSD Vc PrV CR DeV VeA LbA NsA
7. shoe	[du]	_____	St Fr Gl StD Epn DFC WSD Vc PrV CR DeV VeA LbA NsA
8. peach	[bits]	_____	St Fr Gl StD Epn DFC WSD Vc PrV CR DeV VeA LbA NsA
9. snow	[səno]	_____	St Fr Gl StD Epn DFC WSD Vc PrV CR DeV VeA LbA NsA
10. go	[do]	_____	St Fr Gl StD Epn DFC WSD Vc PrV CR DeV VeA LbA NsA
11. tent	[dɛn]	_____	St Fr Gl StD Epn DFC WSD Vc PrV CR DeV VeA LbA NsA
12. tag	[kæk]	_____	St Fr Gl StD Epn DFC WSD Vc PrV CR DeV VeA LbA NsA
13. baker	[bekə]	_____	St Fr Gl StD Epn DFC WSD Vc PrV CR DeV VeA LbA NsA
14. Dan	[mæn]	_____	St Fr Gl StD Epn DFC WSD Vc PrV CR DeV VeA LbA NsA
15. lady	[wed]	_____	St Fr Gl StD Epn DFC WSD Vc PrV CR DeV VeA LbA NsA

EXERCISE 5.2

Stopping (St)	Deletion of Final Consonant (DFC)	Final Consonant Devoicing (DeV)
Fronting (Fr)	Weak Syllable Deletion (WSD)	Velar Assimilation (VeA)
Gliding (Gl)	Vocalization (Vc)	Labial Assimilation (LbA)
Stridency Del (StD)	Prevocalic Voicing (PrV)	Nasal Assimilation (NsA)
Deaffrication (DeA)	Cluster Reduction (CR)	

For the following, first indicate the sound change and then underline the abbreviation of the process or processes that might be occurring.

Target	Form	Snd Change	Potential Processes
1. skip	[kɪ]	_____	St Fr Gl StD DeA DFC WSD Vc PrV CR DeV VeA LbA NsA
2. Kate	[det]	_____	St Fr Gl StD DeA DFC WSD Vc PrV CR DeV VeA LbA NsA
3. ride	[waɪt]	_____	St Fr Gl StD DeA DFC WSD Vc PrV CR DeV VeA LbA NsA
4. pan	[pæm]	_____	St Fr Gl StD DeA DFC WSD Vc PrV CR DeV VeA LbA NsA
5. zoo	[du]	_____	St Fr Gl StD DeA DFC WSD Vc PrV CR DeV VeA LbA NsA
6. dog	[gɔk]	_____	St Fr Gl StD DeA DFC WSD Vc PrV CR DeV VeA LbA NsA
7. glass	[æt]	_____	St Fr Gl StD DeA DFC WSD Vc PrV CR DeV VeA LbA NsA
8. cheese	[ʃid]	_____	St Fr Gl StD DeA DFC WSD Vc PrV CR DeV VeA LbA NsA
9. bigger	[bɪgə]	_____	St Fr Gl StD DeA DFC WSD Vc PrV CR DeV VeA LbA NsA
10. leaf	[jip]	_____	St Fr Gl StD DeA DFC WSD Vc PrV CR DeV VeA LbA NsA
11. show	[so]	_____	St Fr Gl StD DeA DFC WSD Vc PrV CR DeV VeA LbA NsA
12. seat	[dit]	_____	St Fr Gl StD DeA DFC WSD Vc PrV CR DeV VeA LbA NsA
13. match	[mæt]	_____	St Fr Gl StD DeA DFC WSD Vc PrV CR DeV VeA LbA NsA
14. thin	[dɪn]	_____	St Fr Gl StD DeA DFC WSD Vc PrV CR DeV VeA LbA NsA
15. please	[id]	_____	St Fr Gl StD DeA DFC WSD Vc PrV CR DeV VeA LbA NsA

EXERCISE 5.3

Stopping (St)	Deletion of Final Consonant (DFC)	Final Consonant Devoicing (DeV)
Fronting (Fr)	Weak Syllable Deletion (WSD)	Velar Assimilation (VeA)
Gliding (Gl)	Vocalization (Vc)	Labial Assimilation (LbA)
Stridency Del (StD)	Prevocalic Devoicing (PrV)	Nasal Assimilation (NsA)
Deaffrication (DeA)	Cluster Reduction (CR)	

For the following, first indicate the sound change and then underline the abbreviation of the process or processes that might be occurring.

Target	Form	Snd Change	Potential Processes
1. truck	[twʌt]	_____	St Fr Gl StD DeA DFC WSD Vc PrV CR DeV VeA LbA NsA
2. tape	[dep]	_____	St Fr Gl StD DeA DFC WSD Vc PrV CR DeV VeA LbA NsA
3. witch	[wɪs]	_____	St Fr Gl StD DeA DFC WSD Vc PrV CR DeV VeA LbA NsA
4. push	[bʊt]	_____	St Fr Gl StD DeA DFC WSD Vc PrV CR DeV VeA LbA NsA
5. stay	[de]	_____	St Fr Gl StD DeA DFC WSD Vc PrV CR DeV VeA LbA NsA
6. drive	[dwaɪb]	_____	St Fr Gl StD DeA DFC WSD Vc PrV CR DeV VeA LbA NsA
7. lake	[jet]	_____	St Fr Gl StD DeA DFC WSD Vc PrV CR DeV VeA LbA NsA
8. Joe	[do]	_____	St Fr Gl StD DeA DFC WSD Vc PrV CR DeV VeA LbA NsA
9. beetle	[bido]	_____	St Fr Gl StD DeA DFC WSD Vc PrV CR DeV VeA LbA NsA
10. tack	[gæk]	_____	St Fr Gl StD DeA DFC WSD Vc PrV CR DeV VeA LbA NsA
11. nose	[nos]	_____	St Fr Gl StD DeA DFC WSD Vc PrV CR DeV VeA LbA NsA
12. page	[bet]	_____	St Fr Gl StD DeA DFC WSD Vc PrV CR DeV VeA LbA NsA
13. mouth	[maʊt]	_____	St Fr Gl StD DeA DFC WSD Vc PrV CR DeV VeA LbA NsA
14. mine	[maɪ]	_____	St Fr Gl StD DeA DFC WSD Vc PrV CR DeV VeA LbA NsA
15. potato	[tedo]	_____	St Fr Gl StD DeA DFC WSD Vc PrV CR DeV VeA LbA NsA

EXERCISE 5.4

Stopping (St)   Deletion of Final Consonant (DFC)   Final Consonant Devoicing (DeV)
Fronting (Fr)   Weak Syllable Deletion (WSD)   Velar Assimilation (VeA)
Gliding (Gl)   Vocalization (Vc)   Labial Assimilation (LbA)
Stridency Del (StD)   Prevocalic Voicing (PrV)   Nasal Assimilation (NsA)
Epenthesis (Epn)   Cluster Reduction (CR)

For the following, first indicate the sound change and then underline the abbreviation of the process or processes that might be occurring.

Target	Form	Snd Change	Potential Processes
1. smoke	[səmo]	_____	St Fr Gl StD Epn DFC WSD Vc PrV CR DeV VeA LbA NsA
2. get	[de]	_____	St Fr Gl StD Epn DFC WSD Vc PrV CR DeV VeA LbA NsA
3. bunny	[nʌni]	_____	St Fr Gl StD Epn DFC WSD Vc PrV CR DeV VeA LbA NsA
4. shake	[det]	_____	St Fr Gl StD Epn DFC WSD Vc PrV CR DeV VeA LbA NsA
5. train	[twen]	_____	St Fr Gl StD Epn DFC WSD Vc PrV CR DeV VeA LbA NsA
6. gate	[gek]	_____	St Fr Gl StD Epn DFC WSD Vc PrV CR DeV VeA LbA NsA
7. limb	[mɪm]	_____	St Fr Gl StD Epn DFC WSD Vc PrV CR DeV VeA LbA NsA
8. suit	[dut]	_____	St Fr Gl StD Epn DFC WSD Vc PrV CR DeV VeA LbA NsA
9. banana	[næna]	_____	St Fr Gl StD Epn DFC WSD Vc PrV CR DeV VeA LbA NsA
10. cat	[dæt]	_____	St Fr Gl StD Epn DFC WSD Vc PrV CR DeV VeA LbA NsA
11. dish	[dɪs]	_____	St Fr Gl StD Epn DFC WSD Vc PrV CR DeV VeA LbA NsA
12. Debby	[bɛbi]	_____	St Fr Gl StD Epn DFC WSD Vc PrV CR DeV VeA LbA NsA
13. start	[tart]	_____	St Fr Gl StD Epn DFC WSD Vc PrV CR DeV VeA LbA NsA
14. later	[wedə]	_____	St Fr Gl StD Epn DFC WSD Vc PrV CR DeV VeA LbA NsA
15. book	[bʊt]	_____	St Fr Gl StD Epn DFC WSD Vc PrV CR DeV VeA LbA NsA

ANSWER SHEET FOR EXERCISE 5.1

Stopping (St)   Deletion of Final Consonant (DFC)   Final Consonant Devoicing (DeV)
Fronting (Fr)   Weak Syllable Deletion (WSD)   Velar Assimilation (VeA)
Gliding (Gl)   Vocalization (Vc)   Labial Assimilation (LbA)
Stridency Del (StD)   Prevocalic Voicing (PrV)   Nasal Assimilation (NsA)
Epenthesis (Epn)   Cluster Reduction (CR)

Target	Form	Snd Change	Potential Processes
1. shoot	[sut]	ʃ → s	Fr
2. star	[tar]	st → t	StD, CR
3. booth	[but]	θ → t	St
4. rain	[we]	r → w, n → ø	Gl, DFC
5. knees	[nis]	z → s	DeV
6. gate	[det]	g → d	Fr
7. shoe	[du]	ʃ → d	St, Fr, StD, PrV
8. peach	[bits]	b → p, ʧ → ts	Fr, PrV
9. snow	[səno]	sn → sən	Epn
10. go	[do]	g → d	Fr
11. tent	[dɛn]	t → d, nt → n	PrV, CR
12. tag	[kæk]	t → k, g → k	DeV, VeA
13. baker	[bekə]	ɚ → ə	Vc
14. Dan	[mæn]	d → m	LbA, NsA
15. lady	[wed]	l → w, i → ø	Gl, WSD

ANSWER SHEET FOR EXERCISE 5.2

Stopping (St)   Deletion of Final Consonant (DFC)   Final Consonant Devoicing (DeV)
Fronting (Fr)   Weak Syllable Deletion (WSD)   Velar Assimilation (VeA)
Gliding (Gl)   Vocalization (Vc)   Labial Assimilation (LbA)
Stridency Del (StD)   Prevocalic Voicing (PrV)   Nasal Assimilation (NsA)
Deaffrication (DeA)   Cluster Reduction (CR)

Target	Form	Snd Change	Potential Processes
1. skip	[kɪ]	s → θ, p → ø	StD, DFC, CR
2. Kate	[det]	k → d	Fr, PrV
3. ride	[waɪt]	r → w, d → t	Gl, DeV
4. pan	[pæm]	n → m	LbA
5. zoo	[du]	z → d	St, StD
6. dog	[gɔk]	d → g, g → k	DeV, VeA
7. glass	[æt]	gl → ø, s → t	St, StD, CR
8. cheese	[ʃid]	ʧ → ʃ, z → d	DeA, St, StD
9. bigger	[bɪgə]	ɚ → ə	Vc
10. leaf	[jip]	l → j, f → p	St, Gl, StD
11. show	[so]	ʃ → s	Fr
12. seat	[dit]	s → d	St, StD
13. match	[mæt]	ʧ → t	St, Fr, StD
14. thin	[dɪn]	θ → d	St, PrV
15. please	[id]	pl → ø, z → d	St, StD, CR

ANSWER SHEET FOR EXERCISE 5.3

Stopping (St)   Deletion of Final Consonant (DFC)   Final Consonant Devoicing (DeV)
Fronting (Fr)   Weak Syllable Deletion (WSD)   Velar Assimilation (VeA)
Gliding (Gl)   Vocalization (Vc)   Labial Assimilation (LbA)
Stridency Del (StD)   Prevocalic Voicing (PrV)   Nasal Assimilation (NsA)
Deaffrication (DeA)   Cluster Reduction (CR)

Target	Form	Snd Change	Potential Processes
1. truck	[twʌt]	r → w, k → t	Fr, Gl, CR
2. tape	[dep]	t → d	PrV
3. witch	[wɪs]	tʃ → s	Fr, DeA
4. push	[bʊt]	p → b, ʃ → t	St, Fr, StD, PrV
5. stay	[de]	st → d	StD, PrV CR
6. drive	[dwaɪb]	r → w, v → b	Gl, StD, CR, LbA
7. lake	[jet]	l → j, k → t	Fr, Gl
8. Joe	[do]	ʤ → d	Fr, St, StD
9. beetle	[bido]	ḷ → o	Vc
10. tack	[gæk]	t → g	PrV, VeA
11. nose	[nos]	z → s	DeV
12. page	[bet]	p → b, ʤ → t	St Fr StD PrV DeV
13. mouth	[maʊt]	θ → t	St
14. mine	[maɪ]	n → ø	DFC
15. potato	[tedo]	CVCVCV → CVCV	WSD

ANSWER SHEET FOR EXERCISE 5.4

Stopping (St)   Deletion of Final Consonant (DFC)   Final Consonant Devoicing (DeV)
Fronting (Fr)   Weak Syllable Deletion (WSD)   Velar Assimilation (VeA)
Gliding (Gl)   Vocalization (Vc)   Labial Assimilation (LbA)
Stridency Del (StD)   Prevocalic Voicing (PrV)   Nasal Assimilation (NsA)
Epenthesis (Epn)   Cluster Reduction (CR)

Target	Form	Snd Change	Potential Processes
1. smoke	[səmo]	sm → səm, k → ø	Epn, DFC
2. get	[de]	g → d, t → ø	Fr, DFC
3. bunny	[nʌni]	b → n	NsA
4. shake	[det]	ʃ → d, k → t	St, Fr, StD, PrV
5. train	[twen]	r → w	Gl, CR
6. gate	[gek]	t → k	VeA
7. limb	[mɪm]	l → m	NsA, LbA
8. suit	[dut]	s → d	St, StD, PrV
9. banana	[næna]	CVCVCV → CVCV	WSD
10. cat	[dæt]	k → d	Fr, PrV
11. dish	[dɪs]	ʃ → s	Fr
12. Debby	[bɛbi]	d → b	LbA
13. start	[tart]	st → t	StD, CR
14. later	[wedə]	l → w, ɚ → ə	Gl, Vc
15. book	[bʊt]	k → t	Fr

Identifying Assimilation Processes—Exercises and Answers

EXERCISE 5.5

For the following sound changes determine if assimilation is a possibility.

Target	Form	Sound Change	Yes/No	Why
1. goat	[dot]	g → d	_____	_____
2. cake	[tek]	k → t	_____	_____
3. dark	[kark]	d → k	_____	_____
4. car	[tar]	k → t	_____	_____
5. seem	[fim]	s → f	_____	_____

In this exercise a speech sample is provided. By comparing where sound changes do and do not occur determine if the process is that of stopping or assimilation to stops.

Target	Form	Target	Form	Target	Form
1. suit	[tut]	4. seem	[sim]	7. Sue	[su]
2. see	[si]	5. seat	[tit]	8. shoot	[tut]
3. same	[sem]	6. safe	[sep]	9. soon	[sun]

Answer:

EXERCISE 5.6

Atypical Cluster Reduction (ACR) Backing of Stops (BkS) Apicalization (Apl)
Initial Consonant Deletion (ICD) Backing of Fricatives (BkF) Migration (Mgr)
Stops Replacing Glides (SRG) Fricative Replacing Stops (FRS) Denasalization (DeN)
Medial Cons. Substitution (MCS) Devoicing of Stops (DeVl) Metathesis (Met)

For the following, identify the potential processes associated with the sound changes.

Target	Form	Sound Change	Potential Processes
1. sofa	[ofə]	_____	ACR ICD SRG BkS BkF FRS Apl Mgr DeN DeVl Met MCS
2. wake	[dek]	_____	ACR ICD SRG BkS BkF FRS Apl Mgr DeN DeVl Met MCS
3. boat	[pot]	_____	ACR ICD SRG BkS BkF FRS Apl Mgr DeN DeVl Met MCS
4. jelly	[dɛdi]	_____	ACR ICD SRG BkS BkF FRS Apl Mgr DeN DeVl Met MCS
5. ask	[æks]	_____	ACR ICD SRG BkS BkF FRS Apl Mgr DeN DeVl Met MCS
6. nose	[doz]	_____	ACR ICD SRG BkS BkF FRS Apl Mgr DeN DeVl Met MCS
7. boat	[bos]	_____	ACR ICD SRG BkS BkF FRS Apl Mgr DeN DeVl Met MCS
8. suit	[sus]	_____	ACR ICD SRG BkS BkF FRS Apl Mgr DeN DeVl Met MCS
9. skate	[set]	_____	ACR ICD SRG BkS BkF FRS Apl Mgr DeN DeVl Met MCS
10. fun	[sʌn]	_____	ACR ICD SRG BkS BkF FRS Apl Mgr DeN DeVl Met MCS
11. tea	[ki]	_____	ACR ICD SRG BkS BkF FRS Apl Mgr DeN DeVl Met MCS
12. lake	[es]	_____	ACR ICD SRG BkS BkF FRS Apl Mgr DeN DeVl Met MCS
13. sand	[ænd]	_____	ACR ICD SRG BkS BkF FRS Apl Mgr DeN DeVl Met MCS
14. beetle	[biso]	_____	ACR ICD SRG BkS BkF FRS Apl Mgr DeN DeVl Met MCS
15. tin	[θɪn]	_____	ACR ICD SRG BkS BkF FRS Apl Mgr DeN DeVl Met MCS

EXERCISE 5.7

Atypical Cluster Reduction (ACR) Backing of Stops (BkS) Apicalization (Apl)
Initial Consonant Deletion (ICD) Backing of Fricatives (BkF) Migration (Mgr)
Stops Replacing Glides (SRG) Fricative Replacing Stops (FRS) Denasalization (DeN)
Medial Cons. Substitution (MCS) Devoicing of Stops (DeVI) Metathesis (Met)

For the following, identify the potential processes associated with the sound changes.

Target	Form	Sound Change	Potential Processes
1. doe	[ko]	_____	ACR ICD SRG BkS BkF FRS Apl Mgr DeN DeVI Met MCS
2. seed	[ʃig]	_____	ACR ICD SRG BkS BkF FRS Apl Mgr DeN DeVI Met MCS
3. goat	[kok]	_____	ACR ICD SRG BkS BkF FRS Apl Mgr DeN DeVI Met MCS
4. wake	[tek]	_____	ACR ICD SRG BkS BkF FRS Apl Mgr DeN DeVI Met MCS
5. make	[nes]	_____	ACR ICD SRG BkS BkF FRS Apl Mgr DeN DeVI Met MCS
6. you	[ju]	_____	ACR ICD SRG BkS BkF FRS Apl Mgr DeN DeVI·Met MCS
7. van	[dæd]	_____	ACR ICD SRG BkS BkF FRS Apl Mgr DeN DeVI Met MCS
8. zoo	[su]	_____	ACR ICD SRG BkS BkF FRS Apl Mgr DeN DeVI Met MCS
9. star	[sar]	_____	ACR ICD SRG BkS BkF FRS Apl Mgr DeN DeVI Met MCS
10. below	[pido]	_____	ACR ICD SRG BkS BkF FRS Apl Mgr DeN DeVI Met MCS
11. can	[kæd]	_____	ACR ICD SRG BkS BkF FRS Apl Mgr DeN DeVI Met MCS
12. snake	[sek]	_____	ACR ICD SRG BkS BkF FRS Apl Mgr DeN DeVI Met MCS
13. shoe	[u]	_____	ACR ICD SRG BkS BkF FRS Apl Mgr DeN DeVI Met MCS
14. pen	[pɛt]	_____	ACR ICD SRG BkS BkF FRS Apl Mgr DeN DeVI Met MCS
15. fin	[tɪn]	_____	ACR ICD SRG BkS BkF FRS Apl Mgr DeN DeVI Met MCS

ANSWERS TO EXERCISE 5.5

For the following sound changes determine if assimilation is a possibility.

Target	Form	Sound Change	Yes/No	Why
1. goat	[dot]	g → d	Yes	Assimilation to the /t/.
2. cake	[tek]	k → t	No	Change makes them dissimilar.
3. dark	[kark]	d → k	Yes	Velar assimilation possible.
4. car	[tar]	k → t	No	No consonant to assimilate to.
5. seem	[fim]	s → f	Yes	Labial assimilation possible.

In the below exercise a speech sample is provided. By comparing where sound changes do and do not occur determine if the process is that of stopping or assimilation to stops.

Target	Form	Target	Form	Target	Form
1. suit	[tut]	4. seem	[sim]	7. Sue	[su]
2. see	[si]	5. seat	[tit]	8. shoot	[tut]
3. same	[sem]	6. safe	[sep]	9. soon	[sun]

Answer: Due to assimilation. Sound change only occurs when fricative is followed by a stop consonant. Look at minimal pair items 1 and 7; 2 and 5.

ANSWERS TO EXERCISE 5.6

Atypical Cluster Reduction (ACR)   Backing of Stops (BkS)   Apicalization (Apl)
Initial Consonant Deletion (ICD)   Backing of Fricatives (BkF)   Migration (Mgr)
Stops Replacing Glides (SRG)   Fricative Replacing Stops (FRS)   Denasalization (DeN)
Medial Cons. Substitution (MCS)   Devoicing of Stops (DeVI)   Metathesis (Met)

Target	Form	Sound Change	Potential Processes
1. sofa	[ofə]	s → ø	ICD
2. wake	[dek]	w → d	SRG
3. boat	[pot]	b → p	DeVI
4. jelly	[tɛdi]	j → t, l → d	SRG, DeVI, MCS
5. ask	[æks]	C reversal	Met
6. nose	[doz]	n → d	DeN
7. boat	[bos]	t → s	FRS
8. suit	[sus]	t → s	FRS Mgr
9. skate	[set]	CC → C	ACR
10. fun	[sʌn]	f → s	Apl
11. tea	[ki]	t → k	BkS
12. lake	[es]	l → ø, k → s	ICD FRS
13. sand	[ænd]	s → ø	BkF
14. beetle	[biso]	d → s	FRS MCS
15. tin	[θɪn]	t → θ	FRS

ANSWERS TO EXERCISE 5.7

Atypical Cluster Reduction (ACR)   Backing of Stops (BkS)   Apicalization (Apl)
Initial Consonant Deletion (ICD)   Backing of Fricatives (BkF)   Migration (Mgr)
Stops Replacing Glides (SRG)   Fricative Replacing Stops (FRS)   Denasalization (DeN)
Medial Cons. Substitution (MCS)   Devoicing of Stops (DeVl)   Metathesis (Met)

Target	Form	Sound Change	Potential Processes
1. doe	[ko]	d → k	BkS DeVl
2. seed	[ʃig]	s → ʃ, d → g	BkS BkF
3. goat	[kok]	g → k, t → k	BkS Mgr DeVl
4. wake	[tek]	w → t	SRG DeVl
5. make	[nes]	m → n, k → s	FRS Apl
6. you	[du]	j → d	SRG
7. van	[dæd]	v → d, n → d	Apl DeN
8. zoo	[su]	z → s	DeVl
9. star	[sar]	CC → C	ACR
10. below	[pido]	b → p, l → d	DeVl MCS
11. can	[kæd]	n → d	DeN
12. snake	[sek]	CC → C	ACR
13. shoe	[u]	ʃ → ø	ICD
14. pen	[pɛt]	n → t	DeN
15. fin	[ɪn]	f → t	Apl

Assessment of Phonological Disorders

Chapter

6

Robert J. Lowe

ASSESSMENT IS ONE of the major tools of the speech-language pathologist. Like any tool, if used properly it can speed the job at hand. In speech-language pathology, a thorough assessment leads to accurate diagnosis, identification of etiology and complicating conditions, and provides a foundation for intervention. Haphazard assessment leads to wasted time and energy, and eventually to poor diagnostic decisions and inefficient intervention planning.

Assessment for articulation has changed considerably over the past two decades. The profession has moved from simplistic three position, single word tests requiring only a few minutes for administration and scoring, to complicated assessment batteries that may require hours to score and interpret. The change has followed a switch in focus from the phonetic level concentrating on the mechanics of speech production to the phonological level concerned with the organization of the speech sound system. The result is a need for a comprehensive evaluation. Bankson and Bernthal (1982, p. 572) summarize this current view of assessment.

> Articulation assessment should be done with a battery of evaluation instruments. While in the past some clinicians have relied almost exclusively on a single articulation inventory, it has been shown that such a practice provides only a partial picture of an individual's articulatory status and may lead to faulty conclusions and utilization of inappropriate treatment procedures. Rather, in addition to an inventory, articulation assessments should include samples of connected speech, contextual testing, and a measure of speech sound stimulability.

As noted in Chapter 1, the field of phonetics is concerned with the physiological and physical nature of speech sounds. Thus, a phonetic analysis will provide a detailed description of speech sounds focusing on their place, manner, and voicing characteristics. Phonology, however, focuses

131

on the organization of the sound system. A phonological analysis is concerned with how sounds are organized and function within a language. As such, the analysis will determine how sounds change as classes, how sounds are used contrastively (operate as phonemes), and what rules may govern production. In addition, phonology is concerned with how sounds are realized at the surface level, so analysis includes information dealing with the phonetic aspects as well.

Prior to a discussion of what is involved in a phonological analysis, it is necessary to make two distinctions. The first is between phonetic and phonological disorders and the second between evaluation and explanation.

PHONETIC VERSUS PHONOLOGICAL DISORDER

Although we have described phonology as having interests in both underlying and surface representations, clinicians typically make a distinction between what are called phonetic errors and phonological errors. The distinction between the two error types is based on whether or not the sound change maintains or neutralizes a sound contrast. Traditionally, phonetic errors have been referred to as articulation errors. These errors result in production of nonstandard speech sounds but the production still maintains the contrastiveness of the sound system. An example is a lateral lisp used for /s/. Although the /s/ is distorted, its lateralized substitution still functions to contrast with the other sounds in the child's system. Listeners can distinguish between words like ''Sue'' and ''shoe'' or ''see'' and ''tea'' because the lateralized production is still distinctive.

Phonological errors result in a collapse or neutralization of contrast. If the child had substituted a t/s instead of a lateralization, it would be impossible to distinguish between words like ''see'' and ''tea.'' Both words would be realized as [ti]. Thus, we have a loss of contrast in the child's system. This neutralization of contrast can occur despite the child's ability to produce the target sound correctly. As described by Grunwell (1986, p. 272), ''Often an individual with an apparent phonological disability will give evidence of an ability to produce a full range of adequate articulatory movements, and indeed often uses sounds inappropriately in certain contexts and positions in speech while failing to use them appropriately in other contexts and positions.'' Take, for example, the child who substitutes a t/s but uses [s] correctly for the [ʃ] in shoe. This child evidences ability to make the sound correctly but the organization of the sound system is faulty.

In summary, the loss of a phonological contrast indicates a phonological disorder, whereas error productions that still preserve contrasts are considered phonetic in nature. Phonetic errors tend to be distortions of standard productions and thus are often transcribed using diacritics. Phonological errors, on the other hand, are errors that affect the sound system organization and thus tend to be standard productions so that a broad phonetic transcription is adequate to describe them. However, speech errors may have both phonetic and phonological components. A mixture of phonological and phonetic occurs when a speech sound produced in an abnormal manner (phonetic) results in the neutralization of a contrast (phonological). The child who lateralizes both the /s/ and /ʃ/ displays a phonetic error, but this error also neutralizes the contrast between the two speech sounds which introduces a phonological component.

To further complicate matters, the clinician will also have to differentiate between phonological and phonetic errors resulting from motor speech disorders. Disorders such as apraxia and dysarthria can result in phonetic errors as described above and also phonological errors. Perhaps the simplest solution is: Errors that maintain phonemic distinctions regardless of their etiology will be considered phonetic errors. Errors that result in a collapse or neutralization of phonemic contrasts will be considered phonological errors.

EXPLANATION VERSUS DESCRIPTION

In approaching assessment, the clinician can view phonological analysis as simply a description of the child's sound system or as providing a description plus an explanation of the nature of the sound errors. Most clinicians utilize analysis to describe the sound system and give little thought (with the exception of motor speech factors or obvious structural deficits) as to the cause of the child's misarticulations. This approach, however, does little to advance our understanding of the nature of phonological disorders. As presented by Grunwell (1988, p. 222), ''Ideally clinical practitioners (pathologists, therapists, or linguists) should be seekers of explanations, most especially because informed, principled, and accountable diagnoses and remediation should be based upon an understanding of the nature of the disorder or dysfunction.''

Explanation in assessment is not new to speech-language pathology. One of the primary objectives of the voice diagnostic is a determination of etiology and factors that may be maintaining the voice disorder. Assessment of fluency disorders examines learned behaviors and environmental conditions that may have some control over the stuttering behavior. Even the assessment of articulation disorders usually includes an oral-facial examination to rule out the possibility of oral-motor deficits.

If explanation is to be part of assessment, the clinician must look beyond speech sounds and evaluate phenomenon that interact with or function as part of phonology. Grunwell (1992, p. 458) summarizes,

> Because children who are being assessed evidence difficulties in learning to pronounce, phonological and other linguistic assessments must be complemented by information about all the factors that might conceivably impinge upon a child's ability to learn. A multi-dimensional approach is, therefore, essential; this should include anatomical, physiological, and neurological assessments, evaluation of cognitive abilities, and consideration of socioenvironmental factors.

Shriberg and Kwiatkowski (1982a) present a classification system that encourages explanation as well as description. In their system, the term phonological disorders is used as a ''cover term to encompass the entire speech production process, from underlying representations to phonological rules to the behaviors that produce the surface forms of speech'' (p. 228). Their model provides a framework for making distinctions between subgroups of articulation disorders and places an emphasis on explanation by including information on etiology. Their model is displayed in Figure 6.1.

OVERVIEW OF ASSESSMENT

Assuming that phonological assessment is more than a description of sound errors, the evaluation of a child with potential phonological disabilities will try to answer the following questions. (See Table 6.1 for an overview of assessment.)

1. Is there a problem? A phonological disability will result in impaired communication and

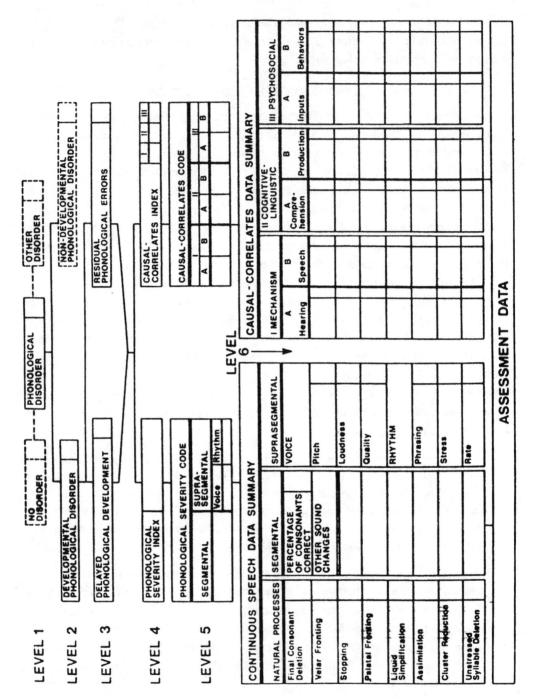

FIGURE 6.1. Diagnostic classification system for phonological disorders.

TABLE 6.1. Overview of Assessment

Is there a problem?	Possible explanatory factors?
Poor intelligibility	Language system
Impaired communication	Cognitive system
Negative reaction to speech	Sensory system
Withdrawal from social interaction	Motor system
Nature of the problem?	Structural adequacy
Severity	Speech models
Phonetic description	Developmental history
Phonological description	Exasperating factors?
Child's capabilities?	Social environment
Phonetic inventory	Trouble words
Syllable structure	Sources of frustration
Contrast system	Need for speech
Stimulability	
Phonetic alternations	
Underlying representations	

the clinician will need to determine to what extent the disability has influenced the child's life. The child's speech may be unintelligible or difficult to understand. As such the speech patterns may interfere with the child's social interactions. Peers may have difficulty understanding the child and react negatively. Repeated clarification requests may result in the child withdrawing from social interactions. If so, treatment will need to address and emphasize the positive aspects of speech.

2. What is the nature of the problem? Having established that a problem exists, it now must be described. How severe is the problem? A severity measure will provide quantitative support for inclusion in an intervention program, as well as baseline information for later use in monitoring progress. In addition to severity, a description of the phonological disability will include a detailed phonetic analysis. This analysis will describe the child's speech sound system in terms of: substitutions, omissions, and distortions. The phonetic information is often presented by word or syllable position and may be categorized by place, manner and voicing features. Along with a phonetic description, phonological aspects are also described possibly including: surface form variability (consistency), phonological processes, distinctive features, phonological rules, and use of phonological strategies.

3. What are the child's capabilities? Although assessments tend to focus on what the client cannot do, valuable information for intervention can be obtained by examining the child's capabilities. This part of the assessment would describe the child's phonetic and syllable structure inventories, system of contrasts, sound stimulability, phonetic alternations, and underlying representations.

4. What are possible explanatory factors? In an attempt to explain why the speech disability has occurred the clinician would evaluate the child's language and cognitive systems, sensory and motor abilities, speech mechanism structural adequacy, speech models (cultural influences, sibling and caretaker speech patterns), and developmental history.

5. What factors exasperate the problem? A phonological disability may be made more difficult by factors in the child's social environment. For example, if there are frequently occurring words that give the child particular trouble it could result in increased frustra-

tion. Examples would be names of siblings or frequently requested items. How others respond to the child can also complicate matters. What prompts encourage the child to clarify productions without frustration and what leads to frustration? Also, is there any teasing about the child's speech? How does the child react? What attitude does the child have about his/her speech? How necessary is speech for the child to communicate needs in or outside the home environment? If the child finds that speech is not necessary to accomplish needs or if the child thinks of speech in negative terms then correction of the speech disability will have a low priority for the child. Changes in the child's home and school environment may become a necessary part of the intervention program if it is to succeed.

REPRESENTATIVE SPEECH SAMPLING

CONNECTED SPEECH

A representative speech sample is one that reflects a child's typical use of speech sounds during everyday activities. For many years speech-language clinicians relied on three position tests as the source for these speech samples. Though convenient, these instruments ignore context (phonetic and situational) in assessment and thus their results are suspect. It has long been known that children make more errors in connected speech than in single word samples. Faircloth and Faircloth (1970) compared sound production in isolated words and connected speech and concluded that the connected speech samples better described the articulatory behaviors of their subject. Other studies found similar results, consistently noting that more errors are recorded in connected speech samples than in single word samples (DuBois and Bernthal, 1978; Healy and Madison, 1987; Johnson, Winny, and Pederson, 1980). Similar findings have been found for phonological processes (Andrews and Fey, 1986; Stoel-Gammon and Dunn, 1985).

Another failing of single word tests is their limited sampling of speech sounds. Often the single word inventories look at one sound in each of three positions (initial, medial, and final). With such a sparse sampling it is impossible to evaluate variability in production or the influence of phonetic context (sound environments, syllable shape, stress).

Healy and Madison (1987) compared sound production in the same words elicited in single word and connected speech samples. Their findings are summarized here:

1. Connected speech samples revealed a significantly higher number of errors than single word samples.
2. Connected speech samples revealed numerically more omission errors, more substitution errors and more distortion errors than single word samples, though the distribution within conditions was similar.
3. Nearly 15% of all errors on connected speech sample were produced at the single word level.
4. Nearly 20% of all errors on connected speech sample were produced as a different error type in single word samples.
5. Thirty-five percent of all errors in connected speech were produced *differently* (emphasis provided) at the single word level. (p. 134.)

Their findings strongly suggest that information on sound production will be missed if the clinician relies solely on either single word or connected speech sampling. Not only were more errors scored in connected speech but the types of errors were different. It is no surprise then, that children pass screening articulation tests only to have the classroom teacher comment that the child still cannot be understood in class.

The occurrence of phonological processes is also affected by the sampling method. In examining phonological process occurrence, Andrews and Fey (1986) compared productions from connected speech sampling and single words. They observed a greater occurrence of processes in the connected speech sampling condition. However, they also noted that three of their 14 subjects used a process in the production of isolated words that was not identified in the connected speech data.

More recently, Morrison and Shriberg (1992) performed a detailed analysis of data from 61 speech-delayed children assessed by both a standardized articulation test and a conversational speech sample. Significant differences were noted on measures from the two sampling conditions. What is interesting is that the findings were not as expected. Vowels, diphthongs, and consonant clusters were produced with more accuracy in conversational speech. In fact, 77% of the subjects had better articulation in the conversational speech sampling than on the articulation test. Established sounds were often produced more accurately in conversational speech while emerging sounds appeared to do better in response to articulation test stimuli.

The data on phonological processes was mixed. The processes of cluster reduction and liquid simplification (gliding and vocalization) were more frequently seen in the articulation test responses, while stopping and final consonant deletion were seen with greater frequency in the conversational speech data. Over half of the subjects had greater than 20% occurrence of stopping in their connected speech samples and no occurrences in the articulation data. It would appear that to adequately evaluate speech patterns for phonological processes both a conventional single word test and a connected speech sample are needed.

A final argument for completing a connected speech sample is the high incidence of language problems associated with phonologically disabled children. As presented by Morrison and Shriberg (1992, p. 271),

> With approximately 80% of this clinical population (speech-delayed) having associated language production problems, and approximately 25% having associated prosody-voice involvement (Shriberg, 1991; Shriberg, et al., 1986; Shriberg, Kwiatkowski, and Rasmussen, 1990), constraints in continuous speech could be associated with many levels of psycholinguistic and motor-speech processing. Conversational speech samples would appear to be the only source of *integrated* speech, language and prosodic analyses needed to assess, plan intervention for, and monitor the progress of these children's individual phonological error patterns.

Obtaining the Sample

Any clinician who has been faced with eliciting a language sample from a shy 4-year-old knows how difficult a task this can be. If the child does not want to talk there is not much hope for obtaining the speech sample. The clinician must learn to shape events so that the child wants to talk. The following guidelines are suggested:

1. Prior to eliciting the speech sample interview the parents to find the child's interests and common uses of speech (communicative intents).

2. Knowing the child's interests, stock the clinic room with toys and objects the child is familiar with and has an interest in.
3. Avoid asking a lot of questions which pressure the child to communicate. Instead, manipulate the environment so that speech is appropriate. For example, when presenting toys to play with, leave the toys on a shelf out of the child's reach. If instead of talking the child points to a toy, deliberately pick up the wrong one, thus opening the door for communication.
4. Structure activities so that the child has opportunities to use speech at different levels of complexity from single word to the limits of the child's language system. A suggested activity is retelling a story using props supplied by the clinician. To elicit specific sounds the clinician might ask the child to help ''clean up'' the room. Scattered about the room would be familiar objects and toys. The clinician would start the activity by bringing out a large box or bag and explaining it is time to clean up and asking the child which toy/object should be bagged first. As the child names the objects they are put away.
5. Provide opportunities to record the child's speech patterns with significant others—mother, father, siblings—in various social activities.

Keep in mind that the goal of the connected speech sampling is to obtain an overall picture of the child's speech system. This includes information about how the child's speech changes with intent, situation, communicative need, and so on. The importance of this cannot be stressed enough. The accuracy of speech production changes with linguistic content and situations. Campbell and Shriberg (1982) examined five phonologically disabled children on their use of comments and topics in discourse. They found that phonological processes occurred significantly less often on comments than on topics. Menyuk (1980) describes the speech of five children observing that speech patterns improved when the children were attempting to communicate important (to them) information. She comments, ''The conclusion that might be reached from these data is that assessment of these children's phonological performance that does not take into account what they can do under appropriate circumstances provides a too narrow picture of their phonological abilities'' (p. 224).

Severity Measure

Figure 6.2 illustrates an analysis form for examining a connected speech sample. The form allows an adult target to child-form comparison, syllable shape inventory, sound change and phonological process analysis by word position. The first column (Item No.) is used to identify the target word from the connected speech sample. In the Target/Form column the adult surface form (target) is compared to the child's production. Column three (Syl) is used to write down the syllable shape used by the child. A target/child-form format could also be used here. The columns marked Subst are used to write in the sound substitutions which will make identification of phonological processes easier. The final column is used to identify phonological processes by number using the key located in the upper portion of the form. Item 25 in the key has been left blank for the examiner to add other processes to evaluate. Using this form a severity measure may be obtained with Shriberg and Kwiatkowski's (1982b) percentage of consonants correct (PCC). The PCC is found by dividing the number of correct consonants by the number of correct plus incorrect consonants and multiplying by 100. Incorrect consonants include

1. deletions of a target consonant;

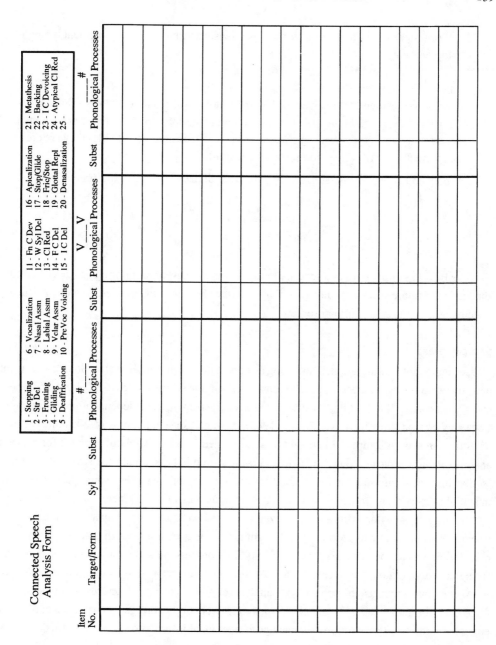

FIGURE 6.2. Connected speech analysis form.

2. substitutions of another sound for a target consonant, including replacement by a glottal stop or a cognate;
3. partial voicing of initial target consonants;
4. distortions of a target sound, no matter how subtle;
5. addition of a sound to a correct or incorrect target consonant, e.g., *cars* said as [karks];
6. initial /h/ deletion (he → [i]) and final n/ŋ substitutions (ring → [rin]) are counted as errors only when they occur in stressed syllables; in unstressed syllables they are counted as correct, e.g., feed her [fidɚ]; running [rʌnin].

Shriberg and Kwiatkowski suggest the following divisions for the PCC scores:

85–100	Mild
65–85	Mild-moderate
50–65	Moderate-severe
<50%	Severe

The PCC has utility both as a severity rating and as a means of monitoring progress. Periodic application to future speech samplings will provide the clinician with an overall value to evaluate effectiveness of the intervention program.

Sample Size

An important consideration in obtaining a connected speech sample is size. Some assessment procedures involving connected speech recommend sample sizes of at least 100 words (Shriberg and Kwiatkowski, 1980) while, for others, the sample size will vary dependent upon minimum frequency criteria (Ingram, 1981). Crary (1983) examined speech patterns of 20 subjects based on 100 word speech samples. Each sample was divided into two 50 word samples for process analysis. Results indicated that the 50 word samples supplied essentially the same information, so that little new information was gained by analysis of both samples. Some processes were missed, but these were processes with a very low frequency of occurrence.

Used in conjunction with a standardized test, a 50 word connected speech sample should provide enough data to perform a valid examination of a child's speech sound system. One potential drawback, however, is that, with only 50 words, some sounds may not reach criteria for inclusion in a phonetic inventory (at least three occurrences per word or syllable position). A larger corpus might also be preferred for analysis of other language structures. To avoid having to go back for another sample, the clinician should probably record as extensive a sampling as possible on the first occasion. In this manner, if additional information is needed it will already be available.

Disadvantages of Connected Speech

Despite the value of connected speech samples, they do have disadvantages. Bernthal and Bankson (1988, p. 206) point out the following disadvantages:

1. Individuals with severe phonological problems may be almost unintelligible, and, thus, it may be impossible to determine what they are attempting to say from a conversational speech sample.
2. Some children may be reluctant to engage in conversational dialogue with an unknown adult.

3. It is an almost impossible task to obtain a spontaneous speech corpus that contains a truly representative sample of English phonemes.

Some of these problems can be reduced or eliminated by controlling the environment and materials in which the sample is collected. To elicit speech the parents or siblings might be involved in the sample collection. To control for phoneme production, having available specific toys or picture stories can increase the likelihood of specific sounds being produced or at least attempted. The clinician might also model specific stories using puppets or other relevant materials and have the child retell the story using the provided props.

STANDARDIZED TESTS

Connected speech sampling is necessary for obtaining a representative speech sample; however, standardized tests offer advantages for the clinician that are hard to ignore. First, it is possible that phonologically disabled children will actively avoid words containing problem sounds (Greenlee, 1974; Ingram, 1975; Schwartz and Leonard, 1982). If this is the case, a spontaneous sample may not reveal speech patterns that need to be addressed in the intervention program. Standardized tests provide a representative sampling of the major English consonants not allowing operation of avoidance/selection strategies.

Second, standardized tests provide quantitative measures of severity. Placement in a remedial program needs justification and typically that means concrete scores that can be compared to a "normal" population and recorded on an individualized education plan. Severity measures will determine if a child qualifies for intervention and also provide baseline information for later comparisons to monitor progress or justify dismissal. There are several phonological assessment instruments available for describing phonological disabilities but only a few have been normed. These include *Assessment Link between Phonology and Articulation: ALPHA* (Lowe, 1986), *Bankson-Bernthal Test of Phonology* (Bankson and Bernthal, 1990), and the *Khan-Lewis Phonological Analysis* (Khan and Lewis, 1986).

A third advantage of standardized tests is time. Most of these tests can be administered in less than 15 minutes. This time is certainly less than that required for obtaining a connected speech sample and scoring time is also typically shorter. Time is a vital consideration especially in school environments where large caseloads put great demands on clinician time.

A fourth advantage is easy comparison between child-form and adult-target. As the target words are known, it eliminates problems of trying to determine what target words are being attempted by the child whose speech may be unintelligible.

Standardized tests are available for both traditional and phonological assessments. Most traditional tests describe the sound system in terms of substitutions, omissions, and distortions in word-initial, medial, and final position. They typically do not address phonological processes, syllable structure, phonological strategies, or effects of phonetic context.

Some traditional tests have been adapted to derive information on phonological processes. Lowe (1986), for example, adapted the *Goldman-Fristoe Test of Articulation* and selected items from the *Templin-Darley Tests of Articulation* for a phonological process analysis. Garber (1986) developed a phonological analysis classification for use with traditional articulation tests. Khan (1986) standardized a phonology test based on items from the *Goldman-Fristoe Test of Artic-*

ulation and Lowe (1986) developed a new phonology test (*ALPHA*) that made available both traditional and phonological analyses.

For more information on use of conventional articulation tests to obtain phonological information see Garn-Nunn (1986) and Garn-Nunn and Martin (1992). For a review of phonological assessment instruments see the Appendix 6.1. Additional information can be found in Bernthal and Bankson (1988), Creaghead, Newman, and Secord (1989), and Edwards and Shriberg (1983).

ANALYSIS OF THE SPEECH SAMPLE

Once the speech sample has been collected through connected speech sampling and standardized testing, the data are examined using various analysis techniques. Stoel-Gammon and Dunn (1985) categorize analysis into two types: independent and relational. An independent analysis examines the child's speech system as self-contained and separate from the adults. A relational analysis compares the child's productions with the adults. Under independent analysis, examples would be phonetic and syllable inventories. Descriptions of phonological processes and sound to target substitutions are examples of relational analyses.

A considerable amount of information can be obtained from the collected data. Figure 6.3 summarizes some of the data that can be collected concerning individual speech sounds. The figure is divided into information that can be obtained concerning sounds made correctly and data on misarticulated or omitted phones. The following subsections elaborate on other forms of analysis that can be performed on the collected sample.

DISTRIBUTION OF PHONES

Analysis systems typically examine sound changes with respect to place, manner, and voicing features, as well as by their distribution in words or syllables. The distributional analysis has traditionally been by word-initial, medial, and final positions, word-initial and final, or by syllable-initial and final positions. Grunwell (1986) suggests use of Syllable Initial Word Initial (SIWI), Syllable Initial Within Words (SIWW), Syllable Final Within Words (SFWW), and Syllable Final Word Final (SFWF).

The problem with these various systems appears to be the medial position, as it is difficult at times to determine if a medial consonant begins or ends the syllable or both (e.g., the medial [p] in the word paper). Grunwell's approach appears to best mirror use of consonants in medial position, though French (1988) warns that use of medial consonants may vary from child to child.

French (1988, p. 42) describes Grunwell's rules for syllabification as follows:

1. Compound words are divided according to their lexical structure, e.g., tea/spoon.
2. Single intervocalic consonants are classified as SIWW, except for [n] which is SFWW, e.g., fa/ther, sing/er. (Grunwell points out that in some cases this rule contradicts the evidence of morphology, as, for example, in wal/king.)
3. A sequence of two intervocalic consonants is divided -C.C-, e.g., cap/tain.
4. A sequence of three intervocalic consonants is divided -C/CC-, unless this results in an unacceptable initial cluster or final consonant, e.g., pen/guin but Ox/ford, since in the

CORRECT PRODUCTION		INCORRECT PRODUCTION

CORRECT PRODUCTION

1. Manner of production.
2. Place of production.
3. Use as a substitution.
4. Contrastiveness.
5. Word or syllable distribution

INCORRECT PRODUCTION

1. Developmental appropriateness.
2. Effect on intelligibility.
3. Part of larger pattern/process.
4. Stimulability.

Deletion

1. Consistency of sound change.
2. Effect of word position.
3. Effect of consonants and vowels.
4. Effect of word shape.

Substitution

1. Type of substitution.
2. Consistency of substitution.
3. Effect of word position.
4. Effect of consonants and vowels.
5. Effect of word shape.

FIGURE 6.3. Overview of information on speech sounds that can be determined from speech sampling.

second example the standard division would yield an initial cluster /sf/ which cannot occur in English.

5. Sequences of four or more consonants are divided as in (4), i.e., -CC/CC, -CC/CCC-.

PHONETIC INVENTORY

A phonetic inventory provides a listing of sounds the child is using without consideration of the targets being attempted. Thus the inventory gives the examiner insight about the motor speech abilities of the child. Figure 6.3 presents typical phonetic inventory forms for word-initial, medial, and final positions. Note that the inventories are arrayed to reflect place (from left to right) and manner (top to bottom). To complete the form, sounds that occur at least three times are circled and considered part of the child's productive inventory. Sounds that occur one or two times are considered marginal (can be marked using parenthesis or underlining). These sounds are not given full status as the clinician may have transcribed incorrectly or the production may have been a fluke. Sound productions that occur at least three times should represent sounds for which the child has productive control. A second criteria is that the sounds occur in at least two different words. This criteria ensures that the correct production was not part of an advanced form, words that better match the adult model than would be expected given the child's use of other segments in other words (Fokes, 1982).

A visual inspection of the completed inventories provides information on the child's preferences for place, manner and word position. Further inspection of phones not marked indicates areas where the child will need growth. This too can be analyzed in terms of place, manner, and word position. Klein (1984) used charts similar to those in Figure 6.4 to score substitutions and deletions as well as the correct productions from traditional articulation tests. Using whole word transcriptions, Klein suggested scoring all speech sounds in the sample in order to obtain a better

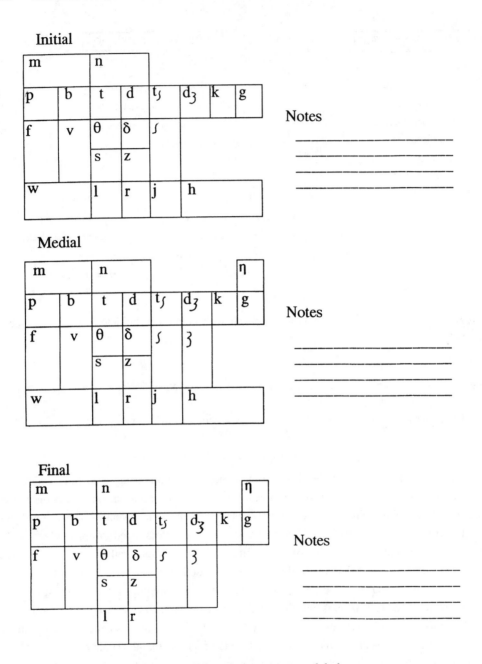

FIGURE 6.4. Phonetic inventory model charts.

overview of the child's sound system. Substitutions or deletions of a sound were scored by entering the symbol of the error below the target sound. Tally marks were then placed to the right of the error to indicate how many times the substitution or deletion occurred. Clusters were scored separately to the side of the charts.

Dinnsen, Chin, Elbert and Powell (1990) examined the phonetic inventories of 40 children between the ages of 40 and 80 months. These children had speech characterized by functional misarticulations with at least six sounds in error across three manner categories as determined from an administration of the *Goldman-Fristoe Test of Articulation* (Goldman and Fristoe, 1986). Their results found considerable variation in terms of the number and types of sounds that occurred. For example, although fricatives occurred in many of the inventories there was no single fricative that occurred in all of them. It was, however, possible to characterize the inventories into five types based on linguistic distinctions involving distinctive features.

The following descriptions of the inventories were adapted from Dinnsen, et al. Table 6.2 shows the typology of phonetic inventories for the 40 functionally disordered children.

Level A. The simplest or most limited type of inventory included nonvowels that were limited to obstruent stops, nasals, and glides. Among the obstruents, there was only a labial/alveolar place of articulation distinction. Specifically, consonants were distinguished from glides by the feature [consonantal]. Among the consonants, obstruents were distinguished from nasals by the feature [sonorant]. A predictable property of all such systems was that nasals constituted the entire set of sonorant consonants. Among the obstruents, labials were distinguished from alveolars by the feature [coronal]. Other predictable properties of such systems were that all obstruents were produced as stops with an anterior point of articulation and without a voicing distinction.

Level B. This level inventory elaborated Level A distinctions by the addition of a voice contrast and, optionally, an additional place of articulation contrast among the obstruents. Thus, Level B inventories were characterized by only two further phonological distinctions related to the features [voice] and [anterior].

Level C. This type inventory elaborated Level B by the addition of a manner of articulation distinction. Level C inventories were typified by the inclusion of fricatives and/or affricates. The features of [continuant] and [delayed release] were relevant to the characterization of Level C inventories.

Level D. The Level D inventory elaborated Level C by the addition of a liquid consonant either [l] or [r]. For all less complex inventories, nasals constituted the full set of sonorant consonants. Nasality was thus a predictable property of sonorant consonants in all simpler inventories. For Level D inventories, however, it was necessary to introduce the feature [nasal] as a distinctive (nonredundant) feature to distinguish the nasal consonants from the liquid consonants.

Level E. The most complex type of inventory (Level E) elaborated Level D by the addition of either a stridency distinction or a lateral/retroflex distinction.

Dinnsen, et al., note that their findings have clinical implications for both assessment and intervention. By comparing a client's inventory with the systems they have identified, it is possible to derive a measure of the relative complexity of the client's system. It would show where the system falls in the developmental sequence. Knowing this would also help in the selection of treatment targets by pinpointing what distinction would be expected to develop next in the sequence.

In addition to consonant inventories, phonetic analysis should include an inventory of vowels. Vowels develop early in the acquisition of the sound system but vowel errors do occur in the speech of phonologically disabled children (see Stoel-Gammon and Herrington, 1990; Pollock and Keiser, 1990; Reynolds, 1990). A vowel inventory can be completed using the vowel quadrangle (see Chapter 1, Fig. 1.2). Like the consonants, the vowel should occur on at least

TABLE 6.2.   Typology of Phonetic Inventories for Forty Functionally Disordered Children

Level	Contrastive Features	Example Inventories
A	[syllable] [consonantal] [sonorant] [coronal]	4: b d m n ŋ w j ʔh
B	[voice]	26: pb td kg m n ŋ w j ʔh
C	[continuant] [delayed release]	1) 13: pb td kg fv m n ŋ w j ʔh 2) 8: pb td kg fv sz ʃ ts dz tʃ dʒ m n ŋ w j ʔh
D	[nasal]	1) 15: pb td kg fvθð ʃ tʃ dʒ m n ŋ l w j ʔh 2) 11: pb td kg tʃ dʒ m n ŋ r w j
E	[strident] [lateral]	1) 39: pb td kg fvθðsz ʃ tʃ dʒ m n ŋ l w j ʔh 2) 17: pb td kg fv sz ʃ ts tʃ dʒ m n ŋ lr w j ʔ 3) 34: pb td fvθðsz ts dz m n l w j ʔ

three occasions and in at least two different words before inclusion in the inventory. Using the quadrangle, vowels meeting criteria could be circled and marginal vowels put in parentheses. A quick visual inspection should suffice to indicate problem areas in terms of tongue advancement and height.

SYLLABLE STRUCTURE AND SHAPE

Another form of independent analysis examines syllable shapes and canonical forms. Syllable shape refers to the arrangement of consonants and vowels within the syllable. Canonical form refers to the sequence of syllables that combine in the formation of words. At the monosyllable level the syllable shape and canonical form would be identical. A syllable shape and form inventory can reveal productive strategies or preferences of the child. For example, the child may only use open syllables in his productions. Or if he/she uses closed syllables, these might occur only with nasals in word-final position. Pollock and Schwartz (1988) present evidence that children show preferences as to what consonants are used in the production of various syllable shapes. Thus, the syllable inventory should include a listing of commonly used syllable shapes (along with a frequency count) and their structural makeup. Children may show positional preferences for segments that would be uncovered by comparing syllable structures with phonetic inventories based on syllable position. Syllables can also be examined in relation to the adult targets possibly revealing syllable maintaining or reduction strategies as discussed in Chapter 5.

SUBSTITUTIONAL ANALYSIS

A conventional form of relational analysis is a comparison of the child's substitutions to adult targets. Substitutional analysis is common to traditional three position articulation tests. Most substitutional analyses are by word position and some include frequency of occurrence information. Figure 6.5 illustrates a substitutional analysis form for word-initial and final positions.

By including data on how many times a substitution could have occurred the analysis can examine consistency as well. Note in Figure 6.5 the [t] replaced /s/ three of four opportunities. The other occurrence saw /s/ correctly produced. This shows the /s/ sound to be somewhat variable in its production providing the examiner with valuable insight for planning therapy. In

TABLE 6.3. Common Syllable and Word Shapes of English

Simple Syllables		Complex Syllables		Polysyllables	
Shape	Example	Shape	Example	Shape	Example
V	a	VCC	ask	VCV	icy
CV	she	CCV	tree	CVCV	daddy
VC	at	CCVC	stop	VCVC	upon
CVC	bat	CVCC	sink	CVCVC	misses
		CCCVC	strap	CVCCVC	pencil
		CCCVCC	stripes	CVCVCV	potato

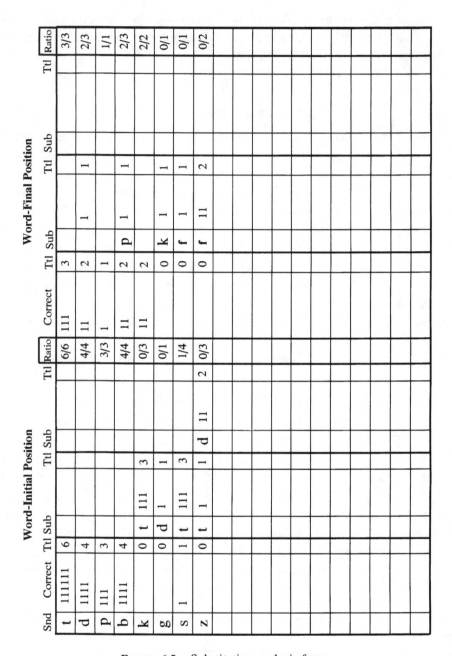

Snd	Word-Initial Position Correct	Ttl Sub	Sub	Ttl Sub	Ratio	Word-Final Position Correct	Ttl Sub	Sub	Ttl Sub	Ratio
t	111111	6			6/6	111	3			3/3
d	1111	4			4/4	11	2	1	1	2/3
p	111	3			3/3	1	1			1/1
b	1111	4			4/4	11	2	p 1	1	2/3
k		0	t 111	3	0/3	11	2			2/2
g		0	d 1	1	0/1		0	k 1	1	0/1
s	1	1	t 111	3	1/4		0	f 1	1	0/1
z		0	t 1 / d 11	2	0/3		0	f 11	2	0/2

FIGURE 6.5.   Substitution analysis form.

cases of variability, the examiner should take the time to look at phonetic context to determine what influences may be operating on the target sounds. A comparison of context where the sound changes to context where the target is correct may yield evidence of assimilation or other contextual information valuable for planning intervention.

The data also show that the word-initial /g/ had only one opportunity to occur. The examiner should note this and go back to elicit a more complete sample in order to fairly evaluate this sound. The same is true for the word-final /g/, /s/, and /p/ sounds.

Note further that the fricatives appear to be produced better in word-final position. In the initial position the fricatives are either omitted or replaced by stops. In word-final position the fricatives are sometimes replaced with other fricatives (e.g., f/s). Knowing this, the examiner might want to make use of word-final context in early attempts at establishing fricatives.

A substitutional analysis can also be completed on vowels. Pollock (1991) discusses use of traditional and phonological test stimuli to examine vowel errors. She makes some pertinent suggestions for supplementing existing stimulus items on conventional tests. The combination of a connected speech sample and conventional test should provide a fairly representative sampling of vowels for examination. Figure 6.6 illustrates a vowel analysis form that allows examination of vowel production in three contexts: closed syllable, open syllable, and multiple syllabic. Space is provided for indicating vowel changes and target items.

ANALYSIS OF PATTERNS

Two forms of pattern analysis are common to the field of speech-language pathology: distinctive features and phonological processes. Both can reveal information about sound changes

	CVC	Snd Changes	CV	Snd Changes	(C)VC(C)V(C)	Snd Changes
i						
I						
e						
ɛ						
æ						
a						
ɔ						
o						
ʊ						
u						
ə ʌ						
ɚ						
ai						
aʊ						
ɔi						
aɚ						
ɛɚ						
ɔɚ						
iɚ						

FIGURE 6.6. Vowel analysis form.

that would be missed with a segmental analysis by identifying the underlying rules that influence sound production. Distinctive features focus on identifying the subphonemic properties that misarticulations have in common. Once these properties are identified they can be targeted in an intervention program with the goal of facilitating production of not just one sound but all the sounds that share the identified features.

Phonological processes identify classes of sounds or sound sequences that change together. A process like stopping might include all of the fricatives, affricates, glides, and liquids. If stopping could be eliminated the result would be a rapid reorganization of the child's sound system.

Distinctive Feature Analysis

A distinctive feature analysis describes speech sound errors on the basis of distinctive feature properties. Costello (1975) describes such a system for the analysis of speech production. The analysis begins with a comprehensive battery of tests including the *Fisher-Logemann Test of Articulation Competence* (1971), *Goldman-Fristoe Test of Articulation* (1969), *McDonald Deep Test of Articulation* (1964), and the *Shelton Sound Production Tasks* (1969). The purpose of these various tests is to determine what sounds most consistently replace target phones. Once this has been established the distinctive feature analysis can be performed.

Costello's analysis makes use of the distinctive feature system described by Singh and Polen (1972) and presented in Chapter 4. Table 6.4 displays the analysis format. The features are listed horizontally with error sounds and their substitutions in a column to the left. The values of the features for each of the sound pairs are then entered across from the phones and below the designated feature. The feature value associated with the target phone is on the right and that of the substitution on the left. Feature values that are dissimilar are circled.

As described by Costello (1975, p. 67), "the examiner then looks down each of the columns vertically to determine if there is a predominant or consistent feature error that accounts for several phoneme errors. Such features are readily visible." As can be seen on Table 6.4, the features of stop/continuant, nonsibilant/sibilant, and front/back show discrepant values. These are the features that would be targeted in an intervention program.

TABLE 6.4. Distinctive Feature Analysis Based on Singh and Polen's (1972) Model

	Front Back	Nonlabial Labial	Nonsonorant Sonorant	Nonnasal Nasal	Stop Continuant	Nonsibilant Sibilant	Voiceless Voiced
t/0	0–0	0–0	0–0	0–0	(0–1)	0–0	0–0
d/	0–0	0–0	0–0	0–0	(0–1)	0–0	1–1
t/s	0–0	0–0	0–0	0–0	(0–1)	(0–1)	0–0
d/z	0–0	0–0	0–0	0–0	(0–1)	(0–1)	1–1
t/	(0–1)	0–0	0–0	0–0	(0–1)	(0–1)	0–0
t/t	(0–1)	0–0	0–0	0–0	0–0	(0–1)	0–0
d/d	(0–1)	0–0	0–0	0–0	0–0	(0–1)	1–1

Phonological Process Analysis

A process analysis is a form of substitutional analysis that extends beyond the segment to include classes of sounds, syllable structures, and phonetic context. Most assessment instruments attempt to identify what processes occur, how often they occur, and how often they could have occurred. In addition, some tests differentiate between developmental and unusual processes, and others examine occurrence of processes by word or syllable position. Figure 6.2 displays an analysis form for a connected speech sample. This form allows examination of processes by word position and provides a frequency count.

Identification criteria—qualitative. Dinnsen (1984) suggests that rules or processes involving substitutions and deletions function to neutralize contrasts and, as such, fall under the category of neutralization rules. For a sound change to qualify as a neutralization rule it must meet three conditions: (*a*) a phonemic contrast must be absent in a particular context, (*b*) there must be evidence of the contrast in some other context, and (*c*) there must be evidence of morphophonemic alternation.

In the first condition it is specified that in at least one phonetic context a particular phonemic contrast is missing. It is from this context that the rule is written. Dinnsen uses the example of word-final devoicing. The operation of this rule neutralizes the voicing contrast in word-final position which means that only voiceless obstruents will appear in that context. The rule could be written as follows:

$$[- sonorant] \rightarrow [-voice] / \_\_\_\_\#$$

A second condition is that there must be evidence of the contrast in some other context. Dinnsen's conditions require that the processes apply optionally. In other words, for a contrast to be lost it must first be established that the contrast exists somewhere in the child's system otherwise, instead of a dynamic rule, we would be dealing with a phonotactic constraint (see Chapter 4). Using the devoicing rule above, other contexts might be word-initial or medial position. As he explains (Dinnsen, 1984, p. 9):

> First, since the function of a neutralization is to neutralize a phonemic contrast, there must be evidence of a contrast somewhere in the system in order for it to be neutralized. The place to look for evidence of the contrast is in some position of the word where the rule presumably does not apply. That is, rules are formulated to apply only in a particular context. The devoicing rule, for example, applies only in word-final position. Consequently, in order to establish that there is, in fact, a voice contrast in the language to be neutralized, one would look to contexts other than those specified by the rule.

The third condition is one of alternation, meaning that morphemes vary in their phonetic realizations dependent upon phonetic context. For example the plural morpheme has three realizations [s], [z], and [əz]. The [s] is used following voiceless stops, the [z] following voiced sounds, and the [əz] following affricates and fricatives. These variations are sometimes referred to as morphophonemic alternations. For a neutralization rule to be identified there must be evidence of alternation between two contexts. In other words, a phoneme has one phonetic realization in one context and another in a different context. Such sound changes point out the dynamic nature of the phonological rule. Again, using Dinnsen's final devoicing example look at the following sample:

Target	Form	Target	Form
duck	[dʌk]	duckie	[dʌki]
pig	[pɪk]	piggie	[pɪgi]

In final position we have operation of the word-final devoicing rule so that the final /g/ in pig is produced as [k]. However, in medial position notice that both the [g] and the [k] phones are produced. This change shows morphophonemic alternation as influenced by word position. Dinnsen points out that the presence of such an alternation reveals some of the properties of the child's underlying representation. In this case, it provides evidence that the child is aware of the voicing distinction and that the underlying representation for pig is probably similar to that of the adult form.

Despite the availability of qualitative criteria they have seen little use in the identification of phonological processes. At present this author is not aware of any published assessment instruments that incorporate such criteria into analysis of children's sound systems. As to why, perhaps the methodology is too sophisticated for the working clinician who is not well versed in linguistics, or perhaps the information is not viewed as making so great an impact on intervention decisions as to warrant the extra effort in analysis.

Identification criteria—quantitative. McReynolds and Elbert (1981) suggested two quantitative criteria for validating the presence of processes. In their criteria they make the point that one occurrence of a sound change does not necessarily signify the presence of a process. After all, by definition a process is a sound change that affects a class of sounds. Their suggested criteria are (*a*) specific errors must have an opportunity to occur in at least four instances, and (*b*) the error has to occur in at least 20% of the items that could be affected by the process. McReynolds and Elbert explain "if the child's sample contained 20 words with final consonants, at least four of the 20 words (20%) had to be produced without a final consonant to list Final Consonant Deletion as a process present in the child's system" (p. 201). McReynolds and Elbert's purpose was to establish that criteria will have an influence on what sound changes are identified as processes; pointing out that a more stringent criteria would not identify as many processes, while a less stringent criteria would identify more.

Hodson and Paden (1983) suggest a more stringent quantitative criteria to determine if a process is in need of intervention. They recommend that a deficient pattern (phonological process) have 40% occurrence before including it in a remedial program. Processes occurring less than this will be monitored but not directly addressed in therapy.

Both of the above criteria apply well to standardized tests where the number of potential occurrences is constant. They are more difficult to apply in the analysis of connected speech samples which vary with each sampling as the clinician would have to evaluate the sample to determine the potential number of occurrences of each process. For connected speech samples the clinician may have to rely on other criteria. For example, to qualify the potential process might have to operate on at least two different sounds and occur at least four times. This criteria

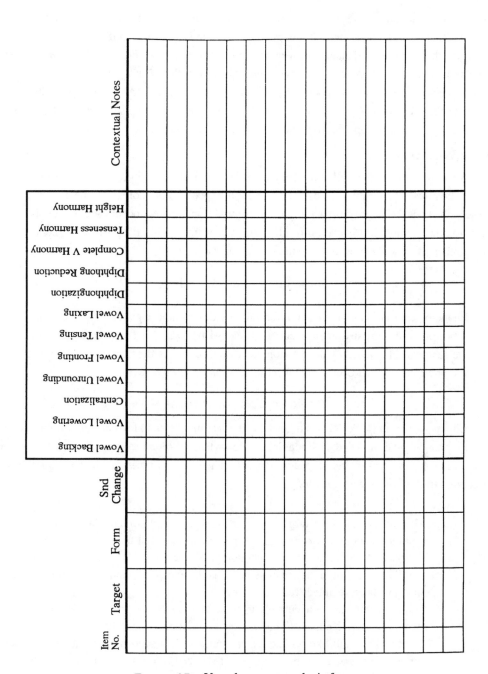

FIGURE 6.7. Vowel process analysis form.

would require that the process affect a class of sounds (two different sounds affected by same process) and occur with enough frequency to have an impact on the child's intelligibility.

Identification of sound change patterns affecting vowels can be performed much in the same way as is done for consonants. The sound changes can be listed in a column on the left and boxes checked to indicate the potential processes (see Figure 6.7). As with consonants, some criteria should be applied to qualify the sound change as a process. A suggested criteria would be the occurrence of the process with more than one vowel and in at least two different syllables.

Phonological Rules

As used in this chapter, rules are detailed explanations of phonological processes. For example, if the process of fronting is observed in a child's speech, a phonological rule can be written to describe under what conditions the process occurs. If the process occurs at every opportunity then no rule is required. However, if fronting only occurs in word-initial position, a phonological rule to that effect will better describe the sound change:

$$\textit{obstruent velars} \rightarrow \textit{alveolar} \, / \, \# \underline{\hspace{1cm}}$$

Phonological rules can be written informally by description (e.g., fronting occurs in word-initial position only), by use of segments (e.g., /k/ → [t] / #_____), or formally by using distinctive features. The value of the phonological rule lies in its description of conditions that allow sound changes. See Chapter 4 for more information on rule writing.

PHONOLOGICAL KNOWLEDGE

Elbert and Gierut (1986) have suggested that assessment should include a description of the child's phonological knowledge. Phonological knowledge "refers to a speaker's competence about the sound system of the language" (p. 49). The different types of knowledge are listed described from most to least knowledge:

Type	Description
1.	All productions of the target sound are correct relative to the adult target.
2.	Child's production of sounds is comparable to the adult target but an occasional error occurs due to an optional phonological rule.
3.	Child's production of sound is same as adults except for immature forms of words that have been retained (fossilized forms).
4.	Child produces target accurately in some word positions but errors still occur in others. The errors appear to be restricted to particular word positions.
5.	Child makes adult like productions in some word positions and some morphemes but errors are observed involving both fossilized forms and positional constraints (Types 3 and 4).
6.	Child never produces sound like the adult model.

Grunwell (1988, p. 237) interprets the descriptions of the different phonological knowledge types as statements "as to what extent the child's pronunciations match up to the adults." She argues that the descriptions do not explain substitutions the child makes when they have no or only partial knowledge of a target phoneme.

Despite Grunwell's misgivings, the information gathered from evaluating phonological knowledge have been applied with some success to the treatment of phonological disorders (Gierut, 1985; Powell, 1991). Chapter 7 will examine phonological knowledge with respect to intervention planning.

To determine Phonological Type, each phoneme must be evaluated in terms of the descriptions presented above. Information from the phonetic inventory and substitutional analysis is used in making the decisions (for more information see Elbert and Gierut, 1986). Decisions concerning phonological type can be entered on the Summary of Analysis Form (Figure 6.8).

STIMULABILITY

Stimulability refers to the child's ability to produce a speech sound under optimal conditions of auditory stimulation and feedback. Diedrich (1983, p. 298) presented a comprehensive review of the literature concerning stimulability and explains that

> the rationale for utilizing stimulability is to determine if there is consistency of a child's performance on two different speech tasks. In one, the stimulus is a spontaneous picture- or word-naming task. In the other, nonsense syllables (or words) are repeated after the examiner. If the child is consistent, similar errors are made on both tasks. The child is said to have low or poor stimulability. If the child is inconsistent, fewer errors are made on the imitative task. The child is now claimed to have high or good stimulability.

Supposedly a child with good stimulability will not need intervention to acquire the speech sound or will acquire the speech sound faster with intervention. As Diedrich points out, there is mixed evidence concerning stimulability and its prognostic value is questionable.

As used in this chapter, stimulability is a means of evaluating contextual factors that may be influencing production. Error sounds are placed in various syllable contexts and presented to the child. The purpose is to determine contexts that facilitate production. This information will be used in the selection of target words during intervention.

Stimulability should assess the effects of syllable position, shape and coarticulation. Some information concerning facilitative environments can be obtained from the phonetic inventory which will reveal where sounds occurred by position. The syllable inventory will show production preferences as well. It is recommended that sounds be evaluated in initial, intervocalic, and final position using CV, VCV, and VC syllable forms. Use of the central unstressed vowel (schwa) with these syllables for part of the assessment is recommended.

In addition, error sound production can be evaluated with the target followed by stops, fricatives, and nasals in CVC contexts again using the schwa as vowel. These contexts will evaluate possible facilitatory effects of phonetic environments. Conventional tests in this area include *McDonald's Deep Test* and the C-PAC (Secord, 1986).

PHONETIC VARIATION

There is an increasing body of evidence to indicate that children produce contrasts among sounds using phonetic distinctions which may or may not be comparable to those used by adults. Some of these distinctions may be perceptible, and others not. For example, Velten's (1943) child produced the words *back* and *bad* as [bæt] and [bæ:t]. The two words were distinguished

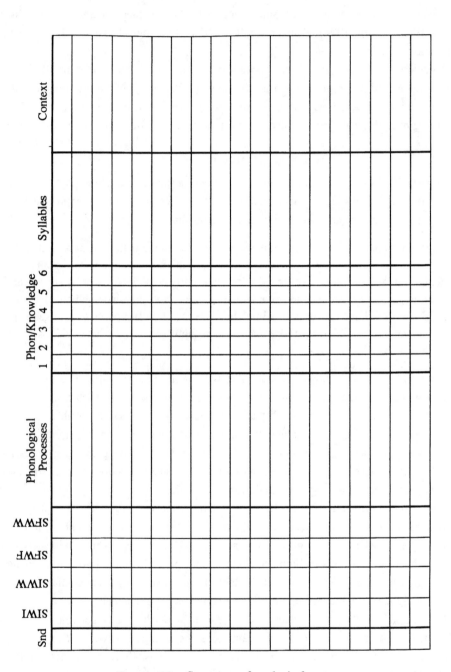

FIGURE 6.8.   Summary of analysis form.

by a lengthening of the vowel in the child's production of *bad*. Weismer, Dinnsen, and Elbert (1981) evaluated three children diagnosed as having omission of final consonants. They measured vowel durations in the children's productions of *cap* and *cab*. Results indicated that some of the children lengthened the vowel for their production of *cab*. This suggests that these children, although they omitted the final consonant, still had some phonological knowledge of the sound as evidenced by their prolongation of the vowel.

Not all differences are as perceptible as vowel length. Gierut and Dinnsen (1986) evaluated two children with similar speech patterns. Based on a phonological analysis both children had a voice contrast in word-medial and final position but not in word-initial position. However, based on an acoustic analysis, the productive knowledge of the contrasts was actually different. One child showed closure duration and VOT values that clearly differentiated between the voiced and voiceless stops. The other child showed no differences in the acoustic measures. Thus, although the phonological assessment would show these two as having the same phonological knowledge for the voicing contrast, in reality a difference existed.

The point to be made is that an auditorily-based assessment may be inaccurate and actually mislead the clinician in making diagnostic and intervention decisions. As we will see in Chapter 7 the state of a child's phonological knowledge can have a significant impact on decisions concerning treatment.

The problem of course is that clinicians typically do not have access to a sound spectrograph nor the time to invest in sophisticated analysis procedures. However, the clinician can at least be aware of potential phonetic differentiations that are perceptible as in the vowel lengthening discussed above and hopefully recognize them when they occur.

How Much Is Enough?

At this point the reader has probably come to the conclusion that any analysis that involves all of the different procedures outlined by this chapter would involve a considerable investment of time. It is not the author's position that all of these procedures are necessary for any given child. For example, if the child has an intact vowel system there would be no need to complete the vowel analysis form. Or, for that matter, if the child only makes a few consonantal errors the clinician could probably settle for a traditional sound by position articulation test.

On the other hand, if the clinician is working with a child who has a severe intelligibility problem as evidenced by multiple consonantal substitutions and omissions, then a thorough assessment of the phonological system is warranted. The author's own preferences for such an assessment battery include the phonetic and syllable inventory, substitutional analysis, phonological process analysis, and categorization of sound errors by phonological type. If vowels are in error then a vowel analysis would also be included.

The clinician is reminded of one of the axioms of the profession—each child is an individual. As such, the clinician must learn to tailor the assessment to fit the child's speech behaviors. Take, for example, the very young child. For children around 2 years of age a traditional sound to target articulation test may yield very little information. Instead, the clinician could rely on speech samples. The sampling would reveal information about the child's sound inventory, classes of sounds present, syllable shapes, match up with adult targets, and, possibly, identification of phonological processes. (For an excellent guide to phonological assessment of young children, the reader is urged to read Stoel-Gammon and Stone, 1991.) The point to be made is that clinicians need to be flexible and aware that different children may require very different approaches when it comes to assessment.

PROFILE OF A PHONOLOGICALLY DISABLED CHILD

Chapter 5 presented characteristics of phonological process use by children with phonological disabilities. It was noted that many of the processes seen in normal development are also present in the speech patterns of phonologically disabled children but their use of the processes differed. Other differences between normal and disordered phonological systems have been identified. Crystal (1981, pp. 47–48) lists the following characteristics as associated with "pure" phonological disabilities not influenced by abnormalities of an anatomical, physiological, or obvious neurological nature:

1. a restricted range and frequency of segments, with consequently fewer potential contrasts and many homophones;
2. a restricted range and frequency of segmental combinations;
3. a restricted range of features, especially affecting place of articulation (often, one place of articulation is predominant);
4. an extremely limited range of fricatives;
5. an extremely limited range of nonnasal sonorants;
6. the likelihood of voiced/voiceless (aspirated/unaspirated or fortis/lenis) confusion;
7. syllable structure tends towards a canonical CVCV form, open syllables being the norm (apart from the use of final nasals);
8. consonant clusters are generally absent;
9. use of the glottal stop as a substitute form is pervasive;
10. the vowel system is relatively well-developed, apart from a tendency to centralize;
11. a relatively wide range of sounds from outside the normal articulatory possibilities of the language.

Stoel-Gammon and Dunn (1985, p. 122) provide additional information in contrasting normal and disordered phonology:

1. static systems that plateau at an early level of development, failing to progress toward mastery;
2. extreme variability in production, without gradual improvement in production;
3. persistence of phonological processes beyond the expected ages of occurrence in normal children;
4. co-occurrence of processes that are observed early in normal acquisition (e.g., Reduplication or Final Consonant Deletion) with correct production of sounds that are normally acquired late in the sequence of acquisition (e.g., liquids, fricatives, clusters); Grunwell (1981) referred to this pattern as *Chronological Mismatch* (see Chapter 5);
5. occurrence of idiosyncratic rules or processes, which rarely occur in normal phonology; these processes significantly reduce intelligibility;
6. restricted use of contrast.

Appendix 6.2 contains a speech sample for practice using the various forms of analysis contained in this chapter. The reader is urged to complete the analysis forms. Only with practice at analysis will the reader fully understand the applications discussed. Assessment involves more than filling out charts; it more closely resembles the solving of a riddle. In this case the riddle is how the child's sound system operates.

EXPLANATIONS AND ASSOCIATED TESTING

Part of the assessment of phonological disability includes a look at factors that may cause, maintain, or in some manner complicate remediation of the disability. Areas such as perceptual dysfunction, hearing loss, structural anomalies, motor speech deficits, and speech models are examples. In an explanation of the etiology of phonological disorders, Grundy (1989) suggests that when children develop associations between objects and the sound patterns representing them, a sound pattern template (SPT) is stored. (The SPT would correspond to the child's internal representation.) Sometimes the SPT is stored accurately and sometimes inaccurately, but in both cases phonological disorders could still develop. Grundy attributes the disorders to productive, perceptual, or organizational problems of speech.

Let us examine this from the viewpoint that the SPT is stored accurately. Grundy (1989) notes there are at least two possible reasons for speech errors to occur. First, ''the connections between the stored SPT and the child's speech production center are faulty and therefore the instructions to the articulators are wrong'' (p. 257). If the instructions are wrong then production will be wrong. Second, the instructions are correct but the speech production is too complex for the child's motor abilities, thus a simpler production is substituted. These two explanations view the disorder as a problem of production where perception and organization are intact.

The speech disorder, however, may be the result of a stored SPT that is inaccurate. Grundy suggests there are at least two possible reasons for this as well. First, the child has simply misperceived the adult form (perceptual problem) and thus the SPT is wrong. Or, second, the child perceives the adult form correctly but doesn't have the capability to store the particular form in his/her present storage system. As a result, the child's system adapts the form to something that can be stored and again production will be based on an inaccurate SPT. This second explanation would explain the phonological disorder as a problem in the organizational mechanism of speech.

Another possibility, not considered by Grundy, is the speech model. If the child's speech model is inaccurate, then the stored SPT will also be inaccurate. Poor speech models not only effect development of the speech disorder but can also operate to maintain the disorder.

Given the above possibilities, the clinician should evaluate several areas that could fall under the heading of associated testing. The purpose of this testing is three-fold:

1. To determine the cause of the speech disorder.
2. To determine conditions that complicate the speech disorder or its remediation.
3. To determine conditions that may maintain the speech disorder.

PERCEPTUAL TESTING

Where possible, it is important to isolate perceptual problems that may be contributing to the speech disorder. As noted, if the child does not accurately perceive the speech model, his/her internal representation will be inaccurate leading to speech errors. Reviews on speech sound discrimination indicate that children with misarticulations often have difficulty discriminating their defective sounds, but may have no difficulty with sounds they produce correctly (Monnin, 1984). Given this relationship it seems reasonable that any evaluation of a child with misarticulations would include some form of sound discrimination testing.

Speech sound discrimination testing addresses the child's ability to distinguish between speech sounds and may also shed some light on the child's understanding of the underlying phonological structures (Winitz, 1984). Unfortunately, speech sound discrimination testing presents some definite problems when it comes to choice of test instrument (see Locke, 1980a, b). At a minimum however, it seems justified that the clinician should determine if the child can distinguish between error sounds and their substitutions at the word level. Thus, minimal pair words might be used in a pointing identification task.

HEARING DISABILITIES

Any evaluation of a child with suspected phonological disability should include, at a minimum, a hearing screening and questions related to "ear problems" on the case history. The main input for speech sound models and feedback is the auditory channel. If that channel is in some manner impaired there will likely be an effect on the speech sound system.

It should be noted that the hearing deficits do not need to be permanent in order to have a deleterious effect on the speech sound system. Shriberg and Kwiatkowski (1982a) report that children referred for phonological deficiencies often have histories of otitis media and effusion (OME). Shriberg and Smith (1983) go so far as to suggest that children with positive histories of middle ear involvement have distinguishable speech patterns. Included in their speech behaviors would be initial consonant deletion and substitutions of one nasal for another.

In summary, the assessment of phonological disability needs to include a screening of current hearing status and a developmental history that considers ear aches, tube placement, etc. The clinician should also be aware that hearing status can fluctuate due to colds and allergies and this may have detrimental affects on the intervention process.

LANGUAGE AND PHONOLOGICAL DISABILITY

Phonological disabilities are often accompanied by delays or disorders in the other components of language (Aram and Kamhi, 1982; Panagos, Quine, and Klich, 1979; Paul and Shriberg, 1982). The language connection appears stronger in children with more involved phonological disability. For example, one subgroup is composed of children who omit consonants and have a limited inventory of phonemes. Panagos (1974) labels these children syllable reducers (not to be confused with the strategy which affects the number of syllables). These children reduce CCV and CVC syllables to CV or VC form. Smit and Bernthal (1983) compare the speech of syllable reducers to children who substitute sounds but preserve the syllable shape. They note that the speech of syllable reducers is usually moderately to severely disordered in comparison to the speech of substituters which is usually rated as mildly to moderately disordered. They also summarize some of the data on these populations pointing out that:

1. In comparison with normal controls, children with substitution errors usually perform more like the normals than like the children with syllable reduction errors.
2. Children with syllable reduction errors tend to have a higher number of articulation errors.
3. Children with syllable reduction errors are slower to respond to intervention, have more

associated neurological abnormalities, have lower IQs, show decrements on measures of auditory processing of linguistic signals, deficits in central auditory processing, and deficits in sensory-receptive functions.

In their own study, Smit and Bernthal observed that the syllable reducers made more expressive syntax errors than substituters or normal controls. They also found that syllable reducers present a different error pattern when imitating syntactic forms. The reducers tended to make more substitutions of functors but they also omitted functors which the syllable maintainers rarely did. They also made more errors on pronouns.

Gross, St. Louis, Ruscello, and Hull (1985) also observed language deficits in phonologically disabled children. They compared language performance in three groups of children: Normal, Residual Error, and Multiple Error. The two articulation groups were differentiated by number of errors with the Multiple Error (ME) group also required to have at least two errors in final consonants (typically omissions). The ME group members had speech patterns similar to the syllable reducers in the Smit and Bernthal study.

The study examined several language measures including mean length of utterance (MLU), percentage of utterances containing noun and verb phrases (completeness), verbs per utterance (complexity), and an overall language error score (LES). Results indicated that the ME group showed no significant difference on MLU but produced significantly less complete and complex utterances than the other two groups. The ME group also had the highest language error scores.

The findings of these two studies and others (Paul and Shriberg, 1982; Shriner, Holloway, and Daniloff, 1969) point out the need for language evaluation to be part of the assessment battery for children with suspected phonological disability. As noted previously, a connected speech sample would have utility for assessment of both phonology and language and would seem all the more warranted given the connection just discussed.

ORAL-FACIAL AND MOTOR EXAMINATION

A standard evaluation of the speech mechanism and oral-motor abilities is to be expected in an assessment of any child with suspected phonological disabilities. Although the speech mechanism is capable of compensating for minor, and even moderate, deficits in structure, the presence of anomalies may complicate speech production and intervention. In some cases (e.g., cleft palate) surgical intervention will be required before remediation of speech production can reasonably be expected.

Oral-motor deficits may also complicate and prolong the intervention process. The prognosis and treatment for children displaying apraxic-like symptoms or dysarthria is quite different from that of the "functional" articulation child. As a step in the assessment of phonologically disabled children the presence of motor speech disorders must be ruled out.

It is beyond the scope of this text to extensively cover the areas of apraxia and dysarthria, however some information is pertinent to distinguish these organic disorders from disorders that have traditionally been called "functional" and which today are called phonological.

Apraxia

Peterson and Marquardt (1990) describe apraxia as an inability to voluntarily program movements due to damage to the anterior dominant hemisphere. A less severe form of apraxia is called dyspraxia and when it occurs in children it is often referred to as developmental apraxia of speech (DAS).

There is some controversy in the field concerning whether or not DAS exists as a clinical entity. Based on this author's experiences, there is no question of the existence of developmental apraxia. Unfortunately, and no doubt one of the reasons for the controversy, DAS is hard to diagnose. As Jaffe (1986) points out, apraxia is defined by a symptom cluster meaning that there are several symptoms of DAS but no one of them must be present to make the diagnosis. In addition, many of the symptoms could be attributed to other disorders. Jaffe presents a comprehensive list of symptoms ascribed to DAS. Some of the symptoms to look for include:

- Presence of oral nonverbal apraxia
- Gross motor incoordination
- Poor imitative skills for articulation
- Inconsistent misarticulations
- Groping trial and error behaviors in attempting speech targets
- Incorrect sequencing on complex diadochokinetic tasks
- Poor response to traditional articulation therapy methods

Dysarthria

Unlike DAS which appears to affect primarily the programming aspects of speech, dysarthria touches all of the speech processes including respiration, phonation, resonance, prosody, and articulation. The distinguishing characteristic of dysarthria is muscular impairment whereas in DAS the muscles are intact.

Dysarthric speech errors tend to be distortions and omissions of consonants. In most forms of dysarthria the errors are made consistently. The examiner, however, should focus on other aspects besides speech in making a differential diagnosis. Factors such as nasality, breathiness, monopitch, voice quality, and speaking rate help distinguish this disorder.

The reader is reminded that identified motor speech deficits in a child does not rule out the possibility of a phonological disorder. Children with motor deficits may also have problems in the organization of their sound system which further complicates speech production. This is also true of children with structural deficits such as cleft palate or velopharyngeal insufficiency. The clinician must isolate which factors are present in order to properly address them in an intervention program.

Speech Models and Developmental History

Case histories tend to be neglected, particularly in school settings where parents are often hard to contact; however, they have much to offer the clinician in terms of identifying potential causes and complicating conditions related to the child's speech system. Standard case histories may identify ongoing ear and hearing related problems, motor deficits, cognitive and linguistic deficits, and environmental factors that may hinder development of the English sound system.

Family History

There is often a positive family history for speech and language disorders. Neils and Aram (1986) evaluated 74 preschool language-disordered children and reported that 45.9% of the subjects had other family members with speech disorders. Related specifically to phonological disabilities, Lewis, Ekelman, and Aram (1989) compared families of 20 normally developing children with the families of children who had severe phonological disabilities. They found that the families of disordered children had significantly more members with speech and language disorders and dyslexia.

In a follow-up study, Lewis (1990) examined the pedigrees of four of the subjects. She found a history of three generations of members with speech/language problems. All of the histories included family members with dyslexia and learning disabilities in addition to the speech/language problems.

Speech Models

A second area to be explored by the case history is speech models. Children without question learn speech from the models they are exposed to. Asking questions related to the presence of other speech problems in the immediate family are not only important but essential in assessment of a child with phonological disability. The child may have many models to learn from including parents, siblings, relatives, neighbors, preschool friends, and even the baby-sitter. It is an important step in assessment to determine the presence of models using nonstandard English.

The presence of nonstandard English is especially relevant in bilingual homes. The child may be faced with the task of sorting out phonological rules from two very different language systems. This can be particularly difficult when the models are not used consistently (switching between languages). Chapter 8 of this text will address phonological deficits associated with cultural variance.

Attitude

As part of the case history a consideration of the child's attitude towards speech may provide some insights for intervention. Ask the parents if there is any teasing because of the speech problems. How has the child reacted? Does the child interact freely or hold back from talking? How aware of the speech errors is the child? Are attempts made at self-correction? Have they noticed any frustration on the child's part? How does the child deal with the communication problem?

Answers to these types of questions will give the clinician an idea of some of the hurdles to be faced in an intervention program. For example, the child may have come to rely on an older sibling to do the talking; as such there is little need to learn how to speak better. Or the child may be so frustrated by past failed efforts to communicate that he/she now views speaking as in some way ''bad.'' The clinician will have to arrange events in therapy to show the child that speech is ''good'' and that there is a ''need'' for communication.

Along these lines Kwiatkowski and Shriberg (1993) have started investigating the influence of two variables, capability and focus, to determine their effect on progress during intervention. Capability variables are divided into two types: linguistic factors and risk factors. The linguistic factors refer to such variables as speech discrimination ability, phonetic inventory, and phonemic inventory. Risk factors include hearing levels, auditory memory, cognitive-linguistic constraints, and psychosocial constraints (e.g., adverse child rearing practices).

Focus also has two variables: motivational events and effort. Motivational events are ''those reinforcers for speech change that occur within the child's natural environment or that are provided by the clinician during intervention'' (Kwiatkowski and Shriberg, 1993, p. 11). Effort refers to the degree to which the child will work for speech change under different levels of the motivational events.

Kwiatkowski and Shriberg are just beginning their research into the potential effects of these variables. Their preliminary findings suggest that capability and focus may be useful in the development of predictive models of speech change.

Problem Words

A final area that can addressed in the case history is particular words and sounds that give the child difficulty. This information helps focus the speech assessment and later will provide

---

Dear Parent:

　　Please complete the following questions as best you can concerning your child's speech behaviors. Your information will help determine what sounds are giving your child problems and what words would be appropriate for use in the therapy program. Return this form to the speech-language pathologist when done. Thank you.

1.　List the sounds you feel give your child the most difficulty. Please indicate at least one word in which you have heard this sound mispronounced.

Sounds   Words

_____   _____

_____   _____

_____   _____

_____   _____

_____   _____

_____   _____

2.　List people who have names your child mispronounces.

3.　List names of pets, toys, favorite foods, TV characters, story characters, etc. that are difficult for your child to pronounce.

4.　List any words in which your child has produced a problem sound correctly.

FIGURE 6.9.　Determining problem sounds and words. A questionnaire for parents.

materials for the intervention program. Figure 6.9 is a worksheet that can be filled out by the parent with help from the clinician. The data will be useful in selecting words that are meaningful and functional for the child.

SUMMARY

We have seen that assessment includes more than a simple inventory of sounds made in initial, medial, and final positions of words. Assessment of phonological disability requires viewing the child's productive speech system as the result of a complex of variables including linguistic, environmental, cognitive, physiological, and phonetic. These variables interact and have an impact on speech development. The clinician must ascertain what the impact is and how it needs to be modified to effect positive change in the child's system.

Without question, the assessment battery described in this chapter will involve a considerable investment in time, but if our profession is to grow, if our knowledge of phonological disabilities and their nature is to move forward, clinicians need to invest that time. Clinicians must move away from a technician frame of reference and toward a clinical-researcher reference. With that move we will see not only improved services for the disabled but an improved profession.

REFERENCES

Andrews N, Fey M. Language, Speech and Hearing Services in Schools 1986;17(3):187–197.

Aram D, Kamhi A. Perspective on the relationship between phonological disorders and language disorders. Seminars in Speech, Language and Hearing 1982;3:101–114.

Bankson N, Bernthal J. Articulation assessment. In Lass N, McReynolds L, Northern J, Yoder D, eds. Speech, language and hearing. Vol. II: Pathologies of speech and language. Philadelphia: W.B. Saunders Company, 1982:572–590.

Bankson N, Bernthal J. Test of phonology. San Antonio: Special Press, Inc., 1990.

Campbell T, Shriberg L. Associations among pragmatic functions, linguistic stress, and natural phonological processes in speech-delayed children. Journal of Speech and Hearing Research 1982;25:547–553.

Crary M. Phonological process analysis from spontaneous speech: the influence of sample size. Journal of Communication Disorders 1983;16:133–141.

Creaghead N, Newman P, Secord W. Assessment and remediation of articulatory and phonological disorders. 2nd ed. Columbus: Merrill Publishing Company, 1989.

Crystal D. Clinical linguistics. New York: Springer-Verlag, 1981.

Diedrich W. Stimulability and articulation disorders. Seminars in Speech and Language 1983;4(4):297–311.

Dinnsen D. Methods and empirical issues in analyzing functional misarticulation. In Elbert M, Dinnsen D, Weismer G, eds. Phonological theory and the misarticulating child (ASHA Monographs No. 22, Ch. 2). Rockville, MD: ASHA, 1984:5–17.

Dinnsen D, Chin S, Elbert M, Powell T. Some constraints on functionally disordered phonologies: phonetic inventories and phonotactics. Journal of Speech and Hearing Research 1990;33:28–37.

Donahue M. Phonological constraints on the emergence of two-word utterances. Journal of Child Language 1986;13: 209–218.

Dubois E, Bernthal J. A comparison of three methods obtaining articulatory responses. Journal of Speech and Hearing Disorders 1978;43:295–305.

Edwards M, Shriberg L. Phonology: applications in communicative disorders. San Diego: College Hill Press, Inc., 1983.

Faircloth M, Faircloth S. An analysis of the articulatory behavior of a speech defective child in connected speech and in isolated word responses. Journal of Speech and Hearing Disorders 1970;25:51–61.

Fokes J. Problems confronting the theorist and practitioner in child phonology. In Crary M, ed. Phonological intervention: concepts and procedures. San Diego: College-Hill Press, 1982:13–34.

French A. What shall we do with "medial" sounds? British Journal of Disorders of Communication 1988;23:41–50.

Garber N. A phonological analysis classification system for use with traditional articulation tests. Language, Speech and Hearing Services in Schools 1986;17(4):253–261.

Garn-Nunn P. Phonological processes and conventional articulation tests: considerations for analysis. Language, Speech and Hearing Services in Schools 1986;17:244–252.

Garn-Nunn P, Martin V. Using conventional articulation tests with highly unintelligible children: identification and programming concerns. Language, Speech and Hearing Services in Schools 1992;23:52–60.

Gierut J. On the relationship between phonological knowledge and generalization learning in misarticulating children [Doctoral Dissertation]. Bloomington, IN: Indiana University, 1985.

Gierut J, Dinnsen D. On word-initial voicing: converging sources of evidence in phonologically disordered speech. Language and Speech 1986;29(2):97–114.

Greenlee M. Interacting processes in the child's acquisition of stop-liquid clusters. Papers and Reports on Child Language Development, Stanford University 1974;6:97–106.

Gross G, St. Louis K, Ruscello D, Hull F. Language abilities of articulatory-disordered school children with multiple or residual errors. Language, Speech and Hearing Services in Schools 1985;16(3):171–186.

Grundy K. Developmental speech disorders. In Grundy K, ed. Linguistics in clinical practice. London: Taylor Francis, 1989:255–280.

Grunwell P. Clinical phonology. 2nd ed. Baltimore: Williams and Wilkins, 1987.

Grunwell P. Phonological assessment, evaluation and explanation of speech disorders in children. Clinical Linguistics Phonetics 1988;2(3):221–252.

Grunwell, P. Assessment of child phonology in the clinical context. In Ferguson C, Menn L, C. Stoel-Gammon C, eds. Phonological development. Timonium: York Press, 1992:457–483.

Healy T, Madison C. Articulation error migration: a comparison of single word and connected speech samples. Journal of Communication Disorders 1987;20:129–136.

Hodson B, Paden E. Targeting intelligible speech. San Diego: College-Hill Press, 1983.

Ingram D. Surface contrast in children's speech. Journal of Child Language 1975;2:287–292.

Jaffe M. Neurological impairment of speech production: assessment and treatment. In Costello J, Holland A, eds. Handbook of speech and language disorders. San Diego: College-Hill Press, 1986:157–186.

Johnson J, Winney B, Pederson O. Single word versus connected speech articulation testing. Language, Speech and Hearing Services in Schools 1980:11:175–179.

Khan L, Lewis N. Khan-Lewis phonological analysis. Circle Pines, MN: American Guidance Service, Inc., 1986.

Klein H. Procedure for maximizing phonological information from single-word responses. Language, Speech, and Hearing in Schools 1984;15:267–274.

Kwiatkowski J, Shriberg L. Speech normalization in developmental phonological disorders: a retrospective study of capability-focus theory. Language, Speech, and Hearing Services in Schools 1993;24(1):10–18.

Lewis B, Ekelman B, Aram D. A familial study of severe phonological disorders. Journal of Speech and Hearing Research 1989;32:713–724.

Lewis B. Familial phonological disorders: four pedigrees. Journal of Speech and Hearing Disorders 1990;55:160–170.

Locke J. The inference of speech perception in the phonologically disordered child. Part I: A rationale, some criteria, the conventional tests. Journal of Speech and Hearing Disorders 1980a;45:431–444.

Locke J. The inference of speech perception in the phonologically disordered child. Part II: Some clinically novel procedures, their use, some findings. Journal of Speech and Hearing Disorders 1980b;45:445–468.

Lowe R. Phonological process analysis using three position tests. Language, Speech and Hearing Services in Schools 1986;17(1):72–79.

Lowe R. Assessment link between phonology and articulation: ALPHA. Moline, IL: LinguiSystems, Inc., 1986.

McReynolds L, Elbert M. Criteria for phonological process analysis. Journal of Speech and Hearing Disorders 1981; 46:197–204.

McDonald E. A deep test of articulation. Pittsburgh: Stanwix House, 1964.

Menyuk P. The role of context in misarticulations. In Yeni-Kimshian G, Kavanagh J, Ferguson C, eds. Child phonology. Vol. I: Production. New York: Academic Press, Inc., 1980:211–226.

Monnin L. Discrimination testing and training: Why? Why not? In Winitz H, ed. Treating articulation disorders: for clinicians by clinicians. Baltimore: University Park Press, 1984:1–20.

Morrison J, Shriberg L. Articulation testing versus conversational speech sampling. Journal of Speech and Hearing Research 1992;35:259–273.

Neils J, Aram D. Family history of children with developmental language disorders. Perceptual and Motor Skills 1986; 63:655–658.

Panagos J. Persistence of the open syllable reinterpreted as a symptom of language disorder. Journal of Speech and Hearing Disorders 1974;39:23–31.

Panagos J, Quine M, Klich R. Syntactic and phonological influences on children's articulation. Journal of Speech and Hearing Research 1979;22:814–848.

Paul R, Shriberg L. Associations between phonology and syntax in speech delayed children. Journal of Speech and Hearing Research 1982;25:536–546.

Peterson H, Marquardt T. Appraisal diagnosis of speech language disorders. 2nd ed. Englewood Cliffs, NJ: Prentice Hall, Inc., 1990.

Pollock K. The identification of vowel errors using traditional articulation or phonological process test stimuli. Language, Speech and Hearing Services in Schools 1991;22(2):39–50.

Pollock K, Keiser N. An examination of vowel errors in phonologically disordered children. Clinical Linguistics Phonetics 1990;4(2):161–178.

Pollock K, Schwartz R. Structural aspects of phonological development: case study of a disordered child. Language, Speech and Hearing Services in Schools 1988;19:5–16.

Powell T. Planning for phonological generalization: an approach to treatment target selection. American Journal of Speech-Language Pathology 1991;1(1):21–27.

Reynolds J. Abnormal vowel patterns in phonological disorder: some data and a hypothesis. British Journal of Disorders of Communication 1990;25:115–148.

Schwartz R, Leonard L. Do children pick and choose? An examination of phonological selection and avoidance in early lexical acquisition. Journal of Child Language 1982;9:319–336.

Secord W. C-PAC: Clinical probes of articulation consistency. Columbus: Merrill Publishing Co., 1986.

Shriberg L, Smith A. Phonological correlates of middle-ear involvement in speech-delayed children: a methodological note. Journal of Speech and Hearing Research 1983;26:293–297.

Shriberg L, Kwiatkowski J. Phonological disorders I: a diagnostic classification system. Journal of Speech and Hearing Disorders 1982a;47:226–241.

Shriberg L, Kwiatkowski J. Phonological disorders III: a procedure for assessing severity of involvement. Journal of Speech and Hearing Disorders 1982b;47:256–270.

Smit A, Bernthal J. Performance of articulation-disordered children on language and perception measures. Journal of Speech and Hearing Research 1983;26:124–136.

Stemberger J. Between-word processes in child phonology. Journal of Child Phonology 1988;15:39–61.

Stoel-Gammon C, Dunn C. Normal and disordered phonology in children. Baltimore: University Park Press, 1985.

Stoel-Gammon C, Stone J. Assessing phonology in young children. Clinical Communication Disorders 1991;1(2):25–39.

Winitz H. Auditory considerations in articulation training. In Winitz H, ed. Treating articulation disorders: for clinicians by clinicians. Baltimore: University Park Press, 1984:21–49.

Velten H. The growth of phonemic and lexical patterns in infant language. Language 1943;19:281–292.

Weismer G, Dinnsen D, Elbert M. A study of the voicing distinction associated with omitted word-final stops. Journal of Speech and Hearing Disorders 1981;46:320–327.

Assessment Link between Phonology and Articulation (ALPHA)

Author: R. Lowe
Date: 1986
Source: LinguiSystems, Inc.
             3100 4th Avenue
             P.O. Box 747
             East Moline, IL 61244–0747
Description: The ALPHA uses a delayed sentence imitation format to elicit 50 embedded target words. The sentences are paired with black and white line drawings to help the client remember the target sentence. The productions are transcribed onto the test protocol using whole word transcription. The productions are then scored for sound changes in word-initial and final position.
Age Range: The ALPHA was designed for administration to children 3 years of age and older.
Norms: A total of 1310 subjects, ages ranging from 3 years, 0 months to 8 years, 11 months made up the normative sample. The normed population was obtained from midwestern cities representing rural, suburban, and inner-city areas. Subjects came from residential areas that included professionals and physical laborers.
Reliability: Test-retest reliability is reported for each of the 15 processes evaluated by the ALPHA. Average reliability ranges from a low of .83 (Syllable deletion) to a high of .99 (Backing). Of these scores 12 of 15 were above .90.
Validity: The ALPHA successfully differentiated between 154 normal and 154 phonologically disabled students (currently enrolled in speech intervention programs) for both phonemes and processes. Scores on the ALPHA also reflect developmental changes as would be expected.
Scoring: The clinician has the options of scoring the productions using a traditional format (substitutions, omissions, distortions), or using a phonological analysis, or both. Fifteen phonological processes are arranged in a scoring matrix across from the transcriptions. Boxes for processes that are not likely to occur for a target word are shaded. A check is placed in the box below the process and across from the sound change to indicate the occurrence of a potential process. The boxes are elongated so that checks on the left side represent word-initial position and checks on the right side indicate word-final position.
Analysis: The ALPHA provides scores for Percent of Occurrence of Processs, Percentile Rank, Standard Score, Standard Deviation Profile, and Total Number of Processes. Administration of the ALPHA takes approximately 10–15 minutes. Scor-

ing time will depend upon which sections are completed, but the whole test can be scored under 30 minutes.

Assessment of Phonological Process—Revised

Author:	B. Hodson
Date:	1986
Source:	Pro-Ed
	8700 Shoal Creek Boulevard
	Austin, TX 78758–6897
Description:	The APP-R is unique in its use of 50 objects, pictures, and body parts to elicit 50 utterances. The child names materials as they are presented. The APP-R was not designed to identify phonological disabilities. Instead, its purpose is to identify priorities in the treatment of unintelligible children. The revised version also includes two screening protocols: *Preschool* and *Multisyllabic*. Picture cards are included for the screening items.
Age Range:	No age ranges are given for the test; however, it has been administered to children as young as 3 years old.
Norms:	Normative data is not supplied as this instrument is designed to identify priorities for intervention.
Scoring:	The APP-R is structured to score over 40 phonological processes. The processes are identified through the child's productions of 50 different target words. Each word is scored for the presence of various processes listed in a matrix format. Unlikely sound changes have their boxes shaded across from the target word.
Analysis:	The APP-R derives a Frequency of Occurrence Score, Percentage of Occurrence, Severity Interval, and Composite Deviancy Score. The manual indicates that elicitation and transcription of the 50 items can be completed within 20 minutes. An additional 30 minutes is required for completing the analysis and summary forms.

Bankson-Bernthal Test of Phonology

Authors:	N. Bankson and J. Bernthal
Date:	1990
Source:	The Riverside Publishing Company
	8424 Bryn Mawr Avenue
	Chicago, IL 60631
Description:	The BBTOP was designed to describe consonant productions and error patterns in preschool and early elementary age children. There are 80 stimulus words elicited using a picture naming format. The child's productions are transcribed onto the test protocol using whole word transcription. A box is available to check if the response was elicited through modelling rather than spontaneous naming. The productions are later scored for errors in word-initial and final position and for phonological processes.
Age Range:	The BBTOP was designed for children in preschool or early elementary. The test

can also be administered to older children with severe phonological/articulation problems.

Norms: Normative data are available for children between the ages of 3 and 6-years-old. The test is described as being normed on a national sample. There are between 120 and 190 children for each year (3, 4, 5, and 6) in the normative samples.

Reliability: The manual reports very good reliability for the test with coefficients for the Word Inventory averaging .96, for Consonants averaging .95, and for Phonological Processes averaging .95. Test-retest reliability scores ranged from .74 for the Consonant Inventory to .89 for the Word Inventory. Test-retest reliability for the Phonological Process Inventory was .84.

Validity: The BBTOP has very good content and construct validity. The manual provides several pages of data supporting the validity of the test instrument.

Scoring: The test protocol uses multiple two-page layouts for scoring. As you open the protocol the right page allows for entering the transcription of the target word and for scoring word-initial and final consonant production. To the right of the transcription is a matrix for the consonant inventory. Under target consonants, highlighted letters F for final and I for initial position indicate the consonant to be scored. If an error occurred, the highlighted letter is to be circled. On the left page 10 phonological processes are scored in the Phonological Process Inventory. Examples of possible productions of the target word are found under the various processes. The examiner is to circle the example that matches the child's production. For both the consonant and process inventories, rows are available at the page bottom to enter total number of errors. Under the Target Word column there is also a box for entering the number of words correct.

Analysis: Each test protocol provides summary charts for initial and final consonants and phonological processes. The bottom half of these charts allow for conversion of raw scores to scaled scores. The protocol cover sheet allows for entering of scores, percentile ranks and standard scores for each of three major categories: Word Inventory, Consonant Inventory, and Phonological Process Inventory. Of these the Word Inventory is unique to the BBTOP. The Word Inventory is a general indicator of phonological accuracy. It would be a useful baseline to monitor progress over time. The test also provides confidence ranges for the three categories.

Khan-Lewis Phonological Analysis

Authors: L. Khan and N. Lewis

Date: 1986

Source: American Guidance Service, Inc.
          Publishers Building
          P.O. Box 99
          Circle Pines, MN 55014–1796

Description: The 44 words from the *Goldman-Fristoe Test of Articulation*—Sounds in Words Subtest—are used as input for phonological process analysis. The words are scored on a multipaged protocol which conveniently lists common sound changes associated with phonological processes.

Age Range: The KLPA is recommended for use in the diagnosis and description of articulation or phonological disorders in preschool children.

Norms: The KLPA was standardized on 852 children between the ages of 2 years, 0 months and 5 years, 11 months. The sample was stratified on the variables of sex, race, or ethnic group (White, Black, and Hispanic) and geographic region.

Reliability: Test-retest reliability coefficients for composite scores range from .93 to .98. Average coefficients for individual developmental phonological processes range from .54 to .95.

Validity: The KLPA has good construct validity. Scores on the test successfully differentiated among children with poor, fair, and good intelligibility. The KLPA also reflects developmental changes.

Scoring: The transcribed word is placed on the KLPA score form where sound changes are scored. The clinician then matches the sound change with sound changes indicated in columns beneath 15 different processes (12 developmental and 3 nondevelopmental).

Analysis: The KLPA provides the following measures: Developmental Phonological Process Rating, Speech Simplification Rating, Percentile Rank, Age Equivalents, and a Composite Score. In addition, the clinician can obtain a Percentage of Occurrence score for individual processes or for total processes. In addition to scores on processes, the KLPA provides for analysis of Phonetic Inventory.

Natural Process Analysis

Authors: L. Shriberg and J. Kwiatkowski

Date: 1980

Source: John Wiley & Sons, Inc.
              605 Third Avenue
              New York, NY 10016

Description: NPA is a procedure for analyzing continuous speech samples for the presence of eight phonological processes. The sample is collected during one or more of these suggested activities: the client describes activities on sequence story cards, tells a story using pictures in a book, talks about interests and experiences, makes comments while engaged in play with familiar and unfamiliar toys, comments on arrangement of small objects and figures, comments on a familiar story being viewed through a toy movie viewer.

Norms: The NPA is not normed; however, the authors provide an extensive Appendix on the acquisition of phonology.

Reliability: Test-retest reliability coefficients are not available for the NPA; however, the text cites a comparison of two administrations for one subject. For that subject 71% of 80 items agreed exactly. Another 21% of items did not agree as data were available on one data set that were not on the other.

Validity: The NPA appears to have good construct validity. It reflects developmental changes and identifies phonological processes that occur in child speech.

Scoring: Between 80 and 100 different words are transcribed onto the NPA provided transcription sheet. These words are later coded for phonological processes using NPA

Coding Sheets. The text provides clear directions for entering the data and coding the sample.

Analysis: The NPA provides information on what processes are being used, what stage in development the processes are in, and what phonetic contexts, if any, influence the occurrence of the process. In addition to processes, the NPA also includes a Phonetic Inventory.

Phonological Assessment of Child Speech

Author: P. Grunwell
Date: 1985
Source: College Hill Press
         4284 41st Street
         San Diego, CA 92105
Description: The PACS describes a set of analysis procedures to analyze a connected speech sample of approximately 100 words. Two dimensions of child speech patterns are evaluated: communicative adequacy and developmental status.
Analysis: PACS provides several measures including a comprehensive phonetic inventory, phonetic analysis of errors, contrasting phone inventory, phonotactic inventory, and phonological process analysis.

Phonological Process Analysis

Author: F. Weiner
Date: 1979
Source: Pro-Ed
         8700 Shoal Creek Boulevard
         Austin, TX 78758–6897
Description: The PPA manual describes it as a speech sampling procedure especially useful in assessing speech of the unintelligible child. Responses to the 136 stimuli of the PPA are elicited from action pictures that sample words both as single words and in the context of sentences. Procedures for elicitation involve delayed imitation and sentence recall.
Age Range: The PPA is most appropriate for children between the ages of 2 and 5 years.
Validity: The PPA would appear to have good construct validity. It identifies phonological processes and reflects developmental changes.
Scoring: The PPA provides a score sheet for each of 16 different processes. Each score sheet lists target words in sequence with the stimulus pictures of the test. The score sheet has space to transcribe the targets in response to direct imitation and sentence recall conditions.
Analysis: Among the measures obtained from the PPA are a Phonetic Inventory, Proportion of Test Processes, and Frequency of Nontest Processes (times process occurred when not specifically being tested). Space is also provided to list processes not specifically sampled by the PPA.

Procedures for the Phonological Analysis of Children's Language

Author: D. Ingram

Date: 1981

Source: University Park Press

300 North Charles Street

Baltimore, MD 21201

Description: The PPACL describes a set of procedures that can be used to complete a comprehensive phonological analysis of stimuli obtained from a spontaneous language sample, phonological diary, or through elicitation and testing. It can analyze for a wide range of phonological processes (28 are described).

Age Range: The PPACL would be most appropriate for children displaying multiple articulation errors.

Validity: The PPACL has apparently good construct validity as it is capable of differentiating between children with and without phonological disability. It is also sensitive to developmental changes.

Scoring: Eight forms are used in the analysis including: lexicon sheet, consonant inventory sheet—lexical types, consonant inventory sheet—phonetic forms, item and replica sheet, child syllable sheet, homonymy sheet, phonological processes sheet, and a summary sheet. The text provides a detailed account of how the scoring is accomplished.

Analysis: The PPACL provides four types of analysis: phonetic inventory, analysis of homonymy, substitution analysis, and phonological process analysis.

Speech Sample at Three Years of Age*

Target	Form	Target	Form	Target	Form
1 cat	[kæt]	21 kitty	[dɪdɪ]	41 did	[dɪd]
2 ladder	[læda]	22 water	[wawə]	42 shovel	[tʌbo]
3 door	[da]	23 yoyo	[jojo]	43 we	[wi]
4 gun	[dʌn]	24 balloon	[bəlu]	44 tub	[tʌb]
5 can	[dæn]	25 ball	[ba:]	45 give	[dɪ:]
6 glass	[dæt]	26 rabbit	[wæbɪ]	46 soap	[dop]
7 zip	[dɪp]	27 house	[haʊʔ]	47 zoo	[du]
8 nose	[no:]	28 choo choo	[dudu]	48 jeep	[dɪp]
9 nose	[nos]	29 dog	[da:]	49 they	[de]
10 shoe	[tu]	30 ice cream	[aɪ:tim]	50 bath	[bæ]
11 dish	[dɪ:]	31 lamp	[læp]	51 chew	[tu]
12 thumb	[tʌm]	32 bunny	[bʌnɪ]	52 teach	[ti]
13 that	[dæt]	33 carrot	[tɛwət]	53 hat	[hæt]
14 fire	[daɪə]	34 monkey	[maki]	54 sit	[dɪt]
15 tie	[taɪ]	35 bye bye	[baɪbaɪ]	55 she	[di]
16 this	[dɪs]	36 drum	[dwʌm]	56 sheep	[dip]
17 why	[waɪ]	37 block	[bak]	57 broom	[bum]
18 teeth	[ti]	38 fishing	[pɪʔɪn]	58 lamb	[læm]
19 nail	[nəo]	39 pencil	[pɛnʔo]	59 push	[pʊʔ]
20 bone	[bon]	40 yellow	[jado]	60 you	[ju]

*Source: Personal communication from Regis Mattock.

7 Intervention

Chapter

Robert J. Lowe and Julia Mount Weitz

SUCCESSFUL INTERVENTION is a process that begins with assessment, continues through the development and implementation of treatment goals, and ends with the maintenance of completed therapy objectives. Information from assessment provides the basis for developing intervention goals and objectives. Assessment data also guides the clinician in selecting appropriate stimulus materials for use with the client. Finally, assessment provides a baseline from which to measure progress during the intervention program. Chapter 6 provided information for performing a comprehensive assessment of a child's phonological system. This chapter begins where assessment ends, by applying the obtained assessment data in the development of an intervention program, and continues on to a review and discussion of language-based approaches as used in the treatment of phonological disorders.

The process of intervention can be summarized by the following sequential steps:

1. Thorough assessment and analysis of the child's phonological system.
2. Identification of target processes based on assessment data and criteria for prioritizing phonological processes for intervention.
3. Identification of target sounds within selected target processes.
4. Development of stimulus materials (word selection) for target sounds.
5. Development of language-based activities that use stimulus materials, emphasize generalization, and develop the child's phonological awareness.

SELECTION OF INTERVENTION TARGETS

PHONOLOGICAL PROCESSES

The comprehensive assessment described in Chapter 6 provides the clinician with the information needed to identify phonological processes for remediation. At a minimum, that information includes a listing of processes that occurred, a percentage of occurrence for each process, and information on the word position distribution of the processes. The clinician's next step is to determine which processes should receive a priority for treatment. The procedure may be to simply choose the processes that are most severe based on the norms of a standardized assessment

175

instrument. However, this approach may not prioritize phonological processes that significantly impair the child's communication. Norms are useful for determining delays in development or eligibility for a remedial program, but they are probably not the best resource for choosing intervention targets. The norms do not take into consideration the social consequences of the disordered phonology and it is these consequences that ultimately motivate the intervention. A better approach is to consider other factors such as impact on intelligibility or the stimulability of the affected sounds in choosing what processes to target.

Various selection criteria have been suggested for identifying target processes. McReynolds and Elbert (1981) presented data that clearly showed the influence of selection criteria on identification of processes for intervention. To be identified as a process, a sound change had to have a 20% or greater rate of occurrence. In addition, there had to be at least four opportunities for the sound change to take place. Use of the criteria reduced the number of identified processes by 50%. McReynolds and Elbert's purpose was to show the impact of selection criteria, not to establish the criteria. At present only Hodson and Paden (1983, 1991) have recommended an actual criteria for identifying processes for intervention. They recommend that a process have an occurrence at or above 40% to qualify for intervention.

Concerning other criteria or guidelines for process selection, Edwards (1983) presents the most comprehensive list. However, she notes that it may not be possible to define a set order in the remediation of processes. Instead, she suggests the following as principles to be considered in making the choices:

1. Choose processes that result in early success, processes that would be relatively easy to remediate.
   a. Select processes that are optional, i.e., their frequency of occurrence is less than 100%.
   b. Select processes that are context-specific or position-specific.
   c. Select processes that affect sounds in the child's phonetic inventory (sounds that child is already capable of producing).
   d. Select processes that affect sounds for which the child is stimulable.
2. Choose processes that are "crucial" for the individual child.
   a. Select processes that are deviant, unusual, or idiosyncratic, e.g., velarization, lateralization, frication of stops, or glottal replacement. Such processes call attention to a child's speech and, therefore, they should be early candidates for therapy.
   b. Select processes that contribute significantly to the child's unintelligibility.
   c. Select processes that result in extensive homonymy.
   d. Select processes that lead to the neutralization of adult contrasts.
   e. Select processes that apply frequently.
3. Choose "early" processes or processes that affect early sounds.
4. Choose processes that interact.
   a. If two or more processes interact to account for a complex substitution, start with a process that occurs alone, as well as "intertwined" with others, and choose a process that will allow you to work on two or three pairs of sounds at once. (The members should differ by just one feature.)
   b. If there are ordered processes, with one "feeding" or producing input for another, begin with the process that is ordered last.

A different approach is advocated by Hodson and Paden (1983, 1991). Based on their assessments of 125 phonologically disordered children, they recognize four general levels of intelligibility each of which has associated phonological processes. Table 7.1 presents the levels (0 through III) and the deficient patterns that characterize them.

Processes associated with the lower levels (0 and I) are considered more detrimental to intelligibility and thus have a priority for remediation over higher level processes. To be considered for remediation, Hodson and Paden also stipulate that the deficient pattern have an occurrence of 40% or above. If this criteria is met, a lower level process is given a priority for intervention over a higher level, even if the higher level process occurs more often.

TARGET SOUND SELECTION

After selection of the processes to be targeted for remediation, the clinician will have to decide which sounds affected by the processes are to be targeted. It may seem contradictory at this point that a book emphasizing phonology would still focus on the treatment of sounds, but the misarticulation and/or omission of speech sounds is what results in communication failure for the phonologically impaired child. To improve the child's speech communication, the child's production of target sounds must approximate accepted standards for the language. It is quite possible, and in fact is still standard practice for many clinicians, to approach remediation of phonological disorders using a traditional sound by sound approach. However, we will see later in this chapter that language-based approaches better reflect what we know about phonology and how children use speech.

TABLE 7.1.   Deficient Patterns According to Intelligibility Levels

Level 0	**Level II**
Omissions	Omissions
Obstruents and Liquids (less frequently,	Cluster Reduction
Glides and Nasals)	Strident phonemes, especially in clusters
Level I	Major Phonemic Substitutes
Omissions	Stopping
Syllables	Liquid Gliding
Prevocalic Singletons, usually Obstruents	Vowelization
(sometimes Sonorants)	**Level III**
Postvocalic Singletons, usually Obstruents	Nonphonemic Alterations
(sometimes Nasals)	Tongue Protrusion (including both Frontal
Cluster Deletion	Lisp and Dentalization)
Major Place Substitutes	Lateralization
Fronting of Velars	Major Phonemic Substitutes
Backing	Affrication or Deaffrication
Glottal Replacement	Minor Place Shifts (including "th" Shifts,
Voicing Alterations	Palatalization or Depalatalization)
Prevocalic Voicing	Vowel Alterations
Prevocalic Devoicing	Devoicing of Final Obstruents
Miscellaneous Patterns	
Reduplication	
Vowel Deviations	
Idiosyncratic (child-specific) rules	

Again we turn to Edwards (1983) for criteria to be used in selecting target sounds. You will notice that the criteria are very similar to those suggested for phonological process selection. Edwards provides the following guidelines for selection of target sounds:

1. Choose target sounds that are in the child's phonetic repertoire.
2. Choose sounds for which the child is stimulable.
3. Choose sounds that should improve intelligibility.
4. Choose frequently occurring sounds.
5. Choose sounds that are acquired early.
6. Choose high-value sounds, that is sounds that will have an impact for the child. For example, sounds that might cause the child embarrassment if used incorrectly.
7. Choose sounds that should be relatively easy to produce in the position of concern.

Hodson and Paden (1983, 1991) suggest a very simple criteria for target sound selection. You use the sound that the child is "ready" to produce. This means that the target sound will be the one the child produces with the least difficulty. To determine this, Hodson and Paden rely heavily on probing the child's phonological system to determine which sounds are stimulable. If the child is not stimulable for a sound then it will not be targeted for intervention until a later time. It is assumed that, as the child is exposed to more stimulable sounds, the more difficult sounds will eventually become stimulable as well. Their results generally support this assumption.

Elbert and Gierut (1986) suggest criteria for choosing target sounds based on a set of predictions. Predictions are projections of what sounds will develop if other sounds are taught. They derived these predictions from their research of the generalization literature. For example, a prediction about sound cognates is that teaching one member of a cognate sound pair will result in improved production of the other member. Elbert and Gierut suggest that basing target selection on predictions will reduce the number of sounds that need to be taught in therapy because teaching certain sounds will essentially "force" the development of others. Following is a listing of the sound changes that can be expected to occur based on Elbert and Gierut's (1986, pp. 105–107) literature review:

PREDICTION: Teaching one member of a cognate sound pair will result in the use of the other sound in the pair.

Example: A child does not produce [s] and [z] correctly.
Treatment: Teach [z] production.
Prediction: Production of [s] will also improve.

PREDICTION: Teaching one allophone will result in the production of other related allophones.

Example: A child does not accurately produce [r], [ɝ] or [ɚ].
Treatment: Teach [ɝ] production.
Prediction: Production of [r] and [ɚ] will also improve.

PREDICTION: Teaching a distinctive feature in the context of one sound will result in the use of that feature in other untreated sounds.

Example: A child does not accurately produce [f, v, s, z, ʃ].
Treatment: Teach [+strident] feature by contrasting [s] with [θ].
Prediction: Untreated sounds with the [+strident] feature [f, v, z, ʃ] will also improve.

PREDICTION: Teaching sounds in the final position of morphemes will result in more accurate production of the sounds in inflected intervocalic contexts.

Example: A child does not produce [s] accurately.

Treatment: Teach [s] word-finally in the context of words like "kiss," "miss," "hiss."

Prediction: Production of [s] will improve intervocalically in words like "kissing," "missing," and "hissing."

PREDICTION: Teaching stops in word-final position will lead to more accurate production in word-initial position.

Example: A child does not produce [k] or [g] in any word position.

Treatment: Teach production of [k] and [g] in word-final position.

Prediction: Production of [k] and [g] in word-initial position will also improve.

PREDICTION: Teaching fricatives in word-initial position will result in more accurate production of fricatives in word-final position.

Example: A child does not produce [f] or [v] in any word position.

Treatment: Teach production of [f] and [v] in word-initial position.

Prediction: Production of [f] and [v] will also improve in word-final position.

PREDICTION: Teaching fricatives will result in more accurate production of stops.

Example: A child does not accurately produce the fricatives [f, v, s] or the stops [d, k, g].

Treatment: Teaching production of [f, v, s].

Prediction: Production of the stops [d, k, g] will also improve.

PREDICTION: Teaching voiced obstruents (stops, fricatives, affricates) will result in accurate production of voiceless obstruents.

Example: A child does not accurately produce [tʃ] or [dʒ].

Treatment: Teach production of [dʒ].

Prediction: Production of [tʃ] will also improve.

PREDICTION: Teaching sounds that are stimulable results in more accurate production than teaching sounds that are not stimulable.

Example: A child does not produce [θ] or [ð] but is stimulable on production of [θ].

Treatment: Teach production of the stimulable sound [θ].

Prediction: Production of [ð] may improve, but production of the [θ] will still be better.

PREDICTION: Sounds that are phonologically "known" will be produced more accurately than sounds that are phonologically "unknown."

Example: A child has knowledge of stops in all positions, but uses an optional rule of word-final deletion. The child does not use affricates in any position.

Treatment: Teach production of affricates, which are phonologically "unknown."

Prediction: Production of stops will be more accurate than production of affricates, even though stops were not treated.

PREDICTION: Teaching sounds of which a child has least phonological knowledge ("unknown" aspects of phonology) will result in changes across untreated aspects of the sound system.

Example: A child uses optional rules affecting production of stops, has a positional constraint against production of liquids word-initially, and has an inventory constraint against production of fricatives. This child has least phonological knowledge of fricatives.

Treatment: Teach production of fricatives.

Prediction: Production of fricatives will improve as well as the other untreated aspects of the sound system, namely, production of stops and liquids.

A system of target selection making use of Elbert and Gierut's predictions, as well as some of Edwards' guiding principles, should yield a viable pool of target sounds for remediation. Some principles, such as ease of production, are incompatible with the predictions, and the clinician will have to decide which approach will best meet the needs of his/her client. For example, if the client shows low motivation for working on his speech, choosing a sound that can be developed easier might have priority over a sound that will lead to more generalization, as initial success at sound change may encourage the child to attempt other target sounds.

CHOOSING STIMULUS WORDS

Perhaps one of the most important decisions to be made by the clinician concerns the stimulus materials that will be used in restructuring the client's sound system. Traditionally, little thought was given to stimulus word selection. Clinicians typically relied on the materials found in a kit or pictures cut from a magazine. As a result, children would practice sound production in words that they might never use in conversation (e.g., butterchurn to practice the [tʃ] sound), or words that might have very difficult phonetic contexts.

With the emphasis shifting to language-based approaches in treatment and away from phonetic approaches, the word level has become the starting point for therapy activities. It is at the word level that sounds make a meaning difference, and it is at the word level that children can perceive the function of sounds in communication. As such, selection of appropriate word stimuli should not be left to chance but done in an informed manner.

Selection of word stimuli requires that the clinician consider several aspects of words. These aspects include phonetic context, meaningfulness, communicative potency, syllable shape and phonetic inventory. These aspects overlap to some extent but will be described in this chapter as separate entities.

Phonetic Context

The inventory and arrangement of consonants and vowels within the word can have a significant influence on its production. Some contexts will facilitate correct production of target sounds while others will make production extremely difficult. Phonetic context can be used to develop a complexity continuum with intervention beginning with easier contexts and gradually progressing into more and more difficult contexts.

Fleming (1971) and Kent (1982) summarize much of the information available concerning phonetic contexts. The general principles are reviewed next.

Stress. Production of target sounds should be easier in stressed syllable contexts. As described by Kent (1982, p. 67), "these syllables help to assure distinctive and well-formed (non-reduced) articulations, and . . . stressed syllables convey a greater acoustic contrast to help the clinician evaluate the sound pattern."

Word or Syllable Position. In general, sounds are easier to produce in word-initial position. However, there is considerable evidence pointing out that individuals may have their own preferences for word position. Some data suggests, for example, that word-final position may be an easier context for the emergence of fricatives (Edwards, 1979, cited in Edwards and Shriberg, 1983; Farwell, 1977; and Ferguson, 1975). Kent also reports on data indicating that for the /s/ sound, word-final context appears to be more facilitating than word-initial.

If the clinician is interested in finding the easiest context, it is best to complete stimulability testing of target sounds in different word positions. The clinician can also look at the child's phonetic inventory to determine if the target appears in specific word positions whether or not it was the intended production. A final option is to look for sounds made with the same or similar manner and where these occur in word contexts.

Adjacent Sounds. Production of a target sound can also be influenced by the sounds that precede and follow it. This influence can be facilitative or inhibiting to accurate sound production. Kent describes two types of facilitative contexts. The first occurs when interaction of articulations of a word minimally interferes with production of the target. The second occurs when the target is very similar to its neighboring sounds. In both cases, it appears that the more minimal the production adjustments needed between the target sound and its neighbors, the easier the context. Gallagher and Shriner (cited in Kent, 1982, p. 70) explain that "large articulatory adjustments seem to place more constraints on the speech production mechanism, and correspondingly, the chance of error for segments within the motoric unit is increased."

Number of Problem Sounds in the Context. The more problem (error) sounds in the context the more difficult that context is for production of a target. If possible, the target sound should initially appear in contexts where it is the only error sound. The remaining sounds in the context should be taken from the child's phonetic inventory taking care to note word position. For example, if the target sound is [s] and it is being targeted in CVC syllables, the clinician might want to try word-final position. That leaves selection of the initial consonant for the target word. Which initial consonant to use can be based on the child's phonetic inventory in that position, as well as on some of the other contextual factors presented in this section.

Presence of the Sound Substitution or Phonetically Similar Phone. The presence of a sound which is acoustically or visually similar to the target will usually interfere with the articulation of that target sound. As Fleming (1971, pp. 363–364) explains, "if a person habitually substitutes /p/ for /f/, he is likely to say 'pup' for 'puff,' particularly since the context begins with the sound he normally says in place of /f/."

Number of Other Sounds and Syllables in the Context. In general, simpler contexts facilitate the production of a target sound. Thus it is generally advisable to begin sound training in one syllable words rather than in polysyllabics or in phrases. Given that the CV is the most natural syllable shape found in the world's languages, it may be the syllable shape of choice when initially beginning therapy.

Hodson and Paden (1983) suggest specific target words to be used during Cycle One of their intervention program. They note that these words offer a starting point and have been found to be successful with a number of their clients. The words are listed in Table 7.2.

Meaningfulness

A second consideration in choosing stimulus words for language-based approaches is meaningfulness. By meaningfulness is meant the degree of familiarity associated with the word by

TABLE 7.2.   Suggested Target Words Used by Hodson and Paden in Cycle One

Final Obstruents	
Final /p/	rope, soap
Final /t/	hat, boat
Final /k/	lock, bike
Consonant-Vowel-Consonant	
/p/ -vowel- /p/	pipe, pop
Syllableness	
Two-syllables	cowboy, baseball
Three-syllables	cowboy hat, baseball bat
Velars	
Final /k/	rock, lock
Initial /k/	car, cow
Final /s/ -clusters	
/ts/	boats
/ps/	ropes, cups
/ks/	books, bikes
Initial /s/ -clusters	
/sp/	spoon, spot
/st/	star, stop
/sm/	smoke, smile
/sn/	snake, snow
/sk/	sky, school
Liquids	
Initial /l/	lock, log
Initial /r/	rock, rug

the child. In general, the more familiar the child is with a word the more likely the child is to include it in his/her active vocabulary. Familiar words are also desirable because they avoid recall errors. Aitchison and Chiat (1984) reported on a study of 90 English children between the ages of 4 and 9 with normal articulation. These children were shown pictures of common (e.g., pig, rabbit, elephant) and uncommon animals (e.g., mongoose, bandicoot, cuscus, raccoon, armadillo) and asked to name them. When an unknown animal was shown, the child was told the proper name and given a short description of it. The pictures of the unknown animals would appear later and the examiners transcribed the child's production of the names.

Results of the study indicated that subsequent productions of the uncommon animal names were often in error. The examiners noted reduction to a CV syllable structure, consonant harmony, omission of unstressed syllables, consonant substitutions, and other errors. It would appear that in learning the new words there was a faulty recall of the names and the children applied many of the simplification rules associated with younger children. The point is that in introducing problem sounds, it would be best to use familiar words so as to avoid the added complication of memory demands.

The other advantage of meaningfulness is that children appear to learn sounds at a faster rate when sounds are embedded within meaningful material. Hillard, Goepfert, and Farber (1976) and Hillard and Goepfert (1979) developed the Semantically Potent Word Approach to articulation intervention. This approach is based on research in the reading literature. Their study of the literature indicated that children more easily learned to read words that were emotionally meaningful to them while at the same time they had difficulty learning to read words found in traditional textbooks. Carrying this over to speech, it stands to reason that children would also have an easier time learning new sounds in words that are meaningful. Thus, words like the child's name or names of pets, friends, favorite activities, and words that are frequently used make for better stimulus materials.

Communicative Potency

Related to meaningfulness is the concept of communicative potency or how functional words are in a child's communication system. Words like "no," "go," and "stop" are communicatively powerful as they allow the child to operate on and manipulate the environment. Short phrases also fall under this category. Phrases like "give me," "that one," and "some more" allow the child to control his/her environment and thus demonstrate the value or power of effective communication. Both the Semantically Potent Word Approach (Hillard, Goepfert, and Farber, 1976) and Communication Centered Instruction (Low, Newman, and Ravsten, 1989) rely on using words that show children how functional (useful) a tool speech is when used accurately.

Phonetic and Syllable Inventory

Perhaps one of the most useful sources of information for choosing stimulus words is the child's phonetic and syllable shape inventories. This information reveals what the child is capable of producing and what forms are preferred. As noted earlier, the phonetic inventory is useful for choosing consonants and vowels that make up the nontarget components of the stimulus words. Their presence in the inventory indicates that the child has the phonetic capability of producing these sounds (especially if using stringent criteria for inclusion). One caution is that the clinician should determine if these sounds can be made upon demand. Although they occur in the inventory this does not necessarily mean that the sounds are controllable at a conscious level by the child.

Syllable shape preferences are a further consideration when developing stimulus words. If a child consistently reduces CVC words to CV syllables, then the clinician should avoid introducing the target sound in CVC syllable shapes because the child has difficulty producing final consonants. The obvious exception to this would be when final consonant deletion is the target process to be remediated. By considering the child's preferences for syllable shape, the clinician can choose words that will minimize complexity and thus increase the likelihood of accurate production of new target sounds.

LANGUAGE-BASED INTERVENTION

Once target sounds and stimulus materials have been chosen, the clinician has several options for intervention programs. As we are viewing errors within a linguistic framework, the programs of choice are language-based. Language-based approaches take the view that a child is phonetically capable of correct sound production but does not use the sounds because of problems in the cognitive organization of the sound system. In other words, the child's errors result from problems in rule learning. Support for this view is evident in the types of errors that children make. Children's sound errors are systematic. In other words, the errors are such that they can be described with rules or more general phonological processes. These rules control how sounds are combined and how they function to contrast with one another. It follows then, that intervention should focus on restructuring or reorganizing the sound system so it functions closer to that of the adults.

Language-based approaches to intervention of phonological disorders have several features in common that distinguish them from phonetic or motor treatment programs.

1. *Intervention begins at the word level.* Language-based approaches focus on the function of speech sounds in language and that function is to differentiate between words. The disorder is considered phonemic in nature not phonetic. Thus, language-based approaches typically begin intervention at the word level and most will focus on the use of sounds in words by contrasting minimal word pairs.

2. *Intervention focuses on development of the phonemic system.* Children with phonological disorders have poorly developed phonemic systems resulting in production of inappropriate homonyms and nonsense words. Expansion of the child's phonemic system will increase the number of contrasts available with a consequent decrease in errors that result in error homonyms and nonsense words.

3. *Activities highlight the communicative function of speech.* Language-based approaches often include activities that emphasize use of speech as a tool where accurate production achieves desired outcomes and error production results in communicative failure. Such activities use natural consequences of clear communication as the reward for use of appropriate speech sounds.

4. *Use of drill is limited.* Although drill work may be part of the language-based approach, it plays a minor role in the development of the target speech sounds. Language-based interventions emphasize a change in the child's phonological system at the covert or underlying level that subsequently result in a change at the phonetic or surface level. Drill work may be used to help the child master the phonetic requirements (motor patterns) of a new speech sound, however actual incorporation of the sound into the phonemic system is accomplished through development of the child's phonological knowledge.

5. *Procedures emphasize rule discovery.* Where phonetic approaches focus on sound production, language-based approaches encourage the child to discover the rules that control production. What this means is that a language-based approach will try to remediate rules for sound changes affecting classes of sounds rather than just one sound at a time. Thus, for the child who evidences the process of stopping, the clinician will focus on the elimination of the stopping process which will affect production of several speech sounds (e.g., [s], [z], and [f]). In contrast, a phonetic approach will focus on one sound at a time emphasizing accurate production. Actual intervention in both approaches may focus on the same sound but the activities, techniques and goals are considerably different.

GOALS OF REMEDIATION

From the foregoing, it follows that the primary goal of remediation is to force the reorganization of the child's sound system so that it matches the adults. A large part of that goal hinges on the child's ability to use sounds in a contrastive manner. In fact, Ingram (1989) views the intervention process as helping the child acquire the ability to use sounds contrastively. He describes this process as eliminating rules that simplify the child's speech while at the same time assisting the child to use more and more sounds contrastively. Ingram describes three aspects of a child's phonology that are a central part of remediation. They are (a) the elimination of instability, (b) elimination of homonyms, and (c) establishment of contrasts. To these we can add a fourth primary objective of intervention, that of generalization.

Elimination of Instability

Ingram observes that children's speech is often unstable, meaning that a given word may be produced with a variety of phonetic forms. He cites Oller and Eiler's (1975) example of a hard-of-hearing girl's production of the word ''pencil.'' The child produced 13 different forms for this one word. As part of the remediation process it would be important to establish one consistent form for the target word. Consistent production will improve the child's intelligibility (because adults will be able to follow the rule system) and also allow the sounds in the word to be contrasted with minimal pair stimuli.

Elimination of Homonyms

Child homonymy results in the production of two or more different adult forms as the same phonetic form. For example, Ingram describes one child, Aaron, who used the form [dado] to represent six different words: butter, ladder, letter, spider, water, and whistle. Homonyms make excellent therapy material as the referents can be used to point out how sounds change the meaning of words. Child homonymy can also be very detrimental to intelligibility so that the clinician might give a priority to elimination of phonological processes that cause the homonyms.

Establishment of Contrasts

The previous goals will eliminate processes associated with words within the child's sample that are unstable and/or result in homonyms. In addition to these, Ingram suggests adding words to the child's active lexicon which contain specific sounds that will expand the child's contrastive system. Which sounds to target can be based on developmental information which usually follows the rule that children will learn more general contrasts first. However, as will be discussed in the section on maximal oppositions, some practitioners suggest choosing targets based on the child's phonological knowledge of the sound system and feature differences.

Generalization

Stimulus and response generalization are desirable events in therapy. Stimulus generalization occurs when learned responses to a particular stimuli can be evoked by other, similar stimuli. For example, stimulus generalization is said to occur when correct articulation following an auditory model carries over and occurs in response to a visual cue (without the auditory model). Response generalization, in contrast, refers to a learned response carrying over to effect untreated behaviors. For example, response generalization occurs if training correct production of the /f/ sound results in improved production of the /v/ sound that was not trained.

Many other kinds of generalization are possible. In traditional therapy for sound production, and especially therapy based upon operant theory, generalization includes production of a newly-learned sound target in untrained words and production of a cognate of the target sound (Elbert, Shelton, and Arndt, 1967), production that extends to a different word position (Elbert and McReynolds, 1978; Rockman and Elbert, 1984), extension to other sounds sharing the same features as the target (Costello and Onstine, 1976; McReynolds and Bennett, 1972), and production of the target sound in longer or more complex utterances, including spontaneous conversation (Elbert, Dinnsen, Swartzlander, and Chin, 1990). Generalization occurs for phonological processes as well. When targeting a particular process, generalization might be thought of as the extension of learning to other phonemes which are affected by the process but which have not been worked with directly.

Generalization of trained responses to untrained consonants is described by Stoel-Gammon and Dunn (1985, p. 173) as "a primary goal of eliminating processes." Language-based approaches assume that generalization will take place if one or more examples of a phonological rule are learned. If not, then every error sound would have to be taught in every word they appeared in. There is considerable evidence that generalization does occur (Compton, 1970; Dunn and Till, 1982; Elbert and Gierut, 1986; and Weiner, 1981); however, Elbert and Gierut (1986) warn that generalization doesn't just happen but must be planned as part of the intervention process.

An opposing view of generalization is presented by Kamhi (1988). He, among others, argues against stimulus generalization, indicating that the traditional concept of generalization assumes "that the learning problem lies in the generalization mechanism rather than in the knowledge base or in noticing the occasions to apply existing knowledge" (p. 308). Citing literature for language disordered children and young children, Kamhi presents evidence to support the belief that language disordered children may take longer (i.e., more trials) to achieve mastery of a rule, but that once mastery is achieved, generalization progresses in the same manner and speed as for normal children. In other words, generalization is dependent upon rule mastery. Kamhi's position is that we must examine the child's knowledge of linguistic rules to explain generalization.

Kamhi suggests that the child's knowledge constitutes a "cognitive system" (Fey, 1988, p. 273) that underlies behavioral manifestations of a linguistic rule. Generalization to connected speech is taken as an indication that "the child has integrated what has been learned about sound production and usage into his or her own phonological system" (Elbert, et al., 1990, p. 694). This knowledge of linguistic rules is deficient when generalization does not take place.

Johnston (1988) points out that the learning of new language rules progresses through several developmental stages and complete mastery of a rule is not an immediate happening. In the final stages of rule learning, automatization is necessary. Accordingly, Johnston advises speech-language pathologists "to distinguish between activities that will promote rule learning and activities that will promote effortless rule utilization" (p. 314). We tend to think of the former as a language or cognitive approach (Masterson, 1993) and the latter as phonetic training, usually employing a drill format. Elbert, Powell, and Swartzlander (1991) contend that both the integration of phonemes into the child's system and automatic production skills are necessary for generalization to occur. In other words, there is still room for some drill work even when taking a language-based approach to intervention.

Several factors have been identified which appear to facilitate generalization. Earlier we reviewed the use of predictions which would lead to greater generalization in choosing target sounds and in the section on instructional procedures we will see that choice of stimuli for minimal pairs also influences the degree of generalization. Dunn (1983) outlines three broad measures for effecting stimulus generalization:

1. Introduce diverse stimuli systematically.
2. Vary activities along a continuum from drill to free play.
3. Vary people and settings.

Diverse stimuli. By diverse stimuli is meant the use of different procedures for evoking target words, e.g., using pictures at one time and objects at another or using open ended sentences or verbal cues. Often overlooked are the kinds of verbal stimuli used to evoke targets. The clinician should incorporate a variety of verbal stimuli, e.g., questions, commands, statements, etc. Dunn (1983) also recommends that words from different grammatical classes be selected.

Varying activities. Dunn (1983) recommends varying activities with some being highly structured and others unstructured. Dunn points out that establishment activities tend to be more structured. By this, Dunn means that the clinician carefully controls antecedent and consequent stimuli when attempting to establish consistent production of the target sound. Once the sound has been established with some consistency, activities designed to promote sound use in conversations are incorporated and these tend to be less controlled. It needs to be stated, however, that even structured activities may incorporate features of naturalism and that naturalistic activities can be structured (Lowe and Mount Weitz, 1992; Shriberg and Kwiatkowski, 1982).

Shriberg and Kwiatkowski (1982) identified and evaluated four intervention structures: Drill, Drill Play, Structured Play, and Play. These intervention structures are differentiated from each other on the basis of (*a*) antecedent instructional events designed to evoke correctly produced target responses from the client; (*b*) subsequent instructional events, those stimuli which occur after the child's response, which focus on response definition (criteria for a correct response); (*c*) antecedent motivational events, such as advancing in a game, which might accelerate learning by heightening the child's interest and receptivity to cues; and (*d*) subsequent motivational events, such as reinforcers. Table 7.3 presents the characteristics of the four different intervention structures.

The researchers found that Drill and Drill Play were the most effective procedures for obtaining correct production of targets. These structures are characterized by (*a*) intervention contexts in which children are instructed about response requirements, (*b*) set response criterion in which motivation prompts the response, and (*c*) feedback with opportunities for correction and contingent reinforcement. They appear to be more effective than those structures that focus more on play and provide incidental teaching opportunities. Clinicians rated Drill Play to be the most effective, most efficient, and the structure that they personally preferred. Children, not unexpectedly, preferred Play most, then Structured Play, followed by Drill Play and, least of all, Drill.

Vary people and places. Another way of achieving generalization is to vary the people who train the child and the settings where training takes place early in the treatment process (Dunn, 1983; Shriberg and Kwiatkowski, 1987). It is not uncommon to train parents to do therapy in the home setting (Shriberg and Kwiatkowski, 1987), to have parents, teachers or peers attend

TABLE 7.3.   Characteristics of Four Different Intervention Structures

Intervention Structure	Antecedent Instructional	Antecedent Motivational	Subsequent Instructional	Subsequent Motivational
Drill	C. stresses response definition and criterion, provides stimuli and cues	None	Feedback; correction opportunities	Contingent reinforcement activity
Drill Play	Same as drill	Play in the form of preparation of materials subsequently used as reinforcers	Same	Same
Structured Play	Stresses fun of motivational events; little emphasis on response definitions; no emphasis on criterion	Same as Drill Play	Same	Same
Play	Emphasis only on activity; no mention of target response, response definition, or criterion	Greater attention to play	No feedback; modeling during play	"Reinforcing" event is noncontingent

therapy, or to have a child practice targets in settings which constitute everyday naturalistic speaking situations for the child (Dunn, 1983). For the most part, only two or three additional teachers or settings are necessary for generalization to occur (Dunn, 1983). One suggestion is to designate significant others in the child's life as listeners. The child can be given various assignments that require delivering information to these listeners who will comply or not comply to the child's requests depending upon the accuracy of the child's speech. This activity involves other people and use of speech outside of the therapy room.

INSTRUCTIONAL PROCEDURES

Instructional procedures are techniques utilized to accomplish the goals of remediation. These procedures are typically incorporated into intervention activities or in some cases function as the activity. Included in such procedures are phonological awareness training, minimal and maximal opposition contrasts, listener confusion, self monitoring and cycles training.

Phonological Awareness Training

Based on the work of Dodd, Hambly, and Leahy (1989) and Leonard, Schwartz, Swanson, and Loeb (1987), described in Chapter 5, it seems apparent that at least some phonologically disordered children have deficits in their phonological knowledge of the sound system. As such, they have difficulty identifying phonetic regularities, segmentation, syllable structures, legal sound sequences, and phonemic contrasts within the language system. Instructional procedures that address these deficits fall under the general heading of phonological awareness training.

Awareness training attempts to focus the child's attention on the underlying structure of language, particularly speech sounds, syllables, and words. Thus, at the segment level, training might entail instruction on how sounds differ, e.g., explaining differences between short sounds (stops) in comparison to long sounds (fricatives). At the syllable level, instruction would focus on the concepts of beginning and ending sounds or on segmenting the syllable into units. At the word level, emphasis might be placed on how sounds differentiate between words. These areas develop the child's metalinguistic awareness which will be crucial for the application of another instructional procedure, that of self-monitoring.

Part of awareness training typically includes some form of ear training or auditory bombardment. Hodson and Paden (1983, 1991) recommend that the child be exposed to amplified speech at the beginning and end of each session. The child wears headphones through which the clinician slowly reads word lists or sentences which contain the child's target sounds. The headphones and amplification are used to help the child focus on the task.

Minimal Opposition Contrasts

Minimal pairs are words that differ by one phoneme which in turn may differ by a few or several distinctive features. Minimal oppositions are minimal pairs in which the contrasting segments differ by only one or two features. For example the words, "tea" and "key" form a minimal pair whose segments differ only in place of production—thus, they form a minimal opposition. For children who substitute a t/k or k/t, these words (tea and key) can be used to contrast the function of phonemes in language. In minimal opposition contrasting, the child is placed in a situation where production of the substitution phoneme results in a communication breakdown. This breakdown focuses attention on the contrastive function of phonemes and creates a need within the child to make a repair. In this case, it is best accomplished by using the target phoneme. The steps associated with minimal opposition contrasting are:

1. Identify a consistent substitution. In our example, this would be the t/k.
2. Identify minimal pair words that are distinguished by the two sounds and appropriate to the child's age and interests. In our example, words like Tea and Key; Top and Cop; Tape and Cape.
3. Familiarize the client with the minimal pair words by describing their attributes, showing their pictures, or providing concrete examples.
4. Display several exemplars of each member of the pair and ask the child to pick up the member the clinician names. This step ensures that the client can distinguish between the items when named.
5. Reverse roles and have the client name the pair member containing his/her target sound.
6. When the child uses the substitution for the target, the clinician should pick up the item that is actually named, not the one intended. This clearly demonstrates a communication breakdown due to inaccurate production.
7. Give the child another opportunity. If the child makes some form of repair the clinician should reward the attempt by picking up the intended item.

There are several variations of minimal opposition contrasting that have been reported in the literature (Blache, 1982; Cooper, 1985; Weiner 1981). Lowe and Mount Weitz (1992) describe a variation where production of both members of the pair are required during the activity. The authors prefer this method because it provides practice in productive differentiation between the two phonemes and also points out that both sounds are appropriate, though in different contexts. It also avoids labelling one of the sounds as the "old way" or "bad way" of talking.

The minimal opposition procedure is most appropriate for clients who are stimulable for the target sound. It may be necessary to provide some phonetic cuing as the child attempts to alter his sound production. Saben and Ingham (1991), investigating the effects of minimal pairs treatment, indicated that their subjects made little progress with minimal opposition contrasting alone, but improved when motoric components were added. Again, this points out the need for some drill work as part of the intervention process.

Maximal Oppositions

Elbert and Gierut (1986) introduced the idea of using maximal oppositions as an instructional procedure. Maximal oppositions are minimal pair words whose segments differ along several features (more than two). For example, the words "can" and "man" form a maximal opposition as the /k/ and /m/ differ in place (velar versus labial), manner (stop versus nasal), and voicing.

Gierut (1989, p. 12) provides the following description for selecting a maximal opposition contrast for her client, J:

> To illustrate, at the onset of treatment, J used only voiced sounds word initially; he did not produce a voicing distinction in this position. In terms of place, J primarily used bilabial sounds initially. Also, he only produced the oral-nasal (i.e., /b, w, j/ vs. / m/) and stop-glide (i.e., /m, b/ vs. /w, j/) manner distinctions. Therefore, it was important that the first maximal opposition be aimed at introducing a voiceless sound produced in a more posterior place of articulation of either the fricative, affricate, or liquid manners. The phoneme /s/ was thus selected for contrast with /m, b, w/, phonemes already used by the child in word-initial position.

Examples of the word pairs are: sad-mad, sat-mat, see-bee, suit-boot, and sail-whale. These word pairs were then used in an imitative phase (child names picture after clinician's model), and a spontaneous phase (child names each picture without a model and sorts them into groups and matches the pairs).

Gierut found that this approach resulted in restructuring of the child's phonological system with considerable generalization. Her subjects generalized correct production of treated sounds to novel words and also learned correct production of untreated phonemes. In a later study, Gierut (1990) compared use of minimal versus maximal opposition contrasting with results favoring use of maximal oppositions. In this study, Gierut also introduced contrasts using major class distinctions (sonorant, consonantal, and syllabic) and found that teaching these types of pairs was as effective or more so than teaching pairs that differed by nonmajor class features (e.g., voicing, nasal, coronal).

Gierut (1991) and Gierut and Neumann (1992) continued research of the minimal pair procedure by comparing the teaching of two unfamiliar phonemes versus traditional minimal pairs in which one of the phonemes is the target and the other a part of the child's phonetic repertoire (the child's substitution). This design points out another way for minimal pairs to differ—through their relationship to the child's pretreatment grammar. The various relationships to grammar are described by Gierut (1992, p. 1050):

> Specifically, the treated phoneme may be unknown to the child, that is, not functional in his or her phonemic inventory. Assuming a relational analysis, the contrasting phone may be its 1:1 corresponding replacement. This comparison is typical of conventional minimal pair treatment (e.g., Weiner, 1981) and establishes an explicit (and potentially homonymous) association between the treated phoneme and the child's grammar. It is also possible to treat an unknown phoneme paired with another known and unrelated phoneme from the child's grammar (Gierut, 1989). In this case, the treated phoneme is again explicitly contrasted with the child's existing system. Finally, two unknown phonemes may simply be compared to each other.

Results of the two studies (Gierut, 1991; Gierut and Neumann, 1992) indicated that minimal pairs comparing two previously unknown phonemes were as effective or more so than teaching one phoneme in comparison to its substitution. This finding was replicated in Gierut (1992). It would seem that if the goal of intervention is to introduce the most phonological change in the least time, the most effective approach is opposition pairs comparing two phonemes previously unknown to a child that also differ by maximal and major class features. Gierut (1992) proposes the hierarchy of minimal pair treatment formats shown in Figure 7.1.

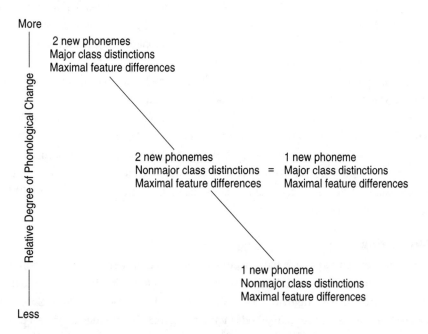

FIGURE 7.1. Hierarchy of minimal pair treatment formats predicting relative degrees of phonological change in the phonemic inventories of disordered systems.

Listener Confusion

Weiner and Ostrowski (1979) investigated the effects of listener uncertainty on articulation. In their study, 15 children between the ages of 3 and 5 years were asked to name various picture stimuli. In the experimental condition the examiner would respond to error productions in one of three manners. Condition EP-1 was correct pronunciation of the picture name. Condition EP-2 was a model of the subject's error and condition EP-3 was a misarticulation different from the subject's response. The examiner's response followed the lead-in phrase "Did you say _____." After hearing the examiner's response the subjects were trained to reply "Yes (or No), I said _____." This last response was then evaluated to determine if phonetic revisions had occurred.

The purpose of the study was to determine how the importance of being understood might affect articulation consistency. Weiner and Ostrowski posited that children should make fewer sound errors when they think they are not being understood because they will be more likely to engage in revision behaviors.

Results of the study supported their hypothesis. In general, the more obvious the misunderstanding, the more likely the children were to engage in revision behaviors. Condition EP-3 (examiner's response is a misarticulation other than what child made) resulted in fewer misarticulations by the subjects than the other two conditions. It would appear that, when the child perceives there has been a miscommunication, he or she will be more likely to alter his or her speech production to make communication clearer. The greater the perceived miscommunication, the more likely the child will engage in some form of revision behavior.

Listener confusion is no doubt part of why minimal and maximal oppositions training has been successful. Dean and Howell (1986) suggest that when communication results in unexpected consequences it introduces conflict which forces the child to cognitively restructure his/her phonological system as seen through his/her use of repair strategies. Behavioral approaches may also owe their success to forced restructuring of the child's phonological system. After all, if feedback to a child's response is negative, it seems reasonable that this too would facilitate a restructuring of the child's phonological system.

The procedure of listener uncertainty or confusion can be incorporated in other activities to encourage revision behaviors on the part of the misarticulating child. An example is to have the child give directions for some activity such as arranging blocks to match a particular array. In following the directions, the clinician can act confused when the articulation is inaccurate. This should prompt revision behavior on the part of the child. In cases of listener confusion, misarticulating children find that their current system of communication is inadequate and this creates a need to change. If that need for change can be capitalized upon, the clinician will be on the road to successful intervention.

Self-Monitoring

Misarticulating children who have been taught to monitor their own production of a target are more likely to achieve generalization to settings outside of the treatment context (Koegel, Kern Koegel, and Costello Ingham, 1986; Shriberg and Kwiatkowski, 1987). Self-monitoring has been taught using a number of methods including having clients judge their own productions; chart their accuracy; determine criteria for response accuracy and apply reinforcement; and use self-instructional and self-cuing techniques (for a review see Dunn, 1983).

Koegel, Kern Koegel, and Costello Ingham (1986) taught children, who had successfully learned to produce target phonemes at the sentence level, to monitor their production of those same sounds in conversations and reading both in and outside of therapy. The children successfully improved their sound production in home and school contexts, as measured by generalization probes. The researchers credited the success of the treatment to the self-monitoring within the natural contexts and in the absence of drill; overtly recording the results of self-monitoring; checks by parents and teachers to be sure the children were monitoring their production; and the application of extrinsic reinforcement for self-monitoring.

To engage in self-monitoring, children need a certain amount of implicit and explicit metalinguistic skill (Shriberg and Kwiatkowski, 1990). "Self-monitoring would seem to require that the child have a linguistic representation of the intended form, have the metalinguistic awareness to detect when features of a surface form differ significantly from those expected in the ambient community, and have the articulatory ability to produce the correctly revised form" (p. 157). Accordingly, children must sometimes receive instruction about metalinguistic categories before engaging in self-monitoring activities (Koegel, Kern Koegel, and Costello Ingham, 1986). Metalinguistic awareness emerges in the preschool years, as evidenced in children's phonetic repairs, and develops gradually, moving from implicit kinds of knowledge to the explicit and conscious manipulation of language.

Shriberg and Kwiatkowski (1990) note that explicit metalinguistic awareness can be trained even in very young children. In a study involving eight preschool children, enrolled in an intervention program for phonological disorders, they observed the spontaneous development of various self-monitoring behaviors. However, the behaviors did not develop unless certain conditions were met. First, the self-monitoring for any particular sound was not likely to occur until after the sound was being made correctly in some contexts and, second, the self-monitoring never occurred at the preword stage for any of the subjects. It appears that exposure to sounds in a management program facilitates self-monitoring behavior.

Cycles Training

Hodson and Paden (1983) introduced the instructional procedure of cycles training. As they describe their program:

> Our overall remediation plan departs significantly from traditional methods. We do not continuously target the phonological pattern until it has reached a predetermined criterion. Rather, we restrict focusing on a pattern to only a few weeks (usually two to four), using a different phoneme or sequence each week. So, several patterns can be targeted inside of a "natural" time block; for example, a semester. (p. 56)

The time required to address each of the child's target patterns (what the child needs to become more intelligible) is referred to as a cycle. The first cycle is referred to as Cycle One. At the completion of Cycle One another cycle is begun which again addresses the child's target patterns. The same sounds, different sounds, or a combination may be addressed for the target patterns during Cycle Two. Most children will require two or three cycles before noticeable intelligibility gains are made.

Cycles training capitalizes on the child's natural ability to generalize and organize the sound system. It appears that exposing the child to several different sounds and patterns during the cycles facilitates reorganization of the child's phonological system. Hodson and Paden report that most of their clients are ready for dismissal within 18 months of beginning their program.

The reader should note that cycles training is only a part of the Hodson and Paden program which also includes comprehensive analysis, consideration of phonetic context, production practice, auditory bombardment, and home assignments. However, it is suggested here that cycles training would have application regardless of other program components. A program, for example, incorporating maximal and minimal opposition training in language-based activities using a cycles training schedule, should yield results similar to those found by Hodson and Paden. The value of cycles training appears to be in exposing the child to various sound patterns which acts to stimulate the reorganization of the phonological system. A similar effect may occur through maximal oppositions training.

DESIGNING PRAGMATICALLY VALID ACTIVITIES

Therapy practices which are variously called "naturalistic," "ecologically valid," or "pragmatically valid" are being used with increased frequency in the treatment of language disabilities (Fey, 1986, 1988; Gallagher, 1991) and can be applied to procedures for phonological disorders as well. The terms "naturalistic" and "ecologically valid" refer to the notion that speech and language should be taught in communication situations that are similar to those encountered in everyday life. Learning in naturalistic contexts should promote the transfer of newly acquired language skills to communication situations outside of therapy (Warren and Rogers-Warren, 1985). In some cases, generalization to new settings will occur without the need for special procedures because of the similarities between the contexts (Fey, 1986).

The term "pragmatically valid" implies something a little different, namely the notion that communication acts have a purpose; that communication occurs within physical, social, and linguistic contexts that alter the nature of the messages themselves; and that participants in a conversation agree to abide by certain conventions for regulating their verbal interaction. The idea that communication acts have a purpose arises from speech act theory (Searle, 1975) which states that utterance acts are produced, that they have a literal meaning (locutionary), a purpose (illocutionary force), and a corresponding (perlocutionary) effect upon the listener. Physical contexts determine what we talk about, what words we use, gestures which might accompany our utterances, how much information the participants share, what can be presupposed, and whether the participants are familiar with the events taking place. The social context determines the relationship between speaker and listener and often determines the formality of the language used. Most of our utterances occur within larger linguistic contexts such as conversations, stories, lessons, pretend play, etc. What we say and how we say it, as well as the amount of information shared by speaker and listener, are often determined by prior linguistic context.

What are the conventions of conversations? Grice (1975) has suggested four: the maxim of quantity stipulates that the speaker will provide a sufficient amount of information for the listener but not more than is required; the maxim of quality dictates that one shall speak the truth, based upon adequate evidence; the maxim of relation specifies that what is contributed will be relevant to the ongoing exchange; and the maxim of manner states that the speaker will attempt to be clear, unambiguous, brief, and orderly in presentation. It is this last maxim that is violated by the presence of a phonological disorder because clarity is affected (Prutting and Kirchner, 1987).

Another term used is "communication-centered" (Low, Newman, and Ravsten, 1989). This term refers to the idea that communication skills can best be taught within prosocial communicative events and activities, "i.e., the pragmatic situation in which language is used and has meaning, is the natural and ideal context for language acquisition" (Low, Newman, and Ravsten, 1989, p. 218), and that enhanced communication between the client and others is the goal of therapy.

For decades, articulation and phonological disorders were treated through drill work. However, Low, Newman, and Ravsten (1989) proposed procedures by which articulation and phonology might be acquired in naturalistic and pragmatically valid communication-centered contexts. As with language instruction, the assumptions are two-fold. First, as Low, Newman, and Ravsten point out, there is evidence that children tend to speak better when their utterances carry more information for the listener (Leonard, 1971; Menyuk, 1980). Second, activities that simulate real-life communication contexts will enable the early transfer or use of newly learned articulation and phonology skills in every day communication. In particular, transfer is not postponed but is instead facilitated during regular therapy activities (Dunn, 1983; Low, Newman, and Ravsten, 1985, 1989).

Low, Newman, and Ravsten proposed a number of principles, placed within a stimulus-response-reinforcement paradigm, to guide their communication-centered methods. The first of these draws on established practice regarding stimulus complexes, namely that the learning situation should be like everyday communicative situations, the ultimate test of the learner's skill. The justification here is that entire complexes of stimuli come to control learned responses and that failure to provide all relevant stimuli in the training situation may cause poor retrieval of the response. A second principle proposed by Low, Newman, and Ravsten is that the response should include the targeted phoneme, be useful to the client, and also be communicatively powerful in the sense that use of the response helps the child control his/her environment. A third principle is directed to the nature of reinforcement, that it should fulfill the purpose conveyed by the client's verbal response. In other words, what the child actually intends happens as a function of correct production. Consequences of this sort are often referred to as "natural reinforcers."

There are additional principles garnered from the literature on pragmatics that can be applied to phonological intervention. These principles are applicable regardless of the theoretical base of instructional procedures (minimal contrasts, maximal contrasts, cycles approach, etc.) which might be used. The principles are appropriate to intervention programs for phonological disorders where no organic or structural components serve to maintain the speech disorder and when target phonemes are stimulable. They can also be adapted to articulation and other disorders of speech. Their application for organic articulation disorders should be considered after establishment of phonemes has been effected to bring about transfer of newly learned skills.

Principles suggested by Lowe and Mount Weitz (1992) will be discussed throughout the remainder of this section and are summarized as:

1. Therapy activities must have **sensemaking** potential and a goal.
2. Therapy activities must provide a coherent relationship between the parts and the whole. Attention to the parts is known as **sensemaking focus.**
3. Acts and utterances which are produced must have a powerful **function** in relationship to the goal.

4. Motivation in therapy evolves from a functional relationship between utterances and the **consequences** associated with the goal and the activity.
5. The target structure in the child's utterances should convey the **new information** in the message.
6. Target sounds should be produced in utterances which convey a variety of **illocutionary functions**.
7. **Motivation** to communicate is essential to creating a need to change how one communicates
8. Target sounds should be used in a variety of novel **semantic-syntactic structures**.

SENSEMAKING

The first principle of pragmatically-valid teaching is that the therapy activity should contribute to sensemaking. This is a term used by Lund and Duchan (1993) to refer to children's ability to understand the nature of events in which they are participants. An activity which is sensible has a point which can be easily interpreted by the client. Once the sense of the event is understood, children see that the event has a goal or children can establish personal goals or an agenda.

Children must be familiar with a particular kind of event if it is to make sense, either from schemata developed from past experience or because of the development in therapy of event scripts. The role of children and others, i.e., what one does in the activity, is clear once sensemaking is established. Children are able to actively participate in therapy activities and can anticipate certain outcomes. Activities that have sensemaking include making craft projects, shopping, searching for hidden items, finding out information, and so on.

There are several ways to apply this concept of sensemaking. In one activity, the client can help put away therapy materials prior to terminating a session. As part of the task the items to be cleared must be named. Presumably, children in therapy have a preexisting schema related to cleaning up and see as their goal or agenda both the clean work area as well as the termination of the session. Children also understand what they must do to clean up. In another activity, which involves pretend play, specifically going to the corner grocery store, children are given a list of items to purchase. If the event makes sense to them, they understand that they must accumulate all of the items on the list and return them to the home area. Games, crafts, preparing snacks, role-playing, and telling stories are other examples of activities which have sensemaking for children because they all have a structure, including a goal which is familiar to children.

SENSEMAKING FOCUS

The idea of ''sensemaking focus'' (Lund and Duchan, 1993) evolves from sensemaking. Sensemaking focus involves directing one's attention to a part of an event or activity. Usually these parts of the activity lead to the ultimate goal that is realized once the activity is finished. The activities given above as examples of sensemaking also have sensemaking focus, individual actions which lead to the culmination of the activity. For instance, in the clean-up activity, the children must put away assorted therapy materials. When playing store, children must read the shopping list, request the items specified, package the items, and so on. Children in therapy focus on each of these actions and they make sense because of their relationship to the broader activity. Individual verbal acts performed in the course of therapy activities also invite sense-making focus, especially when it is those acts which propel the activity toward completion and the activity goal.

FUNCTIONAL UTTERANCES

When children's utterances move them in the direction of their goals, we say that these utterances are functional. They have a purpose, not only with respect to everyday usefulness of words or phrases, but also with respect to their function within the remediation activity. It is a good idea to construct activities which require the use of target responses in order to reach a goal which the children understand. That way, the children's utterances have special meaning in relation to the overall event and become important to the children. The utterances are consistent with the children's agendas and advance their progress toward the goal. In the clean-up example above, the children would have to give directions to other children or the speech-language pathologist regarding which items to remove from the work area; naturally, names for those items would contain the children's target sound(s). The same would be true of grocery shopping insofar as the children request items whose names contain target sounds.

It is not unusual for speech-language pathologists to structure the physical context so that materials are not available to children until they request them. In like manner, when consider-ations of sensemaking, sensemaking focus, and functionalism are incorporated into therapy plans, the production of targeted phonemes fits into the overall scheme and becomes a vehicle for children to reach their goals. These practices are consistent with the recommendation of Low, Newman, and Ravsten (1985, 1989) that utterances be "communicatively powerful," or have an impact on the listener's desire to bring about some outcome. These practices are also consis-tent with the concept of natural reinforcement. Fey (1986) discusses these same principles under the topic of motivation in therapy.

To further understand the relationship between sensemaking, sensemaking focus, and func-tionalism see Table 7.4 for a breakdown of some of the activities included in Lowe and Mount Weitz (1992).

CONSEQUENCES OF ERRORS

Within this pragmatic framework, some consideration must be given to the consequences for failure to produce the target phoneme. We have illustrated how correct production advances children toward their goal in a particular activity. The converse is to delay achievement of a goal when target phoneme production is faulty, i.e., when the child produces substitution pho-nemes or deletes target phonemes. There are many options available when children do not produce a target phoneme, word, phrase, or sentence. In conventional speech therapy practices, it is permissible to do nothing, repeat a trial, provide corrective feedback and opportunities to correct the error, or even penalize the clients.

In a communication framework, two options stand out as appropriate following misuse or failure to use a target. First, the listener indicates to the child that a breakdown has occurred, and there is a misunderstanding of the intention. This is accomplished through use of some form of clarification request. The therapist then gives the child an opportunity to initiate a repair. Repairs involve some kind of revision of the message, in this case, the phonological character-

TABLE 7.4.   Illustrations of Sensemaking, Sensemaking Focus, and Functionalism

Description of Activity	Sensemaking Component	Sensemaking Focus	Functionalism
"Flower Shop"—Children are arranging flowers and flowerpots which have pictures whose names contain target	The children's goal is to arrive at matching displays in their respective shops	Individual flowers and pots are arranged according to some plan	The children have opportunities to verbally direct one another, with utterances containing their targets, of course, and listener acts accordingly
"Hide and Seek"— Children are to find stickers which are hidden under some but not all pictures (minimal pairs)	The children's goal is to collect a large number of stickers and keep them	The children want another child or the clinician to turn over each picture as it is named	The children verbalize their directions, using target phonemes, and the listener complies by turning over the pictures
"I Love It"—Children are to classify items which they like and do not like (perhaps to make up a wish list)	The children's goal is to get pictures of their favorite toys or foods into a special box or to tell a listener what toys, foods, etc., they do/do not like	The children want another child or the clinician to put each picture in the appropriate box	The children verbalize "I love it" or "I don't like it" and the listener puts the picture in the box designated by the speaker

istics of the utterance. The request for repair may be explicit or vague, according to the needs of each child, ranging from the inexplicit "Huh?" or "What?" to something more specific, such as "I don't see anything called [θup]."

Sometimes, particularly in the early stages of therapy for a new sound, children will be unsuccessful in their attempts to revise their messages unaided. In such cases, the clinician's job is to facilitate their ability to phonetically recode. If the child is responsive to modeling stimulation techniques, the clinician can provide a "communicative model" for the child by posing an either/or question, for example, "You need the TEA or the KEY?"

Laufer and Ebin (1991) call this type of prompt a Question in Phonological Mode (QPM) and found that such questions facilitated repairs in 2- and 3-year-old children. An either/or question gives the child an opportunity to try again by offering the choice of reproducing the error or revising his/her communication with help from the model. At the same time, the revision enables the child to better communicate his or her intentions. Most times, the child's production will improve following requests of this type.

A second type of option is available to the clinician when minimal pair contrasts are used because the child's error results in the production of an alternative real word. The clinician simply acts as though the spoken word were the one intended, which lets the child know that the correct intentions have not been conveyed. For example, in the clean-up activity, if a child instructs another to put away the "tea" or "T" while really intending the "key," the listener can actually remove the "tea" or "T," in which case the speaker will usually make a new attempt to realize the goal of the utterance.

UTTERANCES SHOULD CONVEY NEW INFORMATION

In naturalistic activities, the child is typically not told what to say. The messages are constructed by the child to serve his/her goals and usually contain information which is unknown to the listener. We also avoid therapy activities in which the child is asked known-information questions, i.e., questions where the interlocutor already knows the answer and the child is aware of the knowledge state of the listener. Most questions of this type are senseless and only serve the purpose of evoking a target structure or testing the child. Questions of this type can be adapted so that the answer is more informative. Another reason for avoiding known-information questions is evidenced in a study by Campbell and Shriberg (1982) in which speech-delayed children were found to articulate more accurately when they were conveying new and important information. Along the same lines, Leonard (1971, p. 511) points out that a child is more likely to produce error phonemes correctly when the phoneme "is necessary for understanding the message."

ILLOCUTIONARY ACTS

The activity should be constructed so that the consequences of the child's speaking are ones that would naturally follow and which are directly related to the activity. Too often, clinicians respond to correct productions with verbal praise or some tangible reinforcer that has no conversational relationship to the meaning conveyed by the child's utterance. Verbal praise for a production is not a natural consequence. In everyday conversations, an illocution on the part of a speaker usually evokes a corresponding act from the conversational partner. We use a variety of speech acts in our everyday communicative interactions. Unfortunately, this is an important communicative dimension often ignored in therapy situations where many of the tasks only require naming or, worse, imitation.

The goal of a child's utterance should never be to imitate someone else unless, of course, the child wishes to use imitation for some function, such as to tease. Repetition of clinician-generated models and other forms of drill work are avoided since it removes the communicative intention from a child's utterance and is not naturalistic. Occasionally, the child may be told what to say and correct articulation may be modeled, but, to be truly communicative, an imitative utterance should be directed to a third individual who does not have the information (Constable, 1981).

Intervention activities that focus on communication will take advantage of the various speech acts. If the child requests information in the activity, the appropriate response is not to say "Good!" but to supply the information or, if the request is not articulated clearly, then to ask for a clarification. Table 7.5 describes various speech acts and their corresponding consequences as presented in Lowe and Mount Weitz (1992). Where possible the clinician should try to incorporate different speech acts into the communicative requirements of therapy activities.

MOTIVATION

It was assumed in the prior discussion of sensemaking and sensemaking focus that the child would have a desire to engage in the selected activity. The child must agree to the activity and

TABLE 7.5.   Speech Acts and Expected Responses

Speech Acts	Expected Responses
Requests for information in question form	Followed by answers
Requests for action, in the form of commands	Followed by the appropriate objects, actions, or events, or a reason is given for failure to comply
Statements and descriptions	Followed by acknowledgements, other statements and descriptions, agreements, etc.
Greetings	Return greetings
Protests	Compliances, explanations, etc.

desire the outcome. Sometimes the child even initiates the activity. This is one way of "following the child's lead" in therapy. When the clinician follows the child's lead, it sets the stage for effective communication to take place (Warren and Rogers-Warren, 1985). It is also a powerful way of providing motivation for the child's cooperation and use of targeted structures.

One way of motivating the child is to specify the outcome and determine if the child agrees to it. Once the child agrees to the goal, he/she will be more likely to actively participate. When the outcome is unfamiliar to the child, such as making a new craft object, it is wise to present the child with a model of the completed item ahead of time. The model helps the child maintain his/her sense of the event and will encourage participation.

Sometimes giving a child a choice of activities and outcomes will produce higher levels of motivation than using an activity which has been selected beforehand by the clinician. The selection of choices can be based on the child's interests while at the same time taking into consideration the desired response demands.

Often reinforcers are used in speech and language intervention. In operant approaches, reinforcers are used to strengthen a response. In practice, reinforcers are used less systematically to motivate clients to participate in the therapy tasks. The use of stickers and other traditional reinforcers can provide motivation for the child, but these usually detract from the "naturalness" of the activity.

Artificial reinforcers, including tangibles and praise are avoided in pragmatic therapy structures as they detract from the natural rewards associated with efficient communication. Artificial reinforcers rarely occur in the natural environment and, therefore, will have to be systematically faded while more natural consequences take over. Furthermore, there is often no relationship of the artificial reinforcer to the utterance or the ongoing activity. For example, clinicians frequently ask children to name a target word picture and, if produced correctly, the child is allowed to roll dice or use a spinner to play a game. In this context the game and articulation have no direct relationship to one another. When there are no direct links between the child's speech and the consequences, generalization is not facilitated.

The concept of reinforcement has changed in therapy activities which are pragmatic. A current practice is to employ "communicative reinforcers," ones which are natural consequences of various communicative acts. In therapy which is pragmatic, the communicative acts are goal-directed so that correct productions are rewarded by moving the child closer to the activity goal. Motivation and reinforcement are built into the activity.

Target Sounds Used in Semantic-Syntactic Structures

It is best if children use target sounds in semantic-syntactic structures which they have created since constructing sentence frames is a necessary part of communicating in the natural environment. This helps children learn to produce targeted structures within a variety of grammatical contexts. Creation of one's own messages is more demanding cognitively than repeating someone else's sentences since the individual must engage in more psycholinguistic processes. Many authors (see, for example, Clark and Clark, 1977; Crystal, 1987) have indicated that the production of messages involves several steps, some of which include construction of a syntactic outline, generation of an intonation contour, insertion of content words, formation of affixes and function words, and of course the phonological components.

In the early stages of therapy it is desirable to limit syntactic complexity as it will interfere with articulation (Panagos, Quine, and Klich, 1979). However, it is still desirable for the child to create his/her own messages from the very beginning of therapy. As the child gains phonetic control over the sound in simple contexts, the activities can be structured to allow greater opportunity for more creativity in sentence construction and production practice in more complex syntactic structures.

WHOLE LANGUAGE AND CLASSROOM-BASED INTERVENTION

Two relatively recent changes in the delivery of phonological intervention programs have been the incorporation of a whole language philosophy and classroom-based intervention. As described by Norris and Hoffman (1990, p. 72), the whole language philosophy looks at language "as a process involving cognitive, semiotic (i.e., both nonlinguistic and linguistic communications), and social development. These three aspects of development function as an indivisible and integrated system, resulting in language that expresses content, form and use." The whole language philosophy emphasizes that learning "occurs in the process of making sense or meaning out of experience and, therefore, the experiences themselves must be meaningful" (Norris, 1992, p. 11). From a whole language perspective, learning should always be embedded within complex, meaningful experiences and not in isolated drill work. One of those meaningful experiences would certainly involve the school classroom where the child spends a great deal of his/her waking hours.

Whole-Language Approach to Phonology

With respect to phonology, Hoffman, Norris, and Monjure (1990) argue that a child's phonological performance interacts with his/her syntactic, semantic, and pragmatic performance. As such, phonological treatment programs should treat language holistically, as a synergistic system. Hoffman, Norris, and Monjure posited that, by facilitating the growth of higher levels of language, lower levels (e.g., phonological component) would also be stimulated. In a study comparing phonological therapy with a whole-language approach their arguments were supported. Two 4-year-old phonologically delayed children were treated. One child received a phonologically based treatment (minimal pairs) and the other a whole language approach.

For the whole language treatment the child's focus was on communicating to a puppet (listener). With the aid of picture stimuli the clinician told the child a story. The child was then instructed to relate the story to the puppet. Three forms of feedback were used following each of the child's conversational turns. (*a*) Requests for clarification were made when any part of the child's story was unclear, inaccurate or poorly stated. (*b*) Requests to add new events were made when the child left out pertinent information. (*c*) Requests to increase sentence complexity were made if the child attempted to describe more than one event in his utterance.

Results from the study showed that both children had improved phonological performance. The child treated with the phonological approach made small, but greater, increases. However, the big difference between the two children occurred in the language measures. The child treated using the whole language approach made significantly greater gains in overall language. Some of the results included a reduction in the use of sentence fragments, an increased use of complex sentences, and a decrease in use of sentences with either syntactic or verb tense errors.

Given the likelihood of language deficits accompanying moderate to severe phonological disability, whole language treatment offers the clinician an approach for remediation that allows both areas to be targeted. Table 7.6 presents the steps associated with the whole language treatment approach used by Hoffman, Norris, and Monjure.

CLASSROOM-BASED INTERVENTION

A second change in services has been to move away from the use of pull-out models which remove the child with speech disabilities from the classroom for treatment. Instead, the current trend is toward intervention based in the classroom. This is part of a larger pattern seen in special education and is often referred to as an inclusion model of service. With inclusion, children having special needs receive all of their special services within the regular education classroom, rather than being placed in more restrictive educational settings.

Children with phonological disabilities are typically already a part of the regular education classroom. As such, use of the classroom as a therapy room makes sense from a whole language perspective and from the viewpoint that generalization should be improved if practice occurs in real life settings. In the past it was not unusual for clinicians to make use of materials from the

TABLE 7.6.   Therapy Steps Associated with the Whole Language Treatment Approach Used by Hoffman, Norris, and Monjure

Step 1	The clinician points out one event that initiates the story and talks about what the characters are doing and why, using a variety of language models
Step 2	The clinician asks the child to tell that part of the story to a puppet listener
Step 3	If any part of the child's explanation is unclear, inaccurate or poorly stated, the puppet asks for a clarification; the clinician then points out more information and restates the event, using a variety of language models and asks the child to recommunicate the information to the puppet
	or
	The clinician adds a new event that continues the story and continues as described above
	or
	When the story has been told as a sequence of events, the clinician adds elements that attribute motives to the characters actions, causes to events, interpretations of feelings, predictions of future events and inferences

classroom curriculum (e.g., vocabulary words). The delivery of services in the classroom setting is just one further step.

Classroom-based intervention takes advantage of the materials and activities at hand. As described by Masterson (1993, p. 5), "Classroom-based treatment allows the speech-language pathologist to use academic programs as a framework for language intervention services. For the school-age child, textbooks, homework, and classroom discourse can serve as sources from which to draw intervention goals and procedures."

The actual delivery of services will vary depending upon the particular needs of the clients, how many "speech" children are in the classroom, and the collaborative relationship between clinician and classroom teacher. For example, Masterson (1993) suggests that classroom-based intervention is probably more appropriate for children who have conceptually based speech disorders—those who lack specific phonemic contrasts but are capable of the correct articulations. For children needing a motor approach to remediation (repetitive drill on syllables and words) the pull-out model may be more appropriate or may be combined with classroom-based procedures.

How might services be provided in the classroom? Traditionally, clinicians have worked with children in small groups and this may still be appropriate within the classroom. In many cases teachers also work with small groups. One strategy may be for the clinician to work with a small group of "speech" children while the teacher addresses reading or some other subject with the other groups. Another approach is for the clinician to work with the whole class on a speech related task. Masterson (1993) suggests that the area of metaphonology (or metalinguistics) is ideally suited for such teaching, as reading and spelling problems have been associated with deficits in phonological awareness. A good source for materials is Savela and Vilker-Krause (1991) who have developed programs that can be used to develop metaphonological skills in kindergarten and first-grade children.

Another approach is for the clinician to function as a consultant for the classroom teacher. In this role the clinician models techniques for the teacher to use when interacting with children having milder phonological disabilities. This approach allows the clinician extra time for the more severely impaired clients and improves chances for generalization of skills as the teacher will have contact with the child on a daily basis.

Whatever approach is taken, the clinician must be mindful to incorporate as much of the regular education curriculum materials as possible in the intervention program. The child is exposed to these materials on a daily basis which increases the likelihood that new speech behaviors will be carried over into everyday speech. In addition, the materials and activities are part of the larger picture reinforcing the whole language perspective that learning occurs in the context of meaningful experiences.

SUMMARY

This chapter has taken a look at intervention beginning with the analysis of assessment data for development of therapy goals and ending with an overview of various instructional procedures and intervention approaches. The intervention process was seen to involve a number of issues including selection of appropriate targets and stimulus materials, choice of instructional procedures, development of pragmatic activities, and principles of whole language. The chapter viewed phonology as part of the language system, thus intervention emphasized the use of speech to communicate.

Given the number of variables involved in planning and implementing an intervention program it is obviously a complex process. It is surprising that, historically, little time or thought was given to this major professional responsibility of the speech-language clinician. As our knowledge base continues to grow, the clinician of the future must be willing to grow as well. Techniques used 10 years ago may still accomplish the desired outcomes, but as professionals we must strive to use the most efficient methods available for the benefit of our clients.

Part of our professional growth comes from the contributions we make as individuals. Clinicians working with phonologically delayed children have a unique opportunity to study the disorder. We must learn to look beyond the symptoms and try to provide explanations for the disabilities. The clinician must attempt to generate hypotheses on how to approach intervention based on current information and try various techniques and procedures to determine what does and does not work. That information needs to be shared, but, most importantly, the clinician must realize that we are in a constantly changing field, a field of study that is seeing new information released almost on a daily basis. As such, the clinician must take on the perspective and habits of a life-long learner. With such an attitude the clinician will be able to best serve his/her clients.

REFERENCES

Aitchison J, Chiat S. Recall errors and natural phonology. In Thew C, Johnson C, eds. Proceedings of the Second International Congress for the Study of Child Language. Vol. II. New York: University Press of America, 1984:17–26.

Blache S. Minimal word-pairs and distinctive feature training. In Crary MA, ed. Phonological intervention: concepts and procedures. San Diego: College-Hill Press, Inc., 1982:61–96.

Campbell T, Shriberg L. Associations among pragmatic functions, linguistic stress, and natural phonological processes in speech-delayed children. Journal of Speech and Hearing Research 1982;25:547–553.

Clark H, Clark E. Psychology and language. New York: Harcourt Brace Jovanovich, 1977.

Compton A. Generative studies of children's phonological disorders. Journal of Speech and Hearing Disorders 1970;35:315–339.

Constable C. Creating communicative context: analyzing linguistic and non-linguistic event interaction. Paper presented at the meeting of the American Speech, Language and Hearing Association, Philadelphia, 1981.

Costello J, Onstine J. The modification of multiple articulation errors based on distinctive feature theory. Journal of Speech and Hearing Disorders 1976;41:199–215.

Cooper E. The method of meaningful contrasts. In Newman P, Creaghead N, Secord W, eds. Assessment and remediation of articulatory and phonological disorders. Columbus: Merrill Publishing Company, 1985.

Crystal D. The Cambridge encyclopedia of language. Cambridge: Cambridge University Press, 1987.

Dean E, Howell J. Developing linguistic awareness: a theoretically based approach to phonological disorders. British Journal of Disorders of Communication 1986;21:223–238.

Dodd B, Hambly G, Leahy J. Phonological disorders in children: underlying cognitive deficits. British Journal of Developmental Psychology 1989;7:55–71.

Dunn C. A framework for generalization in disordered phonology. Journal of Childhood Communication Disorders 1983;7:46–58.

Dunn C, Till J. Morphophonemic rule learning in normal and articulation-disordered children. Journal of Speech and Hearing Research 1982;25:322–332.

Edwards M. Selection criteria for developing therapy goals. Journal of Childhood Communication Disorders 1983;7(1):36–45.

Edwards M, Shriberg L. Phonology: applications in communicative disorders. San Diego: College-Hill Press, Inc., 1983.

Elbert M, Dinnsen D, Swartzlander P, Chin S. Generalization to conversational speech. Journal of Speech and Hearing Disorders 1990;55:694–699.

Elbert M, Gierut J. Handbook of clinical phonology: approaches to assessment and treatment. San Diego: College-Hill Press, Inc., 1986.

Elbert M, McReynolds L. An experimental analysis of misarticulating children's generalization. Journal of Speech and Hearing Research 1978;21:136–149.

Elbert M, Powell T, Swartzlander P. Toward a technology of generalization: how many exemplars are sufficient? Journal of Speech and Hearing Research 1991;34:81–87.

Elbert M, Shelton R, Arndt W. A task for evaluation of articulation change: I. Development of methodology. Journal of Speech and Hearing Disorders 1967;10:281–288.

Farwell C. Some strategies in the early production of fricatives. Papers and Reports on Child Language Development. Stanford University 1977;12:97–104.

Ferguson C. Fricatives in child language acquisition. Proceedings of the Eleventh International Congress of Linguists. Bologna-Florence, 1975:647–664.

Fey M. Language intervention with young children. Boston: College-Hill Publications, 1986.

Fey M. Generalization issues facing language interventionists: an introduction. Language, Speech, Hearing Services in Schools 1988;19:272–281.

Fleming K. Guidelines for choosing appropriate phonetic contexts for speech-sound recognition and production practice. Journal of Speech and Hearing Disorders 1971;36:356–367.

Gallagher T. Pragmatics of language: Clinical practice issues. San Diego: Singular Publishing Group, Inc.,1991.

Gierut J. Maximal opposition approach to phonological treatment. Journal of Speech and Hearing Disorders 1989;54: 9–19.

Gierut J. Differential learning of phonological oppositions. Journal of Speech and Hearing Research 1990;33:540–549.

Gierut J. Homonymy in phonological change. Clinical Linguistics and Phonetics 1991;5:119–137.

Gierut J. The conditions and course of clinically induced phonological change. Journal of Speech and Hearing Research 1992;35:1049–1063.

Gierut J, Neumann H. Teaching and learning /θ/: a nonconfound. Clinical Linguistics and Phonetics 1992;6:191–20.

Grice H. Logic and conversation. In Cole P, Morgan JL, eds. Syntax and semantics. Vol. 3: Speech acts. New York: Seminar Press, 1975:41–58.

Hillard S, Goepfert L. Articulation training: a new perspective. Language, Speech, Hearing Services in Schools 1979; 10:145–151.

Hillard S, Goepfert L, Farber B. A preschool for communicatively impaired children: an innovative approach. Miniseminar presented to the American Speech and Hearing Association, Houston, 1976.

Hodson B, Paden E. Targeting intelligible speech. San Diego: College-Hill Press Inc., 1983, 1991.

Hoffman P, Norris J, Monjure J. Comparison of process targeting and whole language treatments for phonologically delayed preschool children. Language, Speech, Hearing Services in Schools 1990;21(2):102–109.

Ingram D. Phonological disability in children. 2nd ed. London: Whurr Publishers, 1989.

Johnston J. Generalization: the nature of change. Language, Speech, Hearing Services in Schools 1988;19:314–329.

Kamhi A. A reconceptualization of generalization and generalization problems. Language, Speech, Hearing Services in Schools 1988;19:304–313.

Kent R. Contextual facilitation of correct sound production. Language, Speech, Hearing Services in Schools 1982;13: 66–76.

Koegel L, Kern Koegel R, Costello Ingham J. Programming rapid generalization of correct articulation through self-monitoring procedures. Journal of Speech and Hearing Disorders 1986;51:24–32.

Laufer M, Ebin H. Phonological revision strategies in normally-developing children. Paper presented at the Annual Convention of the American Speech-Language-Hearing Association, Atlanta, November, 1991.

Leonard L. A preliminary view of information theory and articulatory omissions. Journal of Speech and Hearing Disorders 1971;36:511–517.

Leonard L, Schwartz R, Swanson L, Loeb D. Some conditions that promote unusual phonological behavior in children. Clinical Linguistics and Phonetics 1987;1(1):23–34.

Low G, Newman P, Ravsten M. Pragmatic considerations in treatment: communication centered instruction. In Creaghead N, Newman P, Secord W, eds. Assessment and remediation of articulatory and phonological disorders. 2nd ed. Columbus: Merrill Publishing Company, 1989:217–242.

Lowe R, Mount Weitz J. Activities for the remediation of phonological disorders. DeKalb: Janelle Publications, Inc., 1992.

Lund N, Duchan J. Assessing children's language in naturalistic contexts. Englewood Cliffs, NJ: Prentice-Hall, 1993.

Masterson J. Classroom-based phonological intervention. American Journal of Speech-Language Pathology 1993;2:5–9.

McReynolds L, Bennett S. Distinctive feature generalization in articulation training. Journal of Speech and Hearing Disorders 1972;37:462–470.

McReynolds L, Elbert M. Criteria for phonological process analysis. Journal of Speech and Hearing Disorders 1981; 46:197–204.

Menyuk P. The role of context in misarticulations. In Yeni-Komshian GH, Kavanagh JF, Ferguson CA, eds. Child phonology. Vol 1: Production. New York: Academic Press, 1980:211–226.

Norris J. Some questions and answers about whole language. American Journal of Speech-Language Pathology 1992; 1:11–14.

Norris J, Hoffman P. Language intervention within naturalistic environments. Language, Speech, Hearing Services in Schools 1990;21:72–84.

Oller D, Eilers R. Phonetic expectation and transcription validity. Phonetica 1975;31:288–304.

Panagos J, Quine M, Klich R. Syntactic and phonological influences on children's articulation. Journal of Speech and Hearing Research 1979;22:841–848.

Prutting C, Kirchner D. A clinical appraisal of the pragmatic aspects of language. Journal of Speech and Hearing Disorders 1987;52:105–119.

Rockman B, Elbert M. Untrained acquisition of /s/ in a phonologically disordered child. Journal of Speech and Hearing Disorders 1984;49(3):246–253.

Saben C, Ingham J. The effects of minimal pairs treatment on the speech-sound production of two children with phonologic disorders. Journal of Speech and Hearing Research 1991;34:1023–1040.

Savela K, Vilker-Krause N. The efficacy of implementing a kindergarten district-wide metaphonological program. Miniseminar presented at the annual convention of the American Speech-Language-Hearing Association, Atlanta, 1991.

Searle J. Indirect speech acts. In Cole P, Morgan JL, eds. Syntax and semantics. Vol. 3: Speech acts. New York: Seminar Press, 1975:59–82.

Shriberg L, Kwiatkowski J. Phonological disorders. II: A conceptual framework for management. Journal of Speech and Hearing Disorders 1982;47:242–256.

Shriberg L, Kwiatkowski J. Self-monitoring and generalization in preschool speech-delayed children. Language, Speech and Hearing Services in Schools 1990;21:157–170.

Stoel-Gammon C, Dunn C. Normal and disordered phonology in children. Baltimore: University Park Press, 1985.

Warren S, Rogers-Warren A. Teaching functional language: an introduction. In Warren S, Rogers-Warren A, eds. Teaching functional language: generalization and maintenance of language skills. Austin, TX: Pro-ed, 1985.

Weiner F. Treatment of phonological disability using the method of meaningful minimal contrast: two case studies. Journal of Speech and Hearing Disorders 1981;46:97–103.

Weiner F, Ostrowski A. Effects of listener uncertainty on articulatory inconsistency. Journal of Speech and Hearing Disorders 1979;44:487–503.

Phonology and Cultural Diversity

Chapter

8

Adele Proctor

In the last 20 years, American society has moved away from the "melting pot" phenomenon and has reconsidered the cultural and linguistic diversity of its citizens. Educators have promoted positive attitudinal changes about dialects (language variation), developed new views about bilingualism and multilingualism, and recommended new methods for education of culturally and linguistically diverse groups of children (Anderson, 1992; Baca and Amato, 1989; Campbell, Brennan, and Steckol, 1992; Cummins, 1989; Langdon, 1989; Terrell and Hale, 1992). The overall purpose of this chapter is to establish a foundation for understanding phonological issues in the broader context of the cultural and linguistic diversity found in the United States.

There are four specific aims of the chapter. First, to substantiate the importance of assessing phonology relative to dialect (language variation) and acquiring English as a second language, the shifting population trends in the United States will be discussed. Selected definitions of sociological and linguistic terminology will be used to lay the foundation for distinguishing between phonological difference and phonological disorder.

The second aim is to develop a level of awareness among speech-language pathologists (SLPs) that will facilitate the accuracy of their diagnoses and enhance the quality of their remediation efforts. At the most basic level of awareness is the importance of understanding that many phonological variations produced by culturally and linguistically diverse children are **different from** Standard American English (SAE) phonemes, not "deviant," "disordered," "bad," or "wrong." Difference does not mean "right" or "wrong," nor does it automatically mean "in error." For linguistically diverse children, extenuating phonological circumstances must be considered.

Third, selected events in the linguistic history of the United States will be used to discuss the evolution of attitudinal changes about language variation (dialect) and second language acquisition. How and why attitudinal changes about SAE, dialects and acquisition of English as a second language affect phonological assessment strategies will be considered in light of the movement from the "melting pot" concept towards "cultural pluralism."

Finally, the extenuating circumstances that must be considered in adjusting speech evaluations for children from linguistically different backgrounds will be presented. The clinically useful strategies to be recommended for assessment and remediation can be generalized cross-linguistically and were designed with special consideration for the evaluator who is monolingual in Standard American English.

OUR CHANGING SOCIETY

SHIFTING POPULATION TRENDS

The majority or mainstream population of the United States is defined as persons of European descent (White). Currently, persons of European descent compose the largest percentage of the United States population and represent the dominant culture. Minority groups are made up of smaller numbers of persons who are of non-European descent. Labels and definitions for who constitutes majority and minority groups are developed by the United States Census Bureau and are partially based on input from a cross-section of Americans. All decisions regarding which individuals are majority or minority members of the society are based on a process of self-identification (*1990 Census Profile*, 1991).

United States census data indicate that over the last 20 years, there has been a steady increase in the minority population. Since the present and projected demographic changes mainly include African, Latino, Asian, and Native Americans, Cole (1989), among others, has recommended the use of the descriptive term ALANA to collectively refer to these racial/ethnic groups.

An account of the changing demographics in the United States is displayed in Table 8.1. The multicultural population statistics are reported for race and origin (U.S. Department of Commerce, News Release, July 12, 1991 *CB91-215*; *1990 Census Profile, 1991*). The United States census definitions for race, ethnicity, and origin appear to be generally consistent with sociological definitions. For example, Farley (1988, p. 4) defines race as

. . . a grouping of people who (1) are generally considered to be physically distinct in some way such as skin color, hair texture or facial features, from other groupings, and (2) are generally considered by themselves and/or by others to be a distinct group.

Ethnic group refers to "people who are generally recognized by themselves and/or by others as a distinct group, with such recognition occurring on the basis of social or cultural characteristics. The most common of these characteristics are nationality, language and religion" (Farley, 1988, p. 5). Consequently, distinctive physical characteristics are used to define race whereas ethnicity emphasizes social and/or cultural practices relative to nationality. "Origin is defined as ancestry, nationality group, lineage, country of birth of parents or ancestors before arrival in the U.S." (*CB91-215*, p. 19)".

As shown in Table 8.1, racial groups are categorized as White (of European descent, including Canadian, Middle Eastern, Arab), Black (of African descent, including Caribbeans, Nigerians, Haitians), American Indian, Eskimo, Aleut, Asian Americans, Pacific Islanders, and Other (not identified as being in any of the other racial groups).

TABLE 8.1. Multicultural Population Statistics of the United States Race and Origin as Reported by United States Census—1991*

Year	Total	White	Black	American Indian, Eskimo, & Aleut	Asian Americans & Pacific Islanders	Other	Hispanic Origin**
1980	226,545,805	188,371,622	26,495,025	1,959,234	3,500,439	6,758,319	14,608,673
1990	248,709,873	199,686,070	29,986,060	1,420,400	7,273,662	9,804,847	22,354,059
		Percent (%) Increase in Population from 1980–1990					
		6%	13.2%	37.9%	107.8%	45.1%	53.0%
		Population Projections for 2000					
2000	276,382,000	227,634,000	36,177,000	Data not available	Data not yet analyzed	Data not yet analyzed	31,208,000

*Self-identification of population as classified by US Census Bureau. Racial groups are:
  White—or of European descent including Middle Eastern and Mediterranean countries
  Black—Negro, Afro, or African-American, Caribbean, Nigerian, Haitian
  Asian American—Chinese, Filipino, Japanese, Asian Indian, Korean, Vietnamese, Cambodian, Hmong, Laotian, Thai, Bangladesh, Indonesian, Malay, Okinawan, Pakistan, Sri Lanka
  Pacific Islanders—Hawaiian, Samoan, Guamanian, Tongan, Tahitian, N. Meriana, Palauan, Figian
**Origin* is defined as ancestry, nationality group, lineage, country of birth of parents or ancestors before arrival in US. Hispanic origin may be any race (e.g., Mexican, Puerto Rican, Cuban)

Between 1980 and 1990, the rate of growth for the minority population (non-European/non-White) increased at a faster rate than for the majority population. Projections for population trends from the year 1990 to the year 2000, the next decade, are based on census data from the last decade, 1980 to 1990. These population projections also consider immigration, migratory patterns within the country and birth rates among racial groups (Cole, 1989).

Table 8.1 shows that, from 1980 to 1990, there was a 13.2% increase in the Black (African-American) population, a 37.9% increase in American Indian, Eskimo, and Aleut people, a 107.8% increase in Asian American and Pacific Islanders, and a 45.1% increase in the ''Other'' category as compared to a 6% increase in White Americans (European Americans). For the same decade, those who self-identified as being of Hispanic origin increased by 53.0% as compared to the 6% rate of change for White Americans. If projected rates of population growth continue in a similar pattern, by the year 2000, there will be a higher percentage of persons of non-European descent than those of European descent in the United States.

As population trends shift, there is a commensurate need to adjust, adapt, and modify phonological assessment and intervention strategies to accommodate the probability that the ALANA group and others will display a higher proportion of language variation and/or influences of non-native English languages (language differences). For instance, many, but not all, African-Americans speak a social dialect referred to as African-American English (AAE). African-American English (AAE) is also known as Black English (BE), Vernacular Black English (VBE), Black English Vernacular (BEV), Black Vernacular English (BVE), nonstandard Negro English (NNE), Black dialect(s), and Black English dialect. In this chapter, all references to the social dialect spoken by many Americans of African descent will be discussed as AAE. In other words, African-Americans designate a preference for AAE and use AAE to replace what has previously been referred to as BE, VBE, BEV, BVE, or NNE.

With the predicted increase in number of African-Americans, it is expected that there will be a proportionate increase in the frequency of occurrence of social dialects spoken by preschool and school-aged children. With increased projections for Native Americans, those of Hispanic origin and non-European immigrants, it is also anticipated that a greater amount of bi/multilingualism will be found among school children whose family languages will not be derived from an Indo-European language (see Table 8.2). Overall, the current data suggest that the United States population is progressively changing, and a critical variable in the changing demographics is the range and variety of different (diverse) cultures and their associated languages and language varieties.

POPULATION DIVERSITY AND LINGUISTIC DIVERSITY

To a limited degree, the United States tracks the linguistic diversity that accompanies population diversity. Table 8.2 summarizes the 1990 United States census data on linguistic diversity in the United States. These data do not account for language variations (dialects) nor do the data account for the full range of other languages spoken by the population. Linguistic data are collected and specified for only 24 languages with an ''other'' category used for languages not cited in the designated list.

TABLE 8.2. Language Diversity in the US Relative to Number of Households (Based on 1990 CPH-L-96 Census Report)

		Proficiency in English			
Age	Total Population	Speaks English Only	Very Well	Well	Not Well	Does Not
5–17 yrs.	45,342,448	39,019,514	3,934,691	1,480,680	761,778	145,785
18 yrs. & Older	185,103,329	159,581,284	19,927,786	5,829,621	4,065,180	1,699,458
Total All Ages	230,445,777	198,600,798	17,862,477	7,310,301	4,826,958	1,845,243

	Proficiency in Spanish and Other Languages*			
Age	Total Population	Speaks Spanish Only	No One 14 Yrs. or Older Speaks English at Least Very Well	All in Household Speak NonEnglish
5–17 yrs.	45,342,448	4,167,653	1,763,173	4,834,635
18 yrs. & Older	185,103,329	13,177,411	5,978,086	17,513,201
Total All Ages	230,445,777	17,345,064	7,741,259	22,247,838

*Data are collected and classified by the following linguistic categories: German, Yiddish, Other West Germanic, Scandinavian, Greek, Indic, Italian, French, Portuguese, Spanish, Tagalog, Chinese, Hungarian, Japanese, Mon-khmer, Korean, Native North American, Vietnamese Other and unspecified.

There is a total population of more than 45 million between 5 and 17 years old (school-age). In the 5–17-year-old age group, there are more than 6.5 million households considered in the census. Of the 6.5 million, there are either no family members 14 years and older who speak English at least very well or who speak no English. Also, in the 5–17-year-old group, more than 4 million households speak only Spanish. The 1990 census data indicate that 13.9% of the 5–17-year-olds reside in nonEnglish speaking homes.

Of the total population of more than 185 million who are 18 years and older (high school and college age), 13.8% speak a language other than English at home. More than 13 million who are 18 years and older report speaking only Spanish at home. An additional 23.5 million who are 14 years and older report no one in the home speaks English "at least very well." There are more people in the 18-year-old and older sample than below 18 years old. Presumably, the adults influence phonological variation of the children who reside in the same home.

PHONOLOGICAL ISSUES AND CULTURAL DIVERSITY

Phonological issues that evolve as a result of shifting population trends are closely tied to how culture is defined. Culture refers to the collective social customs and behaviors of organized groups of people in that their behavior patterns reflect their belief systems, social practices, art, education, language, religion, and law (Locke, 1992). The language of the cultural group is used to communicate to others and to transmit to the children of the culture common interests, shared beliefs, and shared experiences.

Changes in both sociology and linguistics impact considerably on communication disorders and require us to expand the range of normal in assessment procedures. To appreciate why phonological variation is viewed differently today than in the early part of the 20th century, a brief review of selected historical events that shaped attitudes about Standard American English (SAE) is in order. To demonstrate how changing sociological patterns led to improved understanding of bicultural, bidialectal, and bilingual issues, selected sociolinguistic terminology is interspersed within the context of historical overview in the next section.

FROM THE MELTING POT TO CULTURAL PLURALISM

How American Dialects Evolved

Currently, all languages are seen as being composed of dialects. The standard or prestige dialect (SAE) is the preferred variation, but is no longer viewed as the sole model of correctness, nor is it seen as more logical or better than any other dialect. Among professionals, there should be less social stigmatization associated with dialects, acceptance of a broader range of what constitutes normal and understanding that a difference is not a disorder, abnormal, aberrant or deviant.

The "melting pot" phenomenon that encouraged linguistic and cultural assimilation began during the first major influx of immigrants from Eastern European and Mediterranean countries, around the beginning of the 20th century. Literally, assimilation means "a process of becoming similar" (Cashmore, 1988, p. 25). In the "melting pot" process of assimilation, immigrants pooled their common cultural characteristics, divested themselves of their native language, emphasized the importance of speaking English to their children and sought to develop a new amalgam. Many immigrants became financially successful, were able to educate their children and achieved upward social mobility.

For the first half of the 20th century, immigrants who adapted their native customs to conform to the practices of the dominant culture had a higher probability of economic, political, and social advancement. Linguistic assimilation by use of SAE was perceived as one of the influential variables that fostered success. This social perception about language was consistent with attitudes that extended back to 15th century France, i.e., there is a single correct standard language (Crystal, 1991).

Concurrent with cultural and linguistic assimilation of many European immigrants into the American mainstream, there were other racial and ethnic groups, already residing in the United States for whom assimilation did not or could not occur for a number of reasons. In many states, laws prohibited the formal schooling of African-Americans. People of African descent, as a racial group, experienced a unique American history that included slavery. African-Americans experienced generations of legalized isolation and alienation from the mainstream. The social and linguistic isolation endured by African-Americans fostered the retention of many African-isms in their language (Asante, 1991; Dandy, 1991).

Others, for example, indigenous North Americans, did not view assimilation as a desirable goal and attempted to hold on to their own culture. Still, others were separated by natural boundaries, such as a mountain range or a river, and exclusion from the mainstream occurred due to living in isolated regions (e.g., Appalachian speakers), or because of sociopolitical ideology (e.g., Cajun speakers). For many others, religious beliefs and customs contradicted participation in mainstream society (e.g., the Amish and Mennonites).

Whether by legal mandates against full participation in the mainstream culture or by choice, social and regional isolation resulted in retention of many elements of the nondominant cultures and the maintenance of many linguistic features of the first or indigenous language. Regional and/or social class isolation contributed significantly to the development of different American dialects.

REGIONAL AND SOCIAL DIALECTS

Regional dialects are made up of sound patterns associated with where a person lives. A minimum of 10 different dialect regions have been designated by some dialectologists. However, depending on how dialect is defined and which types of linguistic features are counted, there are considerably more than 10 distinctive regional dialects (Carver, 1989).

Social dialects are associated with one's social class or status, ethnic and/or racial make up. Regional and social dialects may co-occur in the same speaker. For example, an AAE speaker from western Pennsylvania (a designated dialect region) may produce both varieties. Wolfram and Christian (1989) suggest that vowels (V) are more crucial to differentiating regional dialects and consonants (C) play a decisive role in differentiating social dialects.

Theoretically, the degree of mutual intelligibility between speakers distinguishes a dialect from a language and amount of communicative isolation serves as the primary criteria to determine whether or not a linguistic variety is mainly regional or mainly social. The communicative isolation of Black Americans from the dominant culture and mainstream language created the special case of AAE as a social dialect. AAE is not illogical as compared to SAE. It has phonological and grammatical rules that are systematic and speakers apply these rules in a logical manner. Variations within AAE may occur depending on where the speaker lives and the degree of historical interaction with other languages such as American Indian Pidgin, Hawaiian Pidgin, or Caribbean creoles (cf. Dillard, 1972, 1992; Gilbert, 1986).

PIDGINS AND CREOLES: CONVERGENCE AND DIVERGENCE

Pidgins are thought to be developed as languages of utility, i.e., when two or more divergent languages come into contact and their speakers have a need to communicate, varying rules and lexical items are taken from each language to enhance communication. Some pidgins become more formalized and are extended while others die out. When children of pidgin speakers are born and acquire the pidgin of their parents, the language that the children speak is called a creole. A predominant theory about how AAE evolved is called the creole origin hypothesis. The theory proposes that AAE evolved through a process of pidginization to creolization. When AAE speakers use language that is closer to the standard dialect, there is a convergence (decreolization) toward SAE. These speakers will have only a few of the phonological differences in their productive vocabularies. Others, however, in some large urban areas, are thought to be diverging away from SAE. The divergent speakers will exhibit a higher frequency of occurrence of AAE phonological differences.

Table 8.3 shows the eight linguistic features that distinguish AAE from all other regional and social dialects in the country. Of these eight features reported to characterize only AAE, two are found at the phonological level. The other six are morphological or syntactical, but the elements that occur at the grammatical level influence phonological output (Fasold, 1981).

When AAE was examined only for categorical or obligatory rules, the dialect was often misinterpreted as nonsystematic. Categorical or obligatory rules specify exactly how a vowel (V) or consonant (C) should be produced in a specified environment. For example, in an environment where there is no stress (−stress) and no tenseness (−tense), the resulting V will be a schwa [ə]. The optional rule to this specific categorical rule allows for a deletion of the schwa [ə] when it is in the environment before [r]. The result of the optional rules includes words such as "hist(o)ry, gall(e)ry, cel(e)ry, or sal(a)ry" (Fasold, 1990, pp. 244–245). The optional rule accounts for more than one way to say certain words by specifying the environment in which the phoneme may change and remain within a standard range, i.e., intelligible to the listener.

Labov's (1969) study of African-American English (AAE) led to the explication of a third category inclusive of "variable rules." Studies of variable rules of AAE speakers considered both social and linguistic contexts. Variable rules account for the probability that a rule may be applied in environment A or in environment B. However, there is a higher probability that the rule will be applied in environment A than in B. The variable rule notion was one means of demonstrating that there was a logical structuring to AAE and the variable rule concept expanded our understanding of how to consider social factors in defining the normal range of speech production.

From a sociolinguistic perspective, SAE is the prestige dialect that is spoken by the dominant culture and those who hold the economic and political power. However, many regard standard American English as an idealized notion, since there are few of us who produce SAE on a consistent basis and on every occasion that we speak. When speech patterns vary from the

TABLE 8.3.   Eight Linguistic Features that are Unique to Only African-American English (AAE)

Phonological Level

1. Devoicing of voiced stops in stressed syllables
   a. bit → bid
   b. back → bag
2. Reduction of final consonant clusters when followed by a word beginning with a vowel or when followed by a suffix beginning with a vowel
   a. wes' end for west end
   b. bussing for busting

Grammatical Level

1. Present tense, third person –s/–es absence
   a. she run for she runs
   b. she raise for she raises
2. Plural –sl/–es absence on general plurals (as opposed to the same type of absence found on weights and measures)
   a. six doll for six dolls
   b. some boy for some boys
3. Remote time been (expression about something that started in the past and remains significant at present)
   a. Ivory been paid for the tickets
   b. I been seen it coming
4. Possessive –s/–es absence
   a. Glenn hat for Glenn's hat
   b. Waymer car for Waymer's car
5. Copula and auxiliary absence involving is forms (as opposed to the more generally deleted are forms)
   a. she pretty for she's pretty
   b. he home for he's home
6. Use of habitual or distributive be
   a. she be thinking she something
   b. she don't be usually be there

standard, linguists refer to these systematic differences as "variations" or as the "vernacular." Language variation, language difference, the vernacular, and dialect may be used interchangeably. In popular culture, people tend to refer to dialects as "accents." We often hear expressions such as "a Boston accent," which gives information about a speaker's articulation of /r/ or lack of /r/. Dialect is more inclusive than accent. Accent emphasizes pronunciation while dialect includes grammatical features as well (Crystal, 1991).

In the latter part of the 20th century, sociolinguists began to address two primary factors: (*a*) every culture is as equally as valid as every other culture; and (*b*) every language is equally valid as every other language. No language or culture is better than another; differences between and among cultures and languages do not mean that one is better than another.

People of nondominant cultures in the United States argued that their customs, beliefs, and languages were as valid as those of the dominant culture. In the communicative sciences and disorders, there was a resounding call to eliminate the deficit model at all realms of language assessment and intervention. We began to think about articulation in terms of phonological rules and we were encouraged to interpret our speech test results in terms of whether the phonological rules that children used were more representative of languages of their first cultures versus whether their rules were reflective of their knowledge of SAE.

PROGRESSION FROM THE DEFICIT THEORY TO THE DIFFERENCE THEORY

With advances in linguistic sciences and an improved understanding of sociocultural factors, the melting pot philosophy began to give way to a more accepting pluralistic orientation. By the late 1960s, a substantive empirical data set had been amassed and interpreted to demonstrate that there are strong relationships among sociocultural practices, language variation (dialect), and bi/multilingualism (Baratz and Shuy, 1969; Dillard, 1972; Labov, 1972; Wolfram and Fasold, 1974). Increased emphasis was placed on adjusting articulation testing with regard to social dialects and a model for how this could be achieved in the communication disorders was proposed (Seymour and Seymour, 1977; Seymour and Seymour, 1981). Educators began to address the range of linguistic and cultural issues for children with limited English proficiency (LEP) (Cheng, 1987; Mattes and Omark, 1984). Most importantly, there was consensus among the enlightened that the deficit model was unacceptable and oppressive in that it supported a position of linguistic and cultural superiority.

At present, cultural pluralism is an easily accepted notion and one which readily permits us to understand that a single individual may embrace more than one culture and more than one dialect or language. Increased empirical data on first and second language acquisition and developmental sociolinguistics provide a basis for a wider acceptance and an equal value being placed on both cultures and variations/languages of bicultural, bidialectal, and bilingual children (cf. Langdon, 1992; Stockman, 1986). The first culture, first dialect (D_1), or first language (L_1) does not have to be suppressed for the child to learn the rule system of the second dialect (D_2) or second language (L_2). Data further suggested that it was unlikely that a child would exhibit a disorder in D_2 or L_2 if there was no disorder in D_1 or L_1 (cf. Adler, 1990; ASHA, 1983; Baran and Seymour, 1976; Cole and Taylor, 1990; Erickson and Omark, 1981; Jimenez, 1987; Ratusnik and Koenigsknecht, 1976; Seymour and Ralabate, 1985; Taylor and Payne, 1983; Terrell and Terrell, 1983).

The diagnostic category of phonological difference expands the range of an acceptable phonemic production system and reduces the social stigma attached to dialects, because members of the speech community assist in defining the standard (or target phonemes) relative to their own cultural expectations. We also rely on the child's speech community to determine disorder, i.e., if the people in the speech community do not understand the child, it is likely the child has a disorder. A lack of intelligibility by native speakers is a cogent predictor that a phonological disorder is present. The phonological considerations and adjustments that must be made in working with culturally and linguistically different children will be addressed in the next section.

DISTINGUISHING PHONOLOGICAL DIFFERENCE AND PHONOLOGICAL DISORDER

Understanding the relationships between culture and language improves our ability to differentiate phonological patterns associated with language variation from idiosyncratic sound systems that reveal phonological disorders. Relative to cultural diversity and phonological variation, there are two diagnostic categories: (*a*) presence of phonological difference and no disorder; and (*b*) a phonological disorder (misarticulation) in the presence of a phonological difference. A phonological difference exists if the speaker's first dialect (D_1) or first language (L_1) is not SAE. When there is a phonological difference present, the child may shift from D_1 or L_1 to D_2 (SAE) or L_2 (SAE). The process of switching back and forth between D_1-D_2 or L_1-L_2 may involve linguistic borrowing (code mixing) and/or code switching. Borrowing means the individual selects words or concepts learned in one language and uses them in another language. Using a Spanish word in place of an English word can cause confusion on the part of the SAE listener who may interpret the utterance to sound less intelligible or, possibly, interpret the utterance to sound like jargon. However, borrowing, in and of itself, does not reflect a disorder and the presence of borrowing can be determined by recording the child's speech sample and asking a native speaker if s/he can identify any of the sounds or words produced.

The term code switching is used to refer to persons who use both the standard dialect, their regional, and/or their social dialect. This speaker shifts (switches) from one communication code to another depending on the listener and the nature of the communicative situation. Code switching is a normal phenomenon found among people who are fluent in two or more variations/languages. Code switching may occur at the phonological, word, or sentence level. Code switching involves shifting back and forth between the two different variations/languages. The SLP should document whether there is presence of linguistic borrowing and code switching. While the presence of either linguistic phenomenon does not represent a phonological disorder, children exhibiting borrowing or code switching should be monitored until there is clarification that no disorder is present.

A phonological disorder is diagnosed after the SLP has accounted for presence/absence of nondialect structural and neurological problems (e.g., dysarthria or apraxia), and has considered dialectal variations and/or the influence of another language. A disorder is present when the student:

1. is unintelligible or displays reduced intelligibility to the native speakers of the same speech community;
2. misarticulates phonemes that are pronounced the same in both SAE and the first dialect or first language;
3. produces idiosyncratic patterns that are not representative of the processes normally found in the first dialect/language, SAE, or as a function of borrowing or code switching.

The diagnosing of difference versus disorder involves an additional step for the SLP. Instead of completing a single contrastive analysis where the child's speech is compared to the standard dialect (SAE), the SLP will complete a second contrastive analysis to determine if productions are consistent with expectations set for the first dialect or language. To achieve the latter, the SLP will elicit and record the speaker's sample via audio or video tape. The contrastive analysis should be completed to: (*a*) describe the Vs and Cs and/or processes produced by the speaker; (*b*) determine if the phonemes and/or the processes are consistent with SAE; and, if not, (*c*) determine if the phonemes and/or processes are consistent with another dialect or language. If the phonemes and/or processes are consistent with what is expected in D_1 or L_1, but different from SAE, there is a phonological difference present.

STRATEGIES FOR ASSESSING PHONOLOGY OF CULTURALLY AND LINGUISTICALLY DIVERSE CHILDREN

One effective strategy employed in phonological assessment of linguistically diverse populations has been that of using contrastive analysis to sample whether or not the child produces idiosyncratic speech sounds that are not representative of either D_1/L_1 or SAE (D_2/L_2). This approach is effective to the degree that the SLP understands the phonemic similarities and differences between the child's D_1/L_1 and SAE.

Appendix 8.1 is organized to assist those who will find contrastive analysis useful for nonnative English speakers. The transcription system for all consonants, vowels, and glides is shown in conjunction with the diacritics that are used to describe American English and 15 of the most frequently occurring languages in the United States. The phonemic data are adapted from Merritt Ruhlen's (1976) *Guide* and the linguistic selections are based on Mattes and Omark (1984). For each language displayed, the name of the language, the dialect (e.g., American English, French-West Canadian), source from which the phonemic data were obtained, and the classification of the language are given. Ruhlen's *Guide* specifies the glides, consonants, and vowels for each of the languages and are arranged so that they are consistent with positions on the consonant chart and the vowel diagrams.

Remember, just as English has variations, other languages also have varieties (Anderson and Smith, 1987; Tse and Ingram, 1987). For example, the Spanish cited in Appendix 8.1 is Mexican. Different lexical items and phonological processes may be heard from Spanish speakers who are from Puerto Rico, Texas, California, or Madrid. It would be worthwhile to examine Portuguese if you reside in New England or in areas where there are residents from Cape de Verde since it is suggested that Cape Verdean Creole is a combination of Portuguese and African languages.

Todd (1990) suggests that many of the Caribbean creoles and pidgins are Portuguese related. Examination of French may assist with assessing French related Haitian Creole speakers. Many Asian languages, such as Cantonese, Mandarin, Japanese, Korean, and Vietnamese, are tonal in that changing tones (pitch levels) provides phonological and other linguistic information. In a tonal language, the speaker may raise pitch instead of adding a morpheme such as plural −s. If your stimuli elicit plural −s, the speaker who is acquiring English may omit (delete) the −s. Since there are different stress patterns within words in different languages, the type of stress pattern (e.g., phonemic stress) used in the language is also shown in Appendix 8.1.

If interacting with a large number of students from a range of language backgrounds Ruhlen's *Guide* will be invaluable. It contains phonemic information on several hundred languages, presents information on obligatory and optional rules, and also presents patterns of syntactical word order. The *Guide* can serve many purposes, including providing a phonemic database to share with other educators who have difficulty understanding code mixing or code switching or even the concept of phonological difference.

Table 8.4 shows phonological variations that are present in AAE. The presence of AAE will be diagnosed based on the frequency of occurrence and consistency with which the speaker

TABLE 8.4. Phonological Variations for African-American English (AAE)

Position	SAE Form	AAE Form	To SAE Speaker, Sounds Like	
Initial	/str/	/skr/	stream	→ scream
			strap	→ scrap
Initial	/ʃr/	/sr/	shrimp	→ srimp
Initial	/ð/	/d/	this	→ dis
			that	→ dat
Initial	/θ/	/tr/	three	→ tree
			thrust	→ trust
Final	/θ/	/f/	Ruth	→ roof
Final	/ð/	/v/	bathe	→ bave
Final	/nt/	/n/	meant	→ men
			bent	→ Ben
Final	/dnt/	/tn/	didn't	→ dit'n
			shouldn't	→ shut'n
Final	/ŋ/	/n/	sing	→ sin
Final	/sks/	/səs/	masks	→ masses
Final	/skt/	/ks/	asked	→ axt
Final	/sts/	/s/	fists	→ fis
Final	/d/	omission	road	→ row
Final	/g/	omission	log	→ law
Final	/k/	omission	back	→ baa
Final	/t/	omission	boot	→ boo
Final or before consonants	/l/	omission	tool	→ too
			toll	→ toe
			fault	→ fought
			help	→ hep
Final or medial	/r/	omission	four	→ foe
			guard	→ God
			Carol	→ Cal
			carried	→ cad

	Vowels			
	SAE	AAE		
Before nasals	/i/	/e/	pin	→ pen
Before	/r/ or /l/ /ir/	/eh/	beer	→ bear
Before	/r/ /ur/	/ou/	poor	→ pour
Before	/l/ /ɔɪ/	/ɔ/	boil	→ ball
Any position	/aɪ/	/a/	find	→ fond
			time	→ Tom
	/aʊ/	/a/	found	→ fond

produces representative features. There is consistency and regularity of AAE phonological patterns. Some African-American children may use more AAE features than other children. Still other African-American children will produce no AAE features.

Frequently occurring phonological patterns in AAE include: (*a*) the formation of homophones produced by alternating or absent phonemes; and (*b*) sound variations that affect relational meaning and, in some cases, syntactical meaning. Phonological variations common to African American English (AAE), despite region of the country in which the child resides, are shown in Table 8.4.

Table 8.4 should be consulted if the student being tested is African-American or resides in a speech community where AAE is often produced. If a conventional articulation test is administered, be sure to compare test results to Table 8.4 to determine if phonological difference is present. A child who lives in a linguistic environment in which AAE is stable can be expected to exhibit (produce) at least two of the features displayed in Table 8.4.

Data in Table 8.4 are organized to display the position, Initial (I), Medial (M), or Final (F) positions of words, in which the AAE form is produced. Lexical examples are given to describe what the form sounds like in SAE and in AAE. These examples demonstrate homophones that are produced by alternating or deleting phonemes. AAE grammatical forms that affect sound variations are shown in Table 8.5.

Contrastive analysis, however, may not serve all purposes when we take into account the hundreds of languages that are spoken in the world. For example, in Boston alone the documented school children were found to speak 183 languages other than English as their L_1 (Proctor, McLaughlin, and Hutchinson, 1985). Moreover, not all languages have written symbol systems and many other languages have written symbol systems that monolingual English speakers cannot read. Consequently, an additional set of problem solving strategies will also be needed for therapeutic practice.

An important strategic approach to assessment is that the SLP develop sensitivity to and awareness of attitudes and perceptions of the different cultures with whom s/he will interact. Developing sensitivity to different cultures will provide the broad contextual information that will be needed to define and understand the child's speech community. (For greater specificity on selected Asian cultures and languages, see Cheng (1987) and Fang and Ping-an (1992).)

DEVELOPING SENSITIVITY TO CULTURAL DIFFERENCES

Different approaches involving new testing and therapeutic strategies are required to assess the phonological system(s) of children from diverse cultural and linguistic backgrounds. The first strategic approach is for the clinician to be aware that modifications are needed. Second, the SLP should view modifications as challenges, not barriers. The SLP must maintain a nonjudgmental attitude about any child's phonological system until all data have been collected and analyzed. Characterize (define) the speech community by determining family and community perceptions and expectations about the speech sound systems of children. Developing a successful interactive pattern with the speech community and specifying what the speech community accepts as normal will often require that SLPs adjust their perceptions and expectations concerning how long it will take to complete data collection (testing) and analysis. The following

TABLE 8.5.   Additional Linguistic Features of African-American English (AAE)

A. Grammatical Features

1. Third person singular –s. In standard English, the suffix –s is used to identify the present tense of the verb if the subject of that verb is in the third person singular. In AAE (African-American English), however, there is generally no such suffix used to identify third person singular present tense verbs. Therefore, AAE and standard American English (SAE) paradigms are:

Black English		Standard English	
Singular	Plural	Singular	Plural
1. I walk	we walk	1. I walk	we walk
2. you walk	you walk	2. you walk	you walk
3. he walk	they walk	3. he walks	they walk
4. the man walk	the men walk	4. the man walks	the men walk

The absence of this –s is not carelessly deleted by AAE speakers. This suffix is simply not an integral part of the AAE grammatical system.

2. A second feature that is characteristically different in AAE involves –s suffix as an indicator of possession. In SAE, possession is formed by adding an 's as in *boy's coat* or *John's hat*. In AAE, the form is often absent so that possession is indicated simply by word order, as in *boy coat* or *John hat*.

3. The –s suffixes which mark most plurals in SAE are occasionally not required in AAE. Examples such as *five book* and *The other teacher, they'll yell at you*.

4. Absence of the form be. The rules of AAE permit the forms *is* and *are* to be deleted, therefore, AAE forms such as *The boy here* and *He a man* corresponding to *The boy is here* and *He is a man* are realized.

5. Multiple negation. The occurrence of negatives at more than one point in a sentence is characteristic of many nonstandard dialects. Thus, the SAE *He didn't do anything to anybody* is spoken as *He didn't do nothing to nobody*.

6. Habitual be. The form *be* in reference to a habitual or repeated activity is a unique feature of AAE. When *be* is used in a sentence such as *Sometimes he be at school and sometimes he don't* does not have a corresponding SAE grammatical form.

B. Phonological Features

1. Word-final consonant clusters. When words end in certain types of consonant blends, or clusters (two consonant sounds adjacent to each other), phonological rules for AAE allow the final member of the cluster to be deleted. Cluster reduction influences two basic types of clusters. First, clusters in which both sounds of the cluster belong to the same base word can be reduced. Examples are as follows:

SAE	Cluster Reduction	AAE
te*st*	/st/ to /s/	te*s*'
de*sk*	/sk/ to /s/	de*s*'
ba*nd*	/nd/ to /n/	ba*n*'

The second type of cluster reduction affects final -t and -d when the sounds do not belong to the same base word and examples include the following:

SAE	Cluster Reduction	AAE
mi*ssed*	/st/ to /s/	mi*ss*'
ra*mmed*	/md/ to /m/	ra*m*'

C. *Hypercorrection* is a by-product rather than direct evidence of the grammatical and phonological system of AAE. Hypercorrection occurs when the speaker attempts to produce unfamiliar SAE units. This lack of familiarity will result in incorporating items not only where they are appropriate in standard

TABLE 8.5.—*continued*

English but also in inappropriate places. For example, some speakers produce not only –*s* third person forms on the appropriate verbs in standard English (e.g., *He likes the girl*) but on other than third person singular present tense forms resulting in sentences such as *I likes the girl very much.*

Certain types of hypercorrection, also referred to as "malapropism," are evident in vocabularies of AAE speakers. Hypercorrection at the lexical levels is a phenomenon that involves the inappropriate usage of words in an attempt to speak in an educated style or "talkin' proper." Hypercorrection, as a structural and a specific linguistic form, may be overextended or hypercorrection may occur as a result of social circumstances such as an AAE speaker being interviewed for television.

recommendations will facilitate and enhance the quality of assessment and intervention when interacting with bidialectal and/or bi/multilingual children.

A SUCCESSFUL INTERACTIVE DEMEANOR

When the variables of race, ethnicity, origin, and culture are factored into phonological assessments, the assessment process must be adjusted to consider a range of attitudes of a given speech community. For culturally and linguistically diverse children, take the time to develop sensitivity to the different cultural groups represented in the community (Bleile and Wallace, 1992). Also, seek to develop a sense of awareness about the perceptions and attitudes of the different cultural groups regarding speech and oral communication in the child's D_1 and D_2 and/ or L_1 and L_2. Knowledge of the culture will facilitate accuracy of subsequent assessment and intervention plans.

Until the SLP is familiar with the culture and language of the child's speech community, it is rare that a single testing session will be sufficient to complete an entire phonological assessment with accompanying recommendations. The SLP must think of strategies for assessment and prepare for an extended time range in which assessment can be conducted. If remediation is indicated, treatment approaches for culturally/linguistically diverse populations may include important customs not found in conventional American speech therapy. Do not compromise educational equity for time efficiency when you are interacting with culturally and linguistically diverse families.

DEVELOPING SENSITIVITY TO COMMUNITY NEEDS

To develop sensitivity to different cultural groups represented in the community, your first agenda is to get to know the people who will provide collaborative support for you. Consult with colleagues (other teachers or health care leaders) to:

- Determine who the community leaders are for each cultural group
- Determine if there are translators (interpreters) available
  —Who are they?
  —How do you contact them?

If interpreters are not available, ask families to bring a family member or family friend who speaks English when the assessment is scheduled. (Keep in mind that the availability of interpreters will impact on your scheduling.)

Search for alternatives to interpreters by requesting permission to tape record native speakers who may be paraprofessionals in the school system. Categorize your taped samples by language and store for the future. Most high school and university faculty who teach a second language would be happy to make a tape recording for your files.

PROMOTING SERVICES IN THE COMMUNITY

To establish the need for your services, use every possible opportunity to communicate information about the profession of communicative disorders. Since communication is a two-way process, as you develop your own sensitivity about other cultures you must also present information about the nature of communicative disorders.

1. Consult with colleagues and determine if they understand the role of the SLP. Using your best politeness formula, ask if they understand what you do and why.

The following anecdote is used to exemplify the significance of SLPs constantly communicating to others about our profession. After nearly 20 years of clinical practice, research, and teaching, I had not had the experience of a teacher becoming angry with me for completing an oral peripheral exam until I began to work with adolescents who spoke AAE. While consulting in a middle school, a 14-year-old African-American male requested my assistance so that he could improve his speech. After obtaining consent from his guardian, I explained to him what the articulators are and that I would look in his mouth to see if we might find a problem with his articulators. (I suspected apraxia because of a known history of physical abuse.) As I began the oral mechanism exam, the math teacher, also an African-American male, passed the door.

The teacher came in and verbally expressed his anger. Even as an African-American I had never thought of the possibility that someone would associate an oral mechanism exam with the days of slavery when the teeth of humans were examined to partially determine their worth. The teacher did draw this association. I assumed it had not materialized before in my professional life because I had worked with younger children. I, as did other teachers, understood his perspective and it only took about 3 months for me to systematically develop inservice training and to go to different classes to discuss what a speech-language pathologist does and why. There are some attitudes or perceptions that cannot be anticipated, even if you are a member of the same cultural group. However, my experience serves to demonstrate the need for frequent two-way communication. As you ask for information, let the community know what you will be doing and why.

Using your best politeness formula, let them know that some speech problems have organic etiologies or are caused by hearing loss, even slight to mild losses, and that there are many times that you will appear to be testing something other than speech and/or language. Concurrent with providing information to colleagues, there are several other issues on which you will request their assistance.

2. Consult with colleagues and determine which variations and which languages are spoken in the community. Do any of your colleagues (e.g., teacher or teacher's aide) speak the variation or the language? If yes, would s/he be willing to make tape recordings so that you could present some of your testing in the child's native language?

3. Consult with colleagues and determine if the facility in which you are employed has a social worker or determine how you gain access to a social worker who serves the community.
4. Consult with colleagues and determine names of community leaders. (The Director of Head Start is always a good person with whom to make initial contact.)
5. Phone community leaders who have been identified:
    - Introduce yourself by name and explain what you do; i.e., screen/test hearing, language, speech.
    - Explain why you would like to talk to the individual, i.e., need to obtain information on how people in the community feel about hearing, language and speech, and services that they have received in the past.
    - Ask if they have recommendations about speech and the services that they have previously received.
    - Invite members of the community to come in for a visit and/or formalize an opportunity such as an open house for the community to come in and meet with you and your staff.
    - At the end of every conversation, ask for names and telephone numbers of others in the community with whom you might discuss your services.
    - For each individual to whom you speak, send a follow-up letter. For your records, date and keep a written list of all of your phone calls and letters. Written records should contain name, address, phone numbers and date conversation and/or when informative letter was sent. (In cases where persons identified do not have telephones, prepare a separate, brief introductory letter with this same information and mail as you obtain correct addresses.)
6. When you contact an individual:
    - Be sure to ask if you have phoned at a convenient time and determine if you should call back. Checking on whether the other person is able to speak with you at the time you call is not only an appropriate politeness formula, it also reduces your anxiety about whether you have been put off for some unknown cultural reason. Schedule a telephone appointment at another mutually convenient time.

While much of the tedious work involved could be delegated, in cases of interacting with minority people, **please show respect**. This means that the person in charge of hearing, language, and speech must be the one who speaks to the community leaders. As related to African-Americans, do not "dis" (disrespect/show lack of respect for) the community leaders/elders.

If you are not of the same cultural and linguistic group as the individual being tested, keep in mind that members of a community understand this and do not expect you to "act like them." They will appreciate your ability to elicit and try to understand their perspective.

DEFINING THE SPEECH COMMUNITY

The concept of "speech community" means that speech patterns of a given group of people will vary by age, length of time in the United States, frequency with which English is spoken in the home, sound systems of the first language, frequency of contact with the homeland, the geographical region in which people live, and their social status within the community. The process of determining local norms will facilitate defining a specific speech community, i.e., establishing what is an acceptable standard of normal for the native speakers of the language. Bliele and Wallace (1992) provide a creative and clinically useful procedure for defining a speech community.

To define a speech community for African-American children, Bliele and Wallach (1992) administered a standardized articulation test to a group of African-American male and female 3–5-year-olds enrolled in Head Start. Head Start teachers were asked to refer to the SLP children who were intelligible and those who were difficult to understand. A broad phonetic transcription was completed on the results of the standardized test and features common to the less intelligible children were identified as the primary cues that adult AAE speakers used to identify phonological disorder. Results revealed that several nondialect patterns were found among the children reported to have "trouble talking."

The common nondialect patterns found among children in the "trouble talking" group included: (*a*) errors in stops in I and M positions and 1–2 or more stop errors; (*b*) [ʤ] affricate not produced in word-final position; (*c*) two or more fricative errors, but not including [θ]; (*d*) errors on nasals; (*e*) errors of gliding if 4 years or older; (*f*) unable to articulate [r] in at least one position of a word; (*g*) five or greater consonant cluster errors; and (*h*) misarticulation of the [s] cluster.

With regard to AAE, Cole and Taylor (1990) found that three different standardized articulation tests contained items that would be biased against VBE speakers. Of the 141 items on the Templin-Darley Test of Articulation, Second Edition, 29 (21%) were biased. Of the 67 items on the Arizona Articulation Proficiency Scale, 13 (19%) were biased, and of the 91 items on the Photo Articulation Test, 13 (14%) were likely to be biased against the AAE speaker.

Developing Local Norms

Before assessing individuals referred for phonological disabilities, one approach to validating diagnostic results is to develop and maintain a file of local norms, i.e., normal range of phonological differences for children in a given speech community. The following steps will assist in achieving local norms:

1. Explain the concept and purpose of local norms to the speech community. Either individually or at a Parent-Teacher Organization (PTO) meeting, discuss what you would like to accomplish, i.e., compare children with "speech problems" to normal child speakers of similar ages and stages of development. Indicate that not all formal speech tests consider all possible variations. Request referrals for children whom parents and teachers feel have normal speech. It is strongly recommended that you take the time to talk to the speech community about what you are trying to accomplish. Also, be sure to take a sample of the test you will use and show the adults that the "TEST" is not like those on which children receive intelligence quotients (IQ) points or grades.

    You will also have to explain the purpose to your child subjects. Anecdotally, when following the local norms process with two African-American children who were academically sound students and who also spoke Japanese and Spanish fluently, I found them very anxious. Their parents had discussed that I would be testing them. Although it was summer vacation, the children's perception of a test was that there would be some other academic consequence. I permitted them to select who would be first and to allow the second to observe. After both took the test, they received a second explanation of how their results would be used to help other children in their community who might have "speech problems."

2. Administer a standardized articulation test to small groups of children at the same age levels. Select the standardized test that indicates inclusion of minority child speakers in its normative sample. Try to have at least five children in a given age group, although 10 would be an excellent sample size for these purposes. Record responses and explore response forms to determine consistency of production among the children. A brief written consent form may be developed and used to follow-up on the verbal request.

3. Since most standardized articulation tests require a picture naming task, use a phonological process approach and use objects to elicit speech samples from small groups of children of the same age level. Tape record the speech samples and analyze for common processes found among the children (e.g., cluster reduction is a common process found in AAE and should not be viewed as constituting a disorder). To demonstrate a situation in which local norms were obtained, Appendix 8.2 discusses the case of a native Spanish speaker.

4. If you are already familiar with the speech sound system of a community, the *ALPHA* (Lowe, 1986) is a formal measure that will facilitate your ability to explore the relationship between conventional articulation assessment and phonological processes.

The *Assessment of Phonological Processes—Revised (English)* (Hodson, 1986), the *Assessment of Phonological Processes—Spanish* (Hodson, 1986), Mattes' (1986) *Criterion-Referenced Articulation Profile*, and the *Compton Phonological Assessment of Foreign Accent* (1983) are instruments that considered language differences when selecting the normative sample. These commercially available materials will assist with specifying phonological differences, aid with planning individual speech programs, and provide a means of measuring the child's progress.

5. Related variables to consider in testing and adapting tests include:
   - Type of test stimuli
     —consider familiarity with pictures versus use of objects
     —consider visual presentation of stimuli such as color pictures or photographs versus line drawings
     —will speakers of the culture use the same word that is to be elicited by the stimulus in the test tool you select
     —are test items age appropriate and culturally appropriate
     —is the first language read from right to left versus left to right or vertically versus horizontally
     —what would be the most appropriate order in which to present picture stimuli
   - Amount of time for testing—it will take longer
   - Elicitation procedures
     —how will you get the child to talk; will free play with a sibling or a same age peer be helpful
     —will you be able to elicit spontaneous productions versus accepting imitations of your speech
     —should you accept immediate versus elicited imitation
   - Incorporate an interpreter into the testing and therapy sessions
     —consider how you will explain the task to the interpreter

—what and how are instructions to be given to the child

—is the language of instruction appropriate for child's age level

—how can you be sure that the interpreter presents the instructions correctly

- Analysis of results will take longer—ALWAYS TAKE THE TIME TO CONSULT WITH NATIVE SPEAKERS OF THE CHILD'S SPEECH COMMUNITY BEFORE WRITING THE FINAL DIAGNOSIS

STRATEGIES FOR REMEDIATION

The presence of a phonological difference does not rule out the SLP's participation in the child's educational program. Attitude surveys consistently reveal that most adults regard SAE as a realistic educational goal. In fact, many probably think a prime reason we send children to school is to learn SAE (Cecil, 1988; Rickford, 1987; Speicher and McMahon, 1992; Tucker and Lambert, 1969; Weber, 1979). Certainly, ability to communicate in SAE is still closely aligned with employability (Terrell and Terrell, 1983).

For those with phonological differences, it is recommended that we offer options. To offer the options the SLP must develop awareness among speakers of the variation, discuss with parents/guardians, obtain family permission to develop a culturally sensitive program, and request active participation on the part of the family. With availability of computers and home videotape, after the initial family conference, active family participation may occur via disk switching or exchanges of videotape. Children enjoy seeing themselves on television by route of videotape.

As soon as you identify phonological differences, plan a parent conference with the agenda set to explain what is meant by a dialect and the similarities and differences found with SAE. When the difference involves either Spanish or AAE, use the Quick Checklist shown in Table 8.6 to assist in your explanations. This is a process of developing awareness of phonological issues among family members. Discuss cultural attitudes and have students explore how they feel about their speech. Do not pursue working with a language difference without informed consent, just as you would not initiate any other type of remediation without informed consent.

To develop remediation goals when phonological difference is involved, the following process is recommended.

1. Schedule a parent conference. Explain that the child has a language difference NOT a deficit or pathology. Define dialect/language variation. For some, this may require several conferences. Use conference time as an opportunity to educate the adult figures in the child's environment. Of course, parent input is critical so elicit as much information as possible from the family.

2. Depending on degree, consistency and frequency of occurrence of production of AAE, you may plan individual, small group or classroom "Communication Time." Emphasize the fact that people speak differently in different countries; discuss positive values of being able to speak in more than one way. Focus on the fact that people speak differently in different situations and role play the possibilities. Have students develop scripts for different types of social situations. Have students develop narratives of different ways of talking. Talk about how we listen and what are conversational roles in different cultures, role play some of these situations. All of this serves to establish the importance of individual differences and that we can adjust how we speak at different times and in

TABLE 8.6. Quick Checklist

Phonemic Characteristics	a. Syntactic Characteristics	b. Phonemic Characteristics
1a. s/z: example: "fussy" for "fuzzy" b. b/v: example: "best" for "vest" c. ʃ/tʃ: example: "mashes" for "matches" 2. Use of same stressed /a/ for "cat," "father," etc. 3. Difficulty in discrimination and production of the following vowels or vowel combinations: /i/, /ɪ/, & /æ/ 4. Addition of /e/ sound before initial clusters beginning with /s/ Examples: espoon/ spoon; eschool/school 5. s/θ: example: "sanks" for "thanks" NOTE: If the child shows other dialect features, check them in the African-American (AAE) English checklist	1. Use of "in" for "ing" endings; Examples: "They singin–" for "They are singing" 2. Suffixes like "–ed" marking past tense/past participle forms are not pronounced due to consonant reduction rule (see b5) 3. Addition of "–ed" suffix to irregular past tense verbs, i.e., "buyed" for "bought" 4. Absence of "–s" suffix marking 3rd person singular, i.e., "He walk" for "He walks" 5. Use of "have" for "has," i.e., "She have a doll" for "She has a doll" 6. Use of "do" for "does," i.e., "She always do silly things" 7. Use of "don't" for "doesn't," i.e., "She don't go" 8. Absence of person-number agreement with present and past tense forms of verb "to be" (copula), i.e., "You was there; "They is here" 9. Deletion of copula, i.e., "They runnin–" 10. Distributive copula, i.e., "They be singin–" 11. Use of "ain't" for "have/has" and "am/are," i.e., "I ain't gonna do it" 12. Double negatives, i.e., "She didn't do nothin–" 13. Absence of "s" possessive marker: "The girl hat"	1. f/θ: "toofbrush" for "toothbrush;" "teef" for "teeth" (F) 2. t/θ: "trow" for "throw" (I) 3. d/ð: "broder" for "brother" 4. v/ð: "bruvah" for "brother" 5. Consonant reduction in plural forms of words ending in "sp," "st," "sk;" use of "–es" for "–s": i.e., "desses" for "desks;" "tesses" for "tests;" "wasses" for "wasps"

different places. Build in the fact that listening is important—we should listen to ourselves (self-monitor) and listen to others.

3. If you serve as a consultant to a classroom teacher, you can also develop bulletin boards, have children bring information from home, for example, photos of grandparents who are from (*name country*) and speak (name language). Discuss the importance of being able to communicate in more than one way and in more than one language.

4. Individual sessions may be scheduled for those for whom it is unclear if they have a disorder and a difference. This may include structured play to elicit speech samples that can be assessed over several sessions.

5. Drill work may be incorporated into a particular child's program or into small groups with the same dialect (cf. Berger, 1990; Kupfer and Kissel, 1990).

6. The primary remedial strategies recommended here are designed to set the stage for those who are phonologically disordered and lay the foundation for a positive self-image and linguistic attitude for those who have a phonological disorder. For instance, with classroom presentations by the SLP, peers and teachers become familiar with language difference and can become active participants in a given child's remediation.

To effectively provide nonbiased assessments (PL 94–142; PL 95–561), we must develop a better understanding of the logical structures of phonological systems of English based dialects as well as phonological systems of other languages. Moreover, it is necessary to develop a fuller understanding of how social and cultural practices of the students with whom we interact influence different aspects of the child's communicative competence.

Children from the nondominant cultures are likely to produce either variations of American English or language that is influenced by family members who are non-native English speakers (Aitchison, 1991; Wolfram and Christian, 1989). These children may be referred to as bicultural, bidialectal, or bilingual, suggesting the coexistence of two dialects or at least two languages that the same child understands and speaks. However, a traditional phonological screening and/or assessment may reveal that the phonological system which the child is using is mainly the first dialect (D_1) or first language (L_1) and proficiency in the second dialect (D_2) or language (L_2) is limited. In the case of a difference or a disorder, we offer options for change. Appendix 8.3 has been structured to assist in the organization and tracking of language and speech data for culturally and linguistically diverse children. As each of us gains experience, we can anticipate that our creative strategies in communication disorders will consistently include each child's culture as a vital part of any remediation plan.

ACKNOWLEDGMENTS

Sincere appreciation is expressed to Rosalie Lettiere for the organization and design of all tables and graphics in this chapter. Special thanks are extended to Linda Morris, Population Information Assistant, U.S. Bureau of the Census, for the time and effort that she spent on identifying and validating accuracy of data in Table 8.1. Gratitude is also expressed to Phyllis Proctor and Ivory Green who served as speaker informants for AAE and as personal sources of encouragement.

REFERENCES

Adler S. Multicultural clients: implications for the SLP. Language, Speech, and Hearing Services in Schools 1990;21: 135–139.

Aitchison J. Language change: progress or decay? 2nd ed. New York: Cambridge University Press, 1991.

Anderson NB. Understanding cultural diversity. American Journal of Speech-Language Pathology 1992;1:11–12.

Anderson R, Smith BL. Phonological development of two-year-old monolingual Puerto Rican Spanish-speaking children. Journal of Child Language 1987;14:57–78.

Asante MK. African elements in African-American English. In Holloway JE, ed. Africanisms in American culture. Bloomington, IN: Indiana University Press, 1991:19–33.

American Speech-Language-Hearing Association. Position of the American Speech-Language-Hearing Association on social dialects. ASHA 1983;25(1):23–25.

Baca L, Amato C. Bilingual special education: training issues. Exceptional Children 1989;56:168–173.

Baran J, Seymour HN. The influence of three phonological rules of Black English on discrimination of minimal word pairs. Journal of Speech and Hearing Research 1976;19:467–474.

Baratz JC, Shuy RW. Teaching Black children to read. Washington, DC: Center for Applied Linguistics, 1969.

Berger MI. Speak standard, too. Chicago, IL: Orchard Books, 1990.

Bleile KM, Wallace H. A sociolinguistic investigation of the speech of African-American preschoolers. American Journal of Speech-Language Pathology 1992;1:54–62.

Campbell LR, Brennan DG, Steckol KF. Preservice training to meet the needs of people from diverse cultural backgrounds. ASHA 1992;34(12):29–32.

Carver CM. American regional dialects: a word geography. Ann Arbor, MI: University of Michigan Press, 1989.

Cashmore EE. Dictionary of race and ethnic relations. London: Routledge and Kegan Paul, 1988.

Cecil NL. Black dialect and academic success: a study of teacher expectations. Reading Improvement 1988;25(1):34–38.

Census Bureau releases 1990 census counts on specific racial groups. US Department of Commerce News Release CB91–215, Wed., June 12, 1991.

Cheng L-RL. Assessing Asian language performance. Rockville, MD: Aspen Publishers, 1987.

Cole L. E Pluribus Pluribus: multicultural imperatives for the 1990s and beyond. ASHA 1989;31:65–70.

Cole PA, Taylor OL. Performance of working class African-American children on three tests of articulation. Language, Speech, and Hearing Services in Schools 1990;21:171–176.

Compton A. Compton phonological assessment of foreign accent. San Francisco: Carousel House, 1983.

Crystal D. The Cambridge encyclopedia of language. New York: Cambridge University Press, 1991.

Cummins K. A theoretical framework for bilingual special education. Exceptional Children 1989;56:111–119.

Dandy EB. Black communications: breaking down the barriers. Chicago, IL: African-American Images, 1991.

Dillard JL. Black English. New York: Vintage Books, 1972.

Dillard JL. The development of Black English. In Dillard JL. A history of American English. New York: Longman, 1992:60–92.

Erickson JG, Omark DR, eds. Communication assessment of the bilingual bicultural child. Baltimore, MD: University Park Press, 1981.

Farley JE. Majority-minority relations. 2nd ed. Englewood Cliffs, NJ: Prentice Hall, 1988.

Fasold RW. Sociolinguistics of language. Cambridge, MA: Basil Blackwell, 1990.

Fasold RW. The relation between Black and White speech in the south. American Speech 1981;56:163–189.

Feng X, Ping-an H. Articulation disorders among speakers of Mandarin Chinese. American Journal of Speech-Language Pathology 1992;1:15–16.

Gilbert GG. The English of the Brandywine population: a triracial isolate in southern Maryland. In Montgomery MB, Bailey G, eds. Language variety in the south. University, AL: University of Alabama Press, 1986:102–110.

Hodson BW. The assessment of phonological processes—revised (English). San Diego, CA: Los Amigos Research Associates, 1986.

Hodson BW. The assessment of phonological processes—Spanish. San Diego, CA: Los Amigos Research Associates, 1986.

Jimenez BC. Articulation error patterns in Spanish-speaking children. Journal of Childhood Communication Disorders 1987;10:119–123.

Kupfer ML, Kissel J. Bridging the dialect gap. Austin, TX: Pro-Ed, 1990.

Labov W. Contraction, deletion and inherent variability of the English copula. Language 1969;45:715–762.

Labov W. Language in the inner city. Philadelphia, PA: University of Pennsylvania Press, 1972.

Langdon HW. Language disorder or difference? Assessing the language skills of Hispanic students. Exceptional Children 1989;56:160–167.

Langdon HW. Hispanic children and adults with communication disorders: assessment and intervention. Rockville, MD: Aspen Publishers, 1992.

Locke DC. Increasing multicultural understanding: a comprehensive model. Newbury Park, CA: Sage Publications, 1992.

Lowe RJ. The ALPHA (assessment link between phonology and articulation) test of phonology. East Moline, IL: LinguiSystems, 1986.

Mattes LJ. Criterion-referenced articulation profile. San Diego, CA: Los Amigos Research Associates, 1986.

Mattes LJ, Omark DR. Speech and language assessment for the bilingual handicapped. San Diego, CA: College Hill Press, 1984.

1990 Census Profile. Race and Hispanic origin. Suitland, MD: US Department of Commerce Economics and Statistics Administration: Bureau of Census, June, 1991:(2)1–8.

Proctor A, McLaughlin AM, Hutchinson JP. From Creole to English: assessing language difference and language disorder. ERIC: [ED 250 926]. Resources in Education: Languages and Linguistics, 1985.

Public Law 95–561. The Bilingual Education Act. (Title VII of the Elementary and Secondary Act of 1965).

Ratusnik Dl, Koenigsknecht RA. Influence of age on Black preschoolers' nonstandard performance of certain phonological and grammatical forms. Perceptual and Motor Skills 1976;42:199–206.

Rickford J. The haves and the have nots: sociolinguistic surveys and the assessment of speaker competence. Language in Society 1987;16(2):149–178.

Ruhlen M. Guide to the languages of the world. San Diego, CA: Los Amigos Research Associates, 1976. (Several hundred languages are printed in this *Guide*. Order from Los Amigos Research Associates, 7035 Galewood, San Diego, CA 92120; $22.00 per copy.)

Speicher BL, McMahon SM. Some African-American perspectives on Black English vernacular. Language in Society 1992;21:383–407.

Seymour HL, Ralabate PK. The acquisition of a phonologic feature of Black English. Journal of Communication Disorders 1985;18:139–148.

Seymour HN, Seymour CM. A therapeutic model for communicative disorders among children who speak Black English vernacular. Journal of Speech and Hearing Disorders 1977;42:247–256.

Seymour HN, Seymour CM. Black English and standard American English contrasts in consonantal development for four- and five-year-old children. Journal of Speech and Hearing Disorders 1981;46:276–280.

Stockman I. Language acquisition in culturally diverse populations: the Black child as a case study. In Taylor OL, ed. Nature of communication disorders in culturally and linguistically diverse populations. San Diego, CA: College Hill Press, 1986:117–155.

Taylor OL, Payne KT. Culturally valid testing: a proactive approach. Topics in Language Disorders 1983;3:1–7.

Terrell BY, Hale JE. Serving a multicultural population: different learning styles. American Journal of Speech Language Pathology 1992;1:5–8.

Terrell S, Terrell F. Distinguishing linguistic difference from disorders: the past, present and future of nonbiased testing. Topics in Language Disorders 1983;3:1–7.

Todd L. Pidgins and Creoles. London: Routledge, 1990.

Tse S-M, Ingram D. The influence of dialectal variation on phonological acquisition: a case study on the acquisition of Cantonese. Journal of Child Language 1987;14:281–294.

Tucker GR, Lambert WE. White and Negro listeners' reactions to various American-English dialects. Social Forces 1969;47:463–468.

US Office of Education. Education of All Handicapped Children Act (Public Law 94–142). Part II. Implementation of Part B of the Education of the Handicapped Act. Federal Register August 23, 1977;42:250.

Webber R. An overview of language attitude studies with special reference to teachers' attitudes. Educational Review 1979;31:217–232.

Wolfram W. Dialects and American English. Englewood Cliffs, NJ: Prentice Hall, 1991.

Wolfram W, Christian D. Dialects and education: issues and answers. Englewood Cliffs, NJ: Prentice Hall, 1989.

Wolfram W, Fasold RW. The study of social dialects in American English. Englewood Cliffs, NJ: Prentice Hall, 1974.

Appendix 8.1 | Interpretation of Phonetic Descriptions of 15 Different Languages

THE 15 LANGUAGES SELECTED are among the most frequently occurring in the United States. After the name of each language is presented, general information about type of dialect, the bibliographic source of the phonetic information (by author and date) and type of language classification are shown.

Since many languages contain speech sounds that are not produced in English, symbology for glides and diacritics are presented first to assist with interpretation of vowels (V) and consonants (C) shown for the 15 selected languages. Glides are described relative to tongue elevation (high or mid), location (front, central, or back) and degree of lip rounding. Glides, with diacritical markings, can be found on the vowel diagrams that follow. Diacritical markings indicate how individual phonemes (allophones) may vary in different languages.

For the vowel diagrams, the degree of lip rounding, the extent of tongue elevation (high-low) and the portion of the tongue (front, back) participating in producing the speech sound are displayed. The consonant chart uses columns to show place of articulation (e.g., bilabial, labio-dental). Rows are employed to display acoustical classifications of consonants (e.g., stops or fricatives, affricates). The voiceless C always appears directly above its voiced counterpart. For example, the bilabial stop [p] is shown directly above its voiced counterpart [b].

The General Information Categories Included in the Language Descriptions Are as Follows.

Category	Example for English
Name of the language	English
Name of the dialect	American
Source of the phonetic information*	Gleason 1961
Language classification	Indo-European: Germanic: West

*References cited in Ruhlen M. Guide to the languages of the world. San Diego, CA: Los Amigos Research Associates, 1976.

GLIDES

[j]: High front unrounded

[ɥ]: High front rounded

[w]: High back rounded

[ɯ]: High back unrounded

[e̞]: Mid front unrounded

[ə]: Mid central unrounded

[o̞]: Mid back rounded

DIACRITICS

[ʰ]: Aspirated	[ˆ]: Coarticulated	N: Nasal (m, n, ŋ)
[˜]: Nasalized	[ˌ]: Syllabic	L: Liquid (l, r,)
[ˉ]: Long	[ʲ]: Palatalized	G: Glide (j, w)
[ˌ]: Dental	[ʷ]: Labialized	N: North
[ˌ]: Retroflex	[ᵚ]: Velarized	E: East
[ˍ]: Fortis	[ˤ]: Pharyngealized	S: South
[ₒ]: Voiceless	[ɬ]: Voiceless Lateral Fricative	W: West
[ˌˌ]: Breathy Voice	[ɮ]: Voiced Lateral Fricative	C: Central
[ˍ]: Creaky Voice	[ɺ]: Lateral Flap	
[ʔ]: Ejective/Preglottalized	[ ]: Phonetic Transcription	
[ᵍ]: Voiced Click	/ /: Phonemic Transcription	

VOWELS

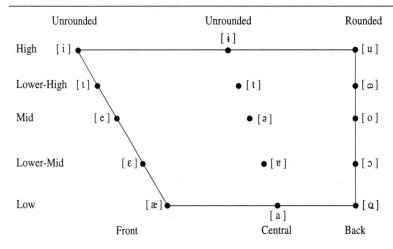

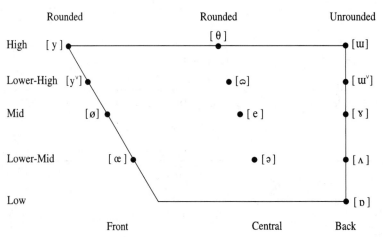

CONSONANTS

	Bilabial	Labiodental	Interdental	Dental	Alveolar	Retroflex	Palatal*	Velar	Labial-Velar	Uvular	Pharyngeal	Glottal
Stops	p b			ṭ ḍ	t d	ṭ ḍ	c ɟ	k g	k͡p g͡b	q ɢ		ʔ
Affricates	pᶠ		t̪ᶿ d̪ᵟ	t̪ˢ d̪ᶻ	tˢ tˡ dᶻ dˡ	č̣ ǰ	č cᶜ ǰ ɟʲ	kˣ ^gˡ				
Fricatives	Φ β	f v	θ ð	s̪ z̪	s z	ṣʃ ẓʒ	ʃ ç ʒ jˆ	x ɣ		χ ʁ	ħ ʕ	h ɦ
Approximants		ʋ		ɹ̪	ɹ	ɻ	j		w			
Nasals	m			ṇ	n	ṇ	ɲ	ŋ	m͡ŋ	N		
Laterals				ḷ	l ɬ	ḷ	ʎ					
Trills				ṛ	r	ṛ				R		
Flaps				ɽ̣	ɾ	ɽ						
Ejectives	pʔ			t̪ʔ	tʔ		cʔ	kʔ	k͡pʔ	qʔ		
Implosives	ɓ ʔb			ḍ ʔb	ɗ ʔd	ʄ	ʔʃ	ɠ ʔg				
Clicks	ʇ			ʅ ꞎ	ʒ	ʗ						

*Includes both palatal and palatoalveolar sounds.

CANTONESE [Chao 1969] [Sino-Tibetan: Sinitic: South] [S China]

```
p  pʰ      ţ  ţʰ      k  kʰ kʷ kʰʷ        l        u   T  ȳ        ū    j  w   high falling
              cˢ  cˢʰ                         e  ø     o   ƶ̄                    mid rising
f              ç              h               ə        ε̄        ō        mid level
m         ṇ         ŋ                                         ā         low falling
          l̩                                                               low rising
                                                                          low level

                                              non-phonemic stress
```

FRENCH (West Canadian) [Ellis 1965] [Indo-European: Italic: Romance: Western]

```
p    t    k          l  y  u
b    d    g          e  ø  ə  o    ẽ  œ̃    õ    ɥ  ɥ  w
f    s    ʃ          ε        ɔ    æ̃
v    z    ʒ          a        ɑ
m    n    ɲ
     l
     r
```

GERMAN [Moulton 1962] [Indo-European: Germanic: West] [Germany]

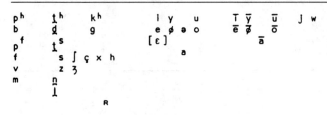

GREEK (Modern) [Householder, Kazazis & Koutsoudas 1964] [Indo-European: Greek]

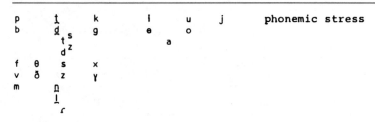

ITALIAN (Standard) [Agard & DiPietro 1969] [Indo-European: Italic: Romance: Western]

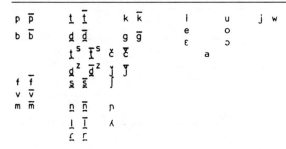

PORTUGUESE (Lisbon) [Head 1964] [Indo-European: Italic: Romance: West]

JAPANESE [Bloch 1950] [Altaic: Japanese]

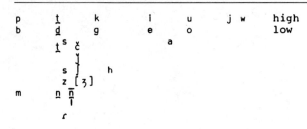

KOREAN (Seoul) [Martin 1951] [Altaic:-]

```
p  pʰ  p?    ṭ  ṭʰ  ṭ?     č  čʰ  č?  k  k?  kʰ  k?      i  u  ɯ      ⊤  ū  ɯ̄      j  w
        s  s?                          h   e[ø]o  ɤ     ē     ō  ɤ̄     non-phonemic stress
m           ṇ                  ŋ          ɛ      ɒ      ɛ̄         ɒ̄
        l
```

MANDARIN [Chao 1968] [Sino-Tibetan: Sinitic: North] [N China]

```
p  pʰ    ṭ  ṭʰ              k  kʰ      i  y   u   j  ɥ  w    high level
        ṭˢ ṭˢʰ ṭˢ ṭˢʰ cˤ cˤʰ            e      o              high rising
f       ṣ       ṣ     ç     χ             a                  low falling
m       ṇ             ç           ŋ                          high falling
        ḷ
        ɻ̩                   [ʀ]                               phonemic stress
```

NAVAJO [Reichard 1951] [Na-Dene: Athapaskan-Eyak: Athapaskan]

```
p    t  tʰ  t?       k  kʰ  kʷ  k?  ?    ɩ       ī      ĩ      ɩ̃̄      ō      j  ?j  [w]
    tˢʰ tˢ?  t'  t'?  čʰ  č?           ɛ   o  ē̄   ō  ɛ̃      õ  ɛ̃̄      ō̄      high
    dᶻ        dˡ      ǰ                    a     ā̃     ã       ã̄          low
    s        ʃ   x  xʷ           h                                        rising
    z        ʒ   ɣ  ɣʷ                                                    falling
[m] ?m       n  ?n
    l  ɬ
```

POLISH (Warsaw) [Schenker 1973] [Indo-European: Slavic: West]

```
p  pʲ    ṭ          k  kʲ       i       u           j  w
b  bʲ    ḍ          g  gʲ       ɛ    ɔ  [ɛ̃]   ɔ̃      penultimate stress
        ṭˢ  č  cʲˤ             a
        ḍᶻ  ǰ  ɉʲ
f  fʲ   ṣ   ʃ  çˤ  x  xʲ
v  vʲ   ẓ   ʒ  ɉʲˤ
m  mʲ   ṇ   ɲ
        ḷ
        r
```

SPANISH (Mexican) [Stockwell & Bowen 1965] [Indo-European: Italic: Romance: Western]

```
p  ṭ  k        l     u   j  w       phonemic stress
b  ḍ  g              e      o
   č          a
f  s  x
m  ṇ  ɲ
   ḷ
   ɾ  r
```

TAGALOG (Manila) [Schachter & Otanes 1972] [Austro-Tai: Austronesian: Indonesian: Hesperonesian: North Indonesian: Philippine]

```
p    t̪    k    ʔ         ɩ        o        T̄       ū    j   w
b    d̪    g              e        o        ē       ō              non-phonemic stress
     [č]                      e               ā
[f]  s         h
m    n̪    ŋ
     l
     ɾ
```

VIETNAMESE (Hanoi) [Thompson 1965] [Austro-Asiatic: Mon-Khmer: Viet-Muong]

```
p    t̪ʰ   t    c    k    ʔ        i         u        j  w  ɰ̃  ɓ̪   high rising
ɓ              ɗ                             ɯ̆           high rising glottalized
f    s̪              x    h        e         o   ɤ       higher mid trailing
     z̪              ɣ             ɛ    ə    ɔ   ʌ                        falling
m    n̪         ɲ    ŋ             æ                     low trailing
     l̪                                                  mid low dropping
                                                        low dropping
```

YIDDISH [Fal'kovich 1966] [Indo-European: Germanic: West]

```
p    t̪    k              l    u    j    initial stress
b    d̪    g              e    o
     t̪ˢ   č         a
f    s̪    ʃ    x
v    z̪    ʒ    ɦ
m    n̪
     l̪
     ɾ         [ʀ]
```

Appendix 8.2 | Word Pairs to Assess Auditory Discrimination of Spanish-English Difference*

Purpose: This particular word list is designed to informally assess auditory discrimination and to determine if there is a need to focus on phonemic discrimination of Spanish-English differences.

Directions: Ask the client to turn around so that s/he cannot see you and no visual cues are given. Tell the client that you will say two words and after each set of two words, please tell you if the two words sound the "same" or "different." The underlined sounds are frequently substituted or interchanged by Spanish speakers who are learning English as a second language.

1. witch/wish _____
2. choose/choose _____
3. use/use _____
4. use/juice _____
5. badge/batch _____
6. chew/juice _____
7. bog/bog _____
8. bale/yale _____
9. tip/dip _____
10. pot/pot _____
11. nice/nice _____
12. tin/sin _____
13. tin/thin _____
14. tin/tin _____
15. toes/those _____
16. so/so _____
17. dip/sip _____
18. dot/sip _____
19. doze/those _____
20. sin/thin _____
21. think/think _____
22. so/though _____
23. them/them _____
24. without/without _____
25. cease/seize _____
26. win/wing _____

---

*By Ann B. Fitzgerald, M.S., CCC-SLP, Speech-Language Pathologist, Waltham-Weston Hospital, Waltham, MA, and Adele Proctor, Sc.D. Ms. Fitzgerald evaluated the client and developed the basis for the test when she was a graduate student and Dr. Proctor was her clinical supervisor.

27. ring/ring _____
28. mat/nat _____
29. wack/wag _____
30. mamm/man _____
31. caught/got _____
32. bat/pat _____
33. wip/wip _____
34. tab/tap _____
35. tide/tide _____

Note: This set of speech stimuli is based on phonological differences between English and Spanish and provides a demonstration of the type of assessment tool that can be developed and on which local norms may be obtained.

BILINGUAL

Spanish-English

DIAGNOSTIC EVALUATION REPORT

NAME: Tony   *DATE OF BIRTH:*   8/17/70
DATE OF EVALUATION: 10/24/89   *AGE:*   19 years
CLINICIAN: Ann B. Fitzgerald
SUPERVISOR: Dr. Adele Proctor

COMPLAINT AND REFERRAL

Tony, a 19-year-old student majoring in English and Philosophy, referred himself for an evaluation because he was concerned about his ability to proficiently produce spoken English. He noted particular difficulty with "tenses," "vowels," and "endings of words." He stated that he does not have as much difficulty with reading and writing, although admitted to occasional ESL (English as a second language) mistakes such as "run-on sentences." Tony indicated that he would like to stay in this country after graduation, and would like to improve his speech production before "going out into the real world."

HISTORY

Tony is a native Spanish speaker who has been in the United States for approximately 8 years. Tony was born in Puerto Rico, but spent most of his young life in Venezuela, where he lived until moving to the United States. His father is originally from Spain and his mother from Puerto Rico. He stated that his family still resides in Venezuela. Although he indicated familiarity with several dialects of Spanish, he did not perceive that his Spanish was more characteristic of a specific regional or social Spanish dialect.

In his case history, Tony indicated that he has been in good health and has had no serious illnesses. He did report, however, a history of ear infections in childhood. Tony also reported recent symptoms of possible cerumen accumulation, particularly in his right ear.

EXAMINATIONS

A. Hearing

A routine pure tone hearing screening was conducted at 20 dB for frequencies of 500 Hz,

1000 Hz, 2000 Hz, and 4000 Hz, in order to assess potential need for further audiological evaluation. Tony passed all frequencies at 20 dB except for 500 Hz in the right ear.

Bilateral otoscopic examination revealed slight cerumen buildup in the right ear.

B. Oral-Peripheral

The oral mechanism appeared adequate for speech production in structure and function. It was noted that a lower right molar was missing. Due to location of the missing molar, speech production should not be adversely affected in either Spanish or English.

C. Language

Language was assessed primarily through informal conversation and picture naming on an articulation test. Tony was observed to have some difficulty in tense usage and morphology. For example, when telling of a situation in which he gave an oral presentation, he stated, "Last summer, I took a course, and we will have to give a presentation." Also, while identifying pictures, he called a drum a "drummer" and a sled a "slider." Tony also had difficulty identifying the pictures "valentine," "top," "seal," "wagon," and "mitten" even after cuing.

D. Speech

The *Fisher-Logemann Test of Articulation Competence* was administered. Tony was asked to name a series of 109 picture stimuli. Each phoneme of English, in each syllabic position and phonetic context was tested. Tony was also asked to read fifteen sentences as part of the sentence test. The sentence test evaluated all singleton consonants, in syllabic structures compatible with English phonology, and every vowel phoneme of English. Tony produced the following errors on the test, and the same misarticulations were also evident in his spontaneous speech:

Consonant Substitutions: dʒ/j, f/θ, fr/θr, -/d, t/θ. (The substitution b/v was noted only in spontaneous speech.)

Vowel Substitutions: i/ɪ, a/æ, ɔ/ə, a/ɔ, u/ʊ. Tony self-corrected his substitution of e/ɛ (however, this substitution was produced frequently in spontaneous speech).

Voicing: s/z, z/s, d/t (b/v was only noted in spontaneous speech).

Occurrence of misarticulations was inconsistent between single words, while others occurred solely in sentences. Some errors occurred in both contexts. Overall, misarticulations were more noticeable in spontaneous speech. Overall, speech intelligibility for English was judged to be good.

It was observed that Tony also had difficulty reflecting the varied quality and length of vowels between stressed and unstressed syllables. For example, he read, "/mɛni θɪŋz/," as, "/mei:ni:θi:ŋz/."

E. Auditory Discrimination

An informal clinician-made test of 35 word pairs reflecting phonemes that Spanish speakers frequently substitute or interchange in English was administered. With his back to the examiner, Tony was asked to state if the pairs presented auditorily were the same or different. Three items were incorrectly identified. Tony stated that "tip/dip" and "doze/those" were the same. Tony also stated that "so/so" was different. He stated later that he thought they were different because he was "picturing" the two words, "sew" and "so" in his head. This suggested that Tony may be trying to "speak" from his knowledge of written English, instead of using a more phonological approach.

The *Wepman Test of Auditory Discrimination,* Form 2A, was administered to assess Tony's ability to recognize differences between phonemes in English. He was presented with 40 pairs of words and asked to indicate similarities and differences between word pairs. Two errors were observed.

The word pair "wreath/reef" was judged to be the same, and the pair "wedge/wedge" was judged to be different.

Each auditory discrimination error corresponded to an articulation error in speech production. Overall, auditory discrimination was judged to be satisfactory.

F. Fluency and Voice

Fluency and voice quality were judged to be unremarkable.

IMPRESSIONS

Tony was very cooperative and enthusiastic throughout the evaluation. He stated, "I even had fun." Tony is motivated to improve his speech production, since he feels that more "eloquent" speech will be beneficial to him in his future career. However, attention should be brought to Tony's statement, "I want my speech to be perfect." He will need assistance in establishing more realistic goals.

Tony's misarticulations were all very characteristic of Spanish-English speakers, and the slight language difficulties observed were related to a language difference. Auditory discrimination difficulty was determined to be a probable contributing factor to misarticulations. Due to Tony's failure to respond to 500 Hz at 20 dB in his right ear, along with recent reported symptoms of possible cerumen accumulation, hearing status was judged to be questionable.

RECOMMENDATIONS

It is recommended that:

1. Tony receive training in spoken English once a week for two hours with focus on auditory discrimination and production of target sounds.

2. Tony receive additional evaluation of tense usage and morphology in English.

3. Tony receive a complete audiological evaluation at _____ University's Hearing, Language, and Speech Clinic.

4. Tony receive assistance in becoming less dependent on written English for speech production.

5. Tony modify his personal goals for producing spoken English to a more realistic framework. Inclusion of information on specific Spanish-English differences in phonology, morphology, syntax, and semantics, in this order, will enhance his ability to adjust goals for spoken English.

Ann B. Fitzgerald
Graduate Student Clinician

Dr. Adele Proctor, CCC/SLP
Associate Professor

File: FORMAT

FORMAT FOR COMPARISON OF ASSESSMENT DATA		
Name:_____ Birthdate:_____ C.A.:_____ Date of Examination_____ Examiner:_____		
	COMPARISON OF EVALUATION DATA	
REVIEW OF RECORDS BEHAVIORS TESTED AND/OR STANDARDIZED TESTS ADMINISTERED	<u>Pre-Test</u> Date:_____ C.A.:_____	<u>Post-Test</u> Date:_____ C.A.:_____

1. HEARING
 	
    Acuity
    Puretone
    Left_____Right_____
    SRT
    Left Right		

Speech Discrimination
 	
    Free-field
    40 dB above threshold
 	
Name of Test/Subtest
Administered:
	____out of a
	possible __
	____one standard
	    deviation
	__above__/below
	the mean
	Percentile____
	Other Score_____
		____out of a
		possible __
		____one standard
		    deviation
		_above/__below
		the mean
		Percentile____
		Other Score____

Memory
_____ meaningless
_____ meaningful
_____   Digits
_____   Nonsense Syllables
_____   Related words
_____   Unrelated words
_____   Commands
	_____normal limits
	Standard Score
	(SS)
	___ ____normal lmts
	___ ____normal lmts
	___ ____normal lmts
	        stage
		_____normal limits
		Standard Score (SS)
		
		___ ____normal lmts
		___ ____normal lmts
		___ ____normal lmts
		        stage

Auditory Attention Name of Test/Subtest Administered:	Type of Score: Remarks:	Type of Score: Remarks:

FORMAT FOR COMPARISON OF ASSESSMENT DATA		
2. RECEPTIVE LANGUAGE _____ Single words _____ Morphology _____ Syntax _____ Story/Narrative Name of Test(s) Administered:	Language Age_____ Remarks:	Language Age_____ Remarks:
Auditory Reception Visual Reception	Type of Score:	Type of Score:
_____Concepts _____Number _____Color	Remarks:	Remarks:
General Informal Observation Understanding of Conversational speech		
Receptive Name of Test(s) Administered: Types of Errors:	Score_____ Percentile_____	Score_____ Percentile_____
Auditory Association Visual Association	Type of Score_____ Type of Score_____	Type of Score____ Type of Score____
3. EXPRESSIVE LANGUAGE Semantics ____Vocabulary ____Verbal Expression ____Word-retrieval Name of Test(s) Administered:	C.A.____ Type of Score___	C.A. ____ Type of Score__
General Impression of Vocabulary, e.g., types of errors	Remarks:	Remarks:

FORMAT FOR COMPARISON OF ASSESSMENT DATA		
Syntax & Morphology Name of Test(s) Administered:	Score_____ Percentile_____	Score_____ Percentile_____

Types of Errors
 	
   Comparison with
   Receptive Test(s):
 	
   Grammatic Closure		

Conversational Speech
    Level of sentence
     structure
 	
   Mean length of utterance
  (MLU)
 	
   D1/L1   D2/L2
   Errors in grammar
	D1/L1
	
	D2/L2
	
	Dialect Related
		D1/L1
		
		D2/L2
		
		Dialect Related

Ability to relate verbal
    information
 	
   From __Language Sample
   From: Name Test(s)/subtests
_____
_____
_____
	C.A. _____
	
	Remarks:
		C.A. ____
		
		Remarks:

FORMAT FOR COMPARISON OF ASSESSMENT DATA															
Articulation Intelligibility Conversational Single Words															
	STIMULABLE						STIMULABLE								
	Position				ISOLATION	SYLLABLE	WORD	Position				ISOLATION	SYLLABLE	WORD
Articulation Profile for single words	I	M	F	BLEND				I	M	F	BLEND			
Error Sounds															
Key: D = Distortion O = Omission A = Addition Phonetically Transcribe = Substitution															
Comments:															

FORMAT FOR COMPARISON OF ASSESSMENT DATA		
Other Aspects of Speech Production: AAE or other dialect/language	Pre-Therapy C.A.	Post-Therapy C.A.

4. ORAL MECHANISM STRUCTURE
 	
Function
  Diadochokinetic
    rate per second
      Lips
      Tongue-tip
      Velum
Sequencing		

Control of Tongue Pointing Lifting Lateralization Protrusion-retraction Intentional sequencing		
5. DEVELOPMENTAL ITEMS	_____level according to_____ norms Remarks:	_____level according to_____ norms Remarks:
Geometric Form Copying		
IMITATION		
Performance Items: Name of Test_____		
6. SIGNIFICANT BEHAVIORS ____ As reported by Parents ____ As reported by Teacher	Remarks:	Remarks:

Figure and Table Credits

Index

Page numbers in *italics* denote figures; those followed by "t" denote tables.